Cultural Food Practices

Diabetes Care and Education Dietetic Practice Group

Cynthia M. Goody, PhD, MBA, RD, and Lorena Drago, MS, RD, CDN, CDE, Editors

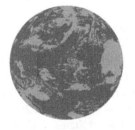

eat right. Academy of Nutrition and Dietetics

10 9 8 7 6

Library of Congress Cataloging-in-Publication Data

Cultural food practices / Diabetes Care and Education Dietetic Practice Group;
Cynthia M. Goody and Lorena Drago, editors.
     p. ; cm.
Includes bibliographical references and index.
ISBN 978-0-88091-433-8 (alk. paper)
1. Diabetes—Diet therapy. 2. Food habits—United States. 3. Minorities—Food—United States.
I. Goody, Cynthia M. II. Drago, Lorena. III. American Dietetic Association. Diabetes Care and
Education Dietetic Practice Group. IV. American Dietetic Association.
[DNLM: 1. Diabetes Mellitus—diet therapy—United States. 2. Diabetic Diet—ethnology—
United States. 3. Cultural Characteristics—United States. 4. Diabetes Mellitus—ethnology—
United States. 5. Food Habits—ethnology—United States. WK 818 C968 2010]
RC662.C85 2010
616.4'620654—dc22   2009024536

Contents

Contents

Chapter 12: Korean American Food Practices   144

Haewook Han, PhD, RD, CSR, Jennifer Kwon, MS, RD, and Linda C. Ro, MS, RD

Chapter 13: Cajun and Creole Food Practices   155

Colette Guidry Leistner, PhD, RD, and Lauren Hirschfeld, MS, RD

Chapter 14: Jewish Food Practices   170

Claudia Shwide-Slavin, MS, RD, BC-ADM, CDE

Chapter 15: Islamic Food Practices   185

Sharon Palmer, RD

About the Editors

Cynthia M. Goody, PhD, MBA, RD, has provided nutrition counseling and education and developed wellness educational programs focused on cardiovascular health, diabetes, food allergies, and weight management in numerous domestic and international settings. A former Peace Corps Volunteer–Guatemala, Cindy has served the Diabetes Care and Education Dietetic Practice Group as a member of its Networking Committee, *OTCE* editor, and chair elect. Goody holds a PhD and MBA from the University of Iowa, as well as an MS in Food Science, Human Nutrition, and Family and Consumer Sciences and a BS in Food, Nutrition, and Dietetics from Iowa State University. She completed a dietetic internship at the University of Iowa Hospitals and Clinics.

Lorena Drago, MS, RD, CDN, CDE, is a registered dietitian, consultant, and certified diabetes educator who specializes in the multicultural aspects of diabetes self-management education. She founded Hispanic Foodways, which offers culturally and ethnically oriented diabetes education tools, programs, and patient education materials. Lorena graduated cum laude from Hunter College of the City University of New York with a Masters of Science degree in Food and Nutrition, and received her BA in Home Economics, Food, and Nutrition from Queens College.

Contributors

Ericka Arrecis, RD, CDE
Woodside, NY

Marisol Avila, RD, CDE
Loma Linda, CA

Kathaleen Briggs Early, PhD, RD, CDE
Yakima, WA

CAPT Tammy L. Brown, MPH, RD,
BC-ADM, CDE
Albuquerque, NM

Eva Brzezinski, MS, RD
San Diego, CA

Ila Champine, RD
Anchorage, AK

Deirdra Chester, PhD, RD
Beltsville, MD

Sophia Cheung, MS, RD, CDE
Boston, MA

Lorena Drago, MS, RD, CDN, CDE
Forest Hills, NY

Karen Fowles, RD
Anchorage, AK

Raquel Franzini Pereira, MS, RD
Maple Grove, MN

Cynthia M. Goody, PhD, MBA, RD
Elmhurst, IL

Colette Guidry Leistner, PhD, RD
Thibodaux, LA

Haewook Han, PhD, RD, CSR
Boston, MA

Lauren Hirschfeld, MS, RD
West Palm Beach, FL

Jamillah Hoy-Rosas, MPH, RD, CDN, CDE
Brooklyn, NY

Janet Jeffrey, MS, RD
Wesley Chapel, FL

LCDR Michelle L. Johnson, MS, RD
Chinle, AZ

Tandalayo Kidd, PhD, RD
Manhattan, KS

Karmeen D. Kulkarni, MS, RD,
BC-ADM, CDE
Salt Lake City, UT

Chantelle C. Kurtz, RD
Farmington, MN

Jennifer Kwon, MS, RD
Bronx, NY

Rosa A. Mo, EdD, RD
West Haven, CT

Sharon Palmer, RD
Duarte, CA

Linda C. Ro, MS, RD
Youngstown, OH

Claudia Shwide-Slavin, MS, RD,
BC-ADM, CDE
New York, NY

CDR Carol Treat, MS, RD, CDE
Anchorage, AK

Diane Veale Jones, MS, RD
Collegeville, MN

Lorraine Weatherspoon, PhD, RD
East Lansing, MI

Ellie Zephier, MPH, RD
Aberdeen, SD

Reviewers

Toby Amidor, MS, RD
Scarsdale, NY

Rita K. Batheja, MS, RD, CDN
Baldwin Habor, NY

Hiba Bawadi, PhD
Jordan

Eva Board, MS, RD, CD
Indianapolis, IN

Constance Brown-Riggs, MSEd, RD, CDE, CDN
Massapequa, NY

Cecelia Butler, MS, RD, CDE
Santa Fe, NM

Teresita Cabrera, MS, RD, CDN
Bronx, NY

Barbara Chang, MS, RD
Cupertino, CA

Wendy (Wenju) Chen, PhD, RD, CNS
Redondo Beach, CA

Kattia Corrales-Yauckoes, MS, RD
Worcester, MA

Jo Jo Dantone-DeBarbieris, MS, RD, CDE
La Place, LA

Marle dos Santos Alvarenga, PhD
São Paulo, Brazil

Jennifer R. Eliasi, MS, RD, CDN
Forest Hills, NY

Fabiola D. Gaines, RD
Orlando, FL

Susan Sau Han Lui, PhD, RD
Happy Valley, Hong Kong, People's Republic of China

Dawna T. Mughal, PhD, RD, FADA
Erie, PA

Gita Patel, MS, RD, CDE
Etna, NH

Christina Ann Persaud, RD
Astoria, NY

Ragini Raghuveer, MSc, MS, RD
Morganville, NJ

Sudha Raj, PhD, RD
Syracuse, NY

Elsa Ramirez-Brisson, MPH, RD
Salinas, CA

Yeong Rhee, PhD, RD
Fargo, ND

Judith C. Rodriguez, PhD, RD, FADA
Jacksonville, FL

Carolyn L. Ross, MS, RD, CDE
Cass Lake, MN

Arne Sorenson, RD, CDE
New Town, ND

Laurie Tansman, MS, RD, CDN
New York, NY

Alyce Thomas, RD
Paterson, NJ

Sonia Tucunduva Philippi, PhD
São Paulo, Brazil

Maomoua Vue, RD, CD, CLC
Onalaska, WI

Natalie A. Webb, MS, RD
Silver Spring, MD

Foreword

Given the changing demographics of the United States, we registered dietitians (RDs) and dietetic technicians registered (DTRs) need to increase our cultural competence to meet the needs of our patients, clients, customers, and students. Accordingly, in its strategic plan, the Academy of Nutrition and Dietetics (formerly the American Dietetic Association) has identified strengthening cultural competence to address health disparities as one of the six strategies to improve the health of Americans. The 2006 Environmental Scan for the Academy identified improvement of cultural competence for RDs and DTRs as an area of importance over the next several years. In 2008 the Academy's House of Delegates identified health disparities as a mega-issue and had a dialogue session on it.

It can be challenging to find ways to incorporate cultural competence into practice. The tools for practitioners have been limited. The Diabetes Care and Education Practice Group's book, *Cultural Food Practices,* edited by Lorena Drago and Cynthia Goody, has responded to this challenge by providing an overview of 15 different cultures/religions; discussing the prevalence of diabetes and type 2 diabetes risk factors in each group; and describing traditional foods, dishes, and health beliefs, current food practices, tips for counseling, and additional resources. The accompanying downloadable PDF files provides 20 culturally specific patient education handouts, including four Spanish translations.

Whether you practice in diabetes or another setting, this book will provide you with a resource you can use to improve your cultural competency and start addressing the health disparities within your own practice area.

Jessie Pavlinac, MS, RD, CSR
President, American Dietetic Association, 2009-2010

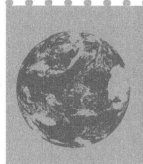

Introduction: Cultural Competence and Nutrition Counseling

Cynthia M. Goody, PhD, MBA, RD, and Lorena Drago, MS, RD, CDN, CDE

In the book, *We Are What We Eat: Ethnic Food and the Making of Americans,* historian Donna Gabaccia asserts, "Food and language are the cultural habits humans learn first and the ones they change with the greatest reluctance" (1). As health care professionals working with people with diabetes, we are quite familiar with this sentiment. We ask our clients:

- "What did you eat?"
- "How much did you eat?"
- "How did the meal affect your blood glucose level?"
- "How was the food prepared?"

The answers inevitably reveal our clients' attachment to the foods of their cultures. In addition to gathering data about eating habits and patterns, we learn about our clients, their views on food, and their devotion to their culture. For example, we learn what kind of meals they enjoyed as children, the foods they share at holidays, and their favorite family recipes.

Understanding the cultural significance of diet not only helps us relate better to our clients, it also helps us be more effective. We can make culturally appropriate recommendations that will resonate with clients much more than a "one-size-fits-all" plan. Then, because the plan fits into their lives, they may be more likely to comply with medical nutrition therapy (MNT).

Diabetes has reached epidemic proportions in the United States, and people from some ethnic and racial groups are disproportionately affected. For many of us in the nutrition profession, an increasing number of our clients have cultural backgrounds different from our own. For this reason, the Academy of Nutrition and Dietetics, American Diabetes Association, and American Association of Diabetes Educators support and encourage practitioners' efforts to develop cultural competence and provide culturally sensitive MNT (2-4). Furthermore, the Commission on Accreditation for Dietetics Education requires that future registered dietitians (RDs) develop their cultural competence and dietetics programs integrate cultural studies into their curricula (5).

In this book, you'll find the tools to help you on your journey toward cultural competence. Written by RDs who are experts in culture and food, as well as in diabetes care, this guide presents traditional and contemporary health beliefs and food patterns for 15 cultural and religious groups. To put this information into the context of MNT, we discuss the importance of courtesy, respect, communication skills, and family dynamics when collaborating with clients. Furthermore, in acknowledgment of the rising popularity of complementary and alternative medicine (CAM), we present commonly used CAM therapies for each group.

The Relationship of Culture to Food and Disease

Culture can be defined as the accumulation of a group's learned and shared behaviors in everyday life. It is the lens we use to view and understand people's beliefs, customs, and knowledge. As we become more familiar with our clients, we gain a deeper understanding of how their cultures create a sense of identity, order, and security in their lives. Through our formal and informal client interactions we see how culture can define social structure, decision-making, and communication styles. We also come to better understand that every culture defines its eating occasions in unique ways (6). This information provides a rich opportunity to employ culturally appropriate behavior, etiquette, and protocol in a way that respects each client.

To understand culture, we first must define ethnicity and race in the context of our professional lives and the world at large. There are no universally accepted definitions of "ethnicity" or "race." Ethnicity is a historically complex concept that typically refers to identity generated within and between social groups. Ethnicity is often referred to as a common ancestry, which may include shared language, nationality, social customs, and/or religion. "Race" is generally used to categorize individuals who share particular physical characteristics, such as skin color, facial features, and hair. Racial categories include African American, American Indian, Asian, and others (7).

RDs are well versed in the science of food and nutrition, but we must also understand that the cultural significance of food goes well beyond daily sustenance (8). Culture influences each person's choices about what to eat, when to eat, how, and with whom. Ethnic and racial groups differ in how they identify foods and how they prepare them, the condiments they use, and the timing and frequency of meals. Foods frequently play an integral role in religious ceremonies and social events. As individuals from other cultures become acculturated to US society, their food practices may change. At the same time, however, they may continue to observe many traditions of their original culture.

Culture also influences everyone's attitudes, beliefs, practices, and values about good health and disease prevention. For example, there are cultural practices regarding the care and treatment of the sick; culture helps individuals decide whom to consult when they are ill; and cultural assumptions affect how both clients and health care professionals see their roles (9). By recognizing that culture shapes how a person defines health, perceives illness, and seeks treatment, we are positioned to provide well-informed MNT that integrates both our scientific understanding of disease and sensitivity to the culturally specific expectations and desires of our clients (10).

As outcomes-driven professionals, RDs must leverage and apply the growing evidence of a positive correlation between understanding a patient's culture, on the one hand, and improved health outcomes (such as client satisfaction and adherence), on the other. Diabetes outcomes may improve when health care providers offer long-term, supportive follow-up that empowers the client, his or her family, and the community at large (11). As members of a helping profession, we are dedicated to the care of individuals. Building on this notion, we are poised for cultural engagement, an active, developmental learning process that requires long-term commitment (7,12).

The Impact of Diabetes on Ethnic and Racial Groups

Dynamic population shifts in the United States and the changing health status of various cultural, ethnic, and racial groups impact the diabetes landscape. Data from the 2000 US Census indicate that non-Hispanic whites were approximately 70% of the total population, whereas individuals identifying themselves as black, Asian, Hispanic, or other comprised 30%. By 2050 the Census Bureau estimates that more than 50% of the population in the United States will identify themselves in a racial or ethnic category other than non-Hispanic white (13).

Approximately 23.6 million children and adults in the United States (7.8% of the population) have diabetes (14). This includes 17.9 million people who have been diagnosed and 5.7 million who are unaware they have the disease (14). In 2007, 1.6 million US residents age 20 years or older were diagnosed with diabetes (14). If present trends continue, one in three people in the United States who were born in 2000 will develop diabetes in their lifetime (15).

Certain ethnic and racial groups are disproportionately diagnosed with diabetes. For example, it is estimated that 13% of African Americans; 10% of Hispanics, and 16.3% of American Indians and Alaska Natives have diabetes, compared with 8.7% of non-Hispanic whites (15,16).

Landmark research has demonstrated creative ways to deliver diabetes care and education. The Diabetes Prevention Program (DPP) was a randomized clinical trial to assess the safety and efficacy of interventions that may delay or prevent development of diabetes in people at increased risk for type 2 diabetes. It included more than 3,200 participants without diabetes who had elevated fasting and postload plasma glucose concentrations. These participants were from diverse backgrounds (55% self-identified as white, 20% were African American, 16% were Hispanic, 5% were American Indian, and 4% were Asian American), and they were randomly assigned to one of three groups: placebo, metformin (850 mg twice daily), or a lifestyle-modification program (17). The lifestyle interventions were culturally tailored to the participants' ethnic groups, and these interventions effectively reduced the incidence of diabetes in participants of all racial and ethnic groups (18). Based on the outcomes from this research, DPP researchers encourage health care professionals to develop therapies to meet the needs of ethnic groups with diabetes.

Cultural Competence and Diabetes Care and Education

As nutrition professionals, one of our greatest strengths is our ability to establish rapport with clients when providing education. We can complement this strength by understanding the influence of culture on health care practices (19). By integrating cultural constructs into diabetes care and education, we may improve diabetes outcomes (19) and better satisfy clients (20). The development of cultural competence is thus essential for every health care provider (21,22).

To effectively encourage clients to make healthier food choices and improve health outcomes, we must understand the food habits, preferences, and practices (eg, holidays, celebrations, and fasting) of the ethnic and racial groups we treat. The result: clients feel that they have been understood and that we respect their beliefs, behaviors, and values.

Cultural competence has been described as a set of congruent attitudes, behaviors, and policies (23). Situated in a system or agency, or among integrated patterns of human behavior, cultural competence constructs include understanding the language, thoughts, communications, actions, customs, beliefs, values, and institutions of ethnic, racial, religious, or social groups (23). These themes are present in the classic Campinha-Bacote model (12) and others, which define cultural competence in terms of recognizing and forming one's attitudes, beliefs, skills, values, and levels of awareness to provide culturally appropriate, respectful, and relevant care and education. Such models emphasize the ability of health care professionals to ask questions, listen carefully, speak simply and respectfully, and involve clients in their own treatment plans (24–26).

Applying the Campinha-Bacote Model of Cultural Competence

As a group of professionals dedicated to food and nutrition, we appreciate and value individuals, families, and communities, and this appreciation is the cornerstone of developing one's cultural competence. When we successfully bridge the differences between our own culture and the cultures of others, we demonstrate and achieve mutual understanding and meet unique needs. Campinha-Bacote's model treats cultural competence as a process, rather than a result, and has five interdependent constructs (12). The following sections describe the components of the model and how health care professionals may apply them when delivering diabetes care and education.

Cultural Awareness

As a first step toward cultural competence, the health care provider examines her own cultural background and asks herself questions about her own values, beliefs, and practices. After all, it is not just the client who has a culture. The health care provider must reflect on her own culture in order to extend beyond it during client outreach. Questions you might ask yourself include the following:

- What assumptions do you make about ethnic and racial groups?
- How might your assumptions and comments make counseling more difficult or less effective?
- Are any of your health-related values, beliefs, and practices related to diabetes? How might they affect the way you provide diabetes care and education?

At the same time that he investigates his personal cultural perspectives, the health care professional also aims to learn about each client's culture, including its effects on values, beliefs, practices, and problem-solving strategies. Asking clients the following questions may help in this process:

- In addition to the questions I have already asked you, is there anything more you like me to know about your diabetes?
- What are some of your health-related values, beliefs, and practices?

Cultural Knowledge

A culturally competent health care professional has broad cultural knowledge, including understanding of the following:

- Relevant cultural norms, values, world views, and practicalities of everyday life
- Cultural variations in family relationships
- Culturally specific health beliefs and practices
- Sociodemographic factors
- Cultural food habits
- Cultural attitudes about health care professionals and when to consult them
- Physical, biological, physiological, and psychological differences among ethnic and racial groups

To acquire cultural knowledge, health care professionals may review research for insight into the following questions:

- What is the prevalence of diabetes in various ethnic and racial cultural groups?
- To what extent does the biomedical model for the causation of diabetes agree or conflict with the client's cultural perspective? Does the client's culture describe or approach diabetes in ways that could affect an individual's reception of the biomedical model?
- What is the client's perspective about who is responsible for his or her diabetes management?
- How does the client perceive a visit with the health care professional to receive diabetes care and education?
- How do food habits and preferences affect the client's ability and willingness to manage his or her diabetes?

Cultural Skill

Progressing from awareness and knowledge, we are prepared to more fully develop cultural skill—the ability to collect culturally relevant information from clients and perform culturally based assessments and interventions. The keys to developing cultural skill are asking open-ended questions and listening to the client's answers. The following are some questions to ask:

- What languages do you speak?
- Would you like us to use an interpreter when we meet?

- What kinds of foods do you like to eat when you feel well? How about when you are not feeling well?
- Which foods do you avoid when you are ill?
- Do you avoid any foods for cultural or religious reasons? Which ones?
- In your opinion, what causes your diabetes?
- How do you think we should manage and treat your diabetes?

Cultural Encounter

A cultural encounter (which may occur in any client interaction) is a process of actively seeking and engaging in cross-cultural exchanges. This process involves obtaining a variety of responses from clients and providing culturally appropriate verbal and nonverbal responses to them. This type of interaction requires a balance of listening, observing, and asking nonjudgmental questions. Individuals see, hear, and feel only what has meaning to them. Nonverbal gestures are relatively easy to observe and understand. The following are suggestions for interacting with clients from different cultures:

- Let clients determine their personal space.
- Observe whether clients make eye contact and understand how to interpret their gaze (eg, in some cultures, direct eye contact is considered rude or confrontational).
- Note how clients use silence.
- Ask open-ended questions; then truly listen to the client's answers (rather than simply waiting for your turn to talk).

Cultural encounters are opportunities to explore cultural food behavior. Encourage clients to bring food labels from home to counseling/education sessions. Also ask them to show you supermarket flyers that advertise ethnic foods and take cell-phone or digital photographs of their meals so you can help them ascertain portion sizes.

The following questions may help you understand the client's food habits and complete the nutrition assessment:

Traditional Foods

- What foods do you commonly eat?
- What are your favorite foods?
- How often do you eat them?
- Which foods do you eat on holidays or special occasions?

Food and Health

- Which foods do you eat to be healthy?
- Which foods do you avoid because you have diabetes?
- Which foods do you eat more of because you have diabetes?
- Have you seen other practitioners to treat your diabetes or conditions related to it? Please describe any treatments or remedies you use.
- We all have favorite remedies that we use when we are sick. Which home remedies do you use?

New Foods

- What foods have you recently eaten for the first time? Why did you start eating them?
- Do you regularly try new foods?
- Which new foods did you dislike? What about them did you not like?

Food Acquisition and Availability

- What foods do you typically buy?
- Where do you buy food?
- Do you have enough food to eat each day?
- Are you able to get the types of food you need?

Food Preparation

- How do you prepare this meal?
- How is this food/dish cooked?
- What recipes do you use?
- What do you usually eat with this food/dish?
- Do you have enough time and equipment to prepare the foods you like?

Food and Socialization

- Who eats meals with you?
- Who do you share holidays with?

Cultural Desire

Cultural desire means we want to be actively involved in cross-cultural encounters and seek greater cultural competence. To succeed in diabetes care and education, health care professionals must acknowledge similarities and differences among cultures and be prepared for interactions unlike those that are typical in their own cultures. For example, you may be more accustomed to asking job-related questions and feel hesitant about "prying" into personal matters, but your clients may be more comfortable if you ask about their families rather than their work. Similarly, you may be trained to measure outcomes in terms of the individual, but your client may be more receptive to knowing how diabetes affects the family. As a general rule of thumb, try to demonstrate a genuine interest in the client first and diabetes second.

*****

This book is one tool that can help you on the road to cultural competence. This journey promises many rewards. In particular, as you become more culturally competent, you and your clients will likely reap the benefits of improved communication and more effective counseling. Enjoy your cultural nutrition exploration!

References

1. Gabaccia DR. *We Are What We Eat.* Cambridge, MA: Harvard University Press; 1998.
2. American Dietetic Association Diversity and Practice Subcommittee. Diversity and Practice Subcommittee Spring 2006 Report. http://www.eatright.org/cps/rde/xchg/ada/hs.xsl/governance_8146_ENU_HTML.htm. Accessed January 27, 2008.
3. American Diabetes Association. Nutrition recommendations and interventions for diabetes—2006. *Diabetes Care.* 2008;31(suppl):S61–S78.
4. American Association of Diabetes Educators. Cultural sensitivity and diabetes education: recommendations for diabetes educators. *Diabetes Educ.* 2007;33:41–44.
5. Skipper A, Young LO, Mitchell B. 2008 accreditation standards for dietetic education. *J Am Diet Assoc.* 2008;108:1732–1735.
6. Makela J. Cultural definitions of the meal. In: Meiselman HL, ed. *Dimensions of the Meal: The Science, Culture, Business, and Art of Eating.* Gaithersburg, MD: Aspen Publishers; 2000:7–18.
7. Davies K. Addressing the needs of an ethnic minority diabetic population. *Br J Nurs.* 2006;15:516–519.
8. Barer-Stein TB: *You Eat What You Are: People, Culture, and Food Traditions.* 2nd ed. Willowdale, Canada: Firefly Books; 1999.
9. Sucher KP, Kittler PG. *Food and Culture.* 5th ed. Belmont, CA: Wadsworth; 2007.
10. Kleinman A, Eisenberg L, Good B. Culture, illness, and care: clinical lessons from anthropologic and cross-cultural research. *Ann Intern Med.* 1978;88:251–258.
11. DeCoster VA, Cummings SM. Helping adults with diabetes: a review of evidence-based interventions. *Health Social Work.* 2005;30:259–264.
12. Campinha-Bacote J. A model and instrument for addressing cultural competence in health care. *J Nurs Educ.* 1999;38:203–207.
13. US Census Bureau. U.S. Interim Projections by Age, Sex, Race, and Hispanic Origin. March 18, 2004. http://www.census.gov/ipc/www/usinterimproj. Accessed January 27, 2008.

14. Centers for Disease Control and Prevention. National Diabetes Fact Sheet: General Information and National Estimates on Diabetes in the United States, 2007. Atlanta, GA: US Department of Health and Human Services; 2008.

15. Centers for Disease Control and Prevention. National Diabetes Fact Sheet: General Information and National Estimates on Diabetes in the United States, 2005. Atlanta, GA: US Department of Health and Human Services; 2005.

16. Indian Health Service, Division of Diabetes Treatment and Prevention. Diabetes in American Indians and Alaska Natives: Facts at-a-Glance. June 2008. http://www.ihs.gov/medicalprograms/diabetes. Accessed September 25, 2008.

17. Knowler WC, Barrett-Connor E, Fowler SE, Hamman RF, Lachin JM, Walker EA, Nathan DM; Diabetes Prevention Program Research Group. Reduction in the incidence of type 2 diabetes with lifestyle intervention or metformin. *N Engl J Med.* 2002;346:393–402.

18. Diabetes Prevention Program Research Group. The Diabetes Prevention Program: baseline characteristics of the randomized cohort. *Diabetes Care.* 2000;23:1619–1629.

19. Liburd LC, Namageyo-Funa A, Jack L, Gregg E. Views from within and beyond: illness narratives of African-American men with type 2 diabetes. *Diabetes Spectrum.* 2004;17:219–224.

20. Williams JH, Auslander WF, de Groot M, Robinson AD, Houston C, Haire-Joshu D. Cultural relevancy of a diabetes prevention nutrition program for African-American women. *Health Promot Pract.* 2006;7:56–67.

21. Bethancourt JR. Cultural competence: marginal or mainstream movement? *N Engl J Med.* 2004;351:953–955.

22. Juckett G. Cross-cultural medicine. *Am Fam Physician.* 2005;72:2267–2274.

23. Nettles A. Call to action. *Diabetes.* 1999;25:2–3.

24. Boyle MA, Holben DH: *Community Nutrition in Action: An Entrepreneurial Approach.* 4th ed. Belmont, CA: Wadsworth/Thompson Learning; 2006.

25. Harris-Davis E, Haughton B. Model for multicultural nutrition counseling competencies. *J Am Diet Assoc.* 2000;100:1178–1185.

26. Lynch EW, Hanson MJ: *Developing Cross-Cultural Competence: A Guide for Working With Children and Their Families.* 3rd ed. Baltimore, MD: Brookes Publishing; 2004.

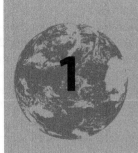

American Indian Food Practices

CAPT Tammy L. Brown, MPH, RD, BC-ADM, CDE, Ellie Zephier, MPH, RD, and LCDR Michelle L. Johnson, MS, RD

Introduction

According to the US Census 2000 report, "We the People: American Indian and Alaska Natives in the United States," 4.3 million Americans (1.5% of total US population) identify themselves as American Indian or Alaska Native (AI/AN) (1). Just over half of these individuals claim AI/AN ancestry only. The AI/AN population is younger than the US population as a whole. Thirty-three percent of the AI/AN population is younger than 18 years, and 5.6% is age 65 years or older. This compares with 26% and 12.4%, respectively, of the total population (1,2).

There are 562 culturally diverse, federally recognized tribes in 35 states in the United States. The Indian Health Service (IHS), a federal agency established in 1955 under the US Public Health Service (USPHS), is the principal health care provider and advocate for the people in these tribes. The provision of health services to federally recognized AI/AN populations grew out of a special relationship between the federal government and Indian tribes. Numerous treaties, laws, Supreme Court decisions, and executive orders have given form and substance to this government-to-government relationship. This relationship distinguishes American Indians and Alaska Natives from all other racial and ethnic groups in the United States. The mission of the IHS is to partner with AI/AN people to raise their physical, mental, social, and spiritual health to the highest level possible. IHS is a decentralized health care system, administered through 12 area offices, 46 hospitals, and more than 500 IHS tribal and urban outpatient facilities. Approximately 1.9 million American Indians and Native Alaskans reside on or near reservations served by IHS or tribally operated health centers, health stations, Alaska Native village clinics, and residential treatment centers. More than 600,000 American Indians and Native Alaskans are served by 34 urban programs, ranging from community health to comprehensive primary health care services (2).

In the half century since the creation of the IHS, the health and longevity of the AI/AN people have improved through advances in medicine, nutrition, and preventive health care. However, despite these significant gains, American Indians and Alaska Natives continue to experience disproportionate rates of morbidity and mortality, when compared with other Americans, from tuberculosis, alcoholism, diabetes, unintentional injuries, homicide, and suicide (3).

Chronic diseases, including cardiovascular disease, cancer, and diabetes mellitus, have replaced infectious diseases as the predominant causes of death and disability in AI/AN people. When IHS was established, diabetes was not among the leading causes of death in this population. Today, it ranks among the top four (3).

Diabetes mellitus is a fairly recent phenomenon in the AI/AN population. Reported cases were extremely rare in the first half of the 20th century. However, in the 1940s and

1950s, physicians treating Indian people noted occasional cases of a condition that resembled diabetes. Because diabetes complications were not observed, the doctors concluded this was a "benign chemical abnormality." As incidence increased and complications became more common, it became apparent that this "benign chemical abnormality" was indeed diabetes (4). By the 1970s, medical providers throughout the IHS were reporting an increasing prevalence of diabetes (predominantly type 2 diabetes) in AI/AN populations, and it soon became obvious that diabetes was a growing epidemic throughout all tribes.

Much of what we now know about diabetes in AI/AN communities comes from ongoing cooperative studies with the Pima Indian tribe. (See discussion in Risk Factors for Type 2 Diabetes section later in this chapter.) Since 1965 the National Institutes of Health (NIH) have maintained research facilities in Phoenix, Arizona, and at the Gila River Indian community (Sacaton, AZ) to carry out studies with volunteers from the Pima Indian community. The Pima Indians of Arizona have the highest rates of diabetes in the world—more than 50% of adults have been diagnosed with type 2 diabetes. The studies that were conducted in the Pima communities in the 1960s and 1970s have taught the United States and the world much about type 2 diabetes.

Diabetes Prevalence

American Indians and Alaska Natives have the highest prevalence rates of diabetes of all the racial and ethnic groups in the United States—16.3% of AI/AN adults have been diagnosed with diabetes, compared with 8.7% of non-Hispanic whites (5). Type 2 diabetes is the most common type of diabetes in AI/AN individuals, whereas type 1 diabetes is rare. Prevalence of type 2 diabetes is highest among Native Americans of full-blood heritage (6,7). The reasons for the high prevalence of type 2 diabetes in AI/AN are not fully understood.

Although the prevalence of diabetes is increasing in the US population as a whole, the increase in the AI/AN population has been especially dramatic. Diabetes prevalence is increasing in all tribal communities and in all age groups. It is more prevalent among females than males. Between 1997 and 2004, the prevalence of diagnosed diabetes increased by 45% in all major regions served by IHS (8,9).

Rates of diagnosed diabetes vary across the 12 IHS administrative areas. In 2004, the age-adjusted diabetes prevalence in AI/AN adults was greatest (26.7%) in the Tucson, Arizona, area and lowest in the Alaska area (6.1%). However, in the same year, the rate of increase in age-adjusted prevalence of diabetes in AI/AN adults was highest in the Alaska area (55%) and lowest in the Tucson area (12%) (10,11). (See Chapter 2 for more information on Alaskan Natives.)

In the general US population, diabetes prevalence increases in adults in their 30s. In contrast, prevalence in the AI/AN population increases in a younger age group, individuals in their 20s (7,8). Prevalence of diabetes among AI/AN adults ages 25 to 34 years increased 160% between 1990 and 2004 (10,11).

Alarmingly, the prevalence of diagnosed type 2 diabetes has also increased among AI/AN children and adolescents. Prevalence in AI/AN adolescent ages 15 to 19 years increased by 128% between 1990 and 2004 (10,11). This is troubling because youths and young adults with diabetes may experience many more years of disease burden than those who are diagnosed later in life, and they are at greater risk for serious and costly complications earlier in life (10,11).

Between 1999 and 2004, diabetes mortality was more than three times greater in the AI/AN population than in the general US population. Diabetes mortality is also increasing. From 1992 to 1999, diabetes mortality increased 62% in the AI/AN population, compared with a 10% increase in the general US population (5,12,13).

Cardiovascular disease (CVD) is the number one cause of death of AI/AN adults, and AI/AN individuals with diabetes are 3 to 4 times more likely to develop CVD than those without diabetes (5,13). The prevalence of diabetic retinopathy in American Indians and Alaska Natives is 2.2 times greater than in the general US population (5,13). Similarly, diabetes eye diseases are disproportionately high in AI/AN populations, with some tribes reporting prevalence as high as 50% (13).

The rate of diabetes-related kidney failure is 3.5 times higher among American Indians and Alaska Natives than in the general US population (13). There is some good news about kidney disease, however. Since 1993, the incidence of end-stage renal disease (ESRD) among American Indians and Alaska Natives has declined, even as prevalence of diabetes has increased. The change in ESRD incidence is greatest among adults older than 55 years (incidence has decreased by 26% in those younger than 55 years, by 40% in those between the ages of 55 and 64 years, and by 39% in those age 65 years and older). The decline in new cases may be due to the reduction of risk factors and improvements in diabetes care practices in Indian communities (14).

Risk Factors for Type 2 Diabetes

Genetic, environmental, and behavioral factors increase the risk of diabetes in American Indians and Alaska Natives. These factors include a hereditary predisposition to diabetes, insulin resistance, obesity, increasingly sedentary lifestyles, exposure to diabetes in utero, and the effects of living in adverse social and physical environments (11).

Over the last several centuries, the social, cultural, economic, and lifestyle patterns of AI/AN communities have changed drastically as a result of depopulation, resettlement, colonization, and assimilation. Many tribes were forcibly removed from their homelands and resettled in areas designated as Indian reservations (15). Resettlement disrupted traditional food acquisition practices such as farming, gathering, hunting, and fishing. Dietary patterns also changed with the introduction of new foods, such as government-supplied sugar, flour, salt pork, and beef. Today, federal food assistance programs, such as Food Distribution Programs on Indian Reservations (FDPIR) and Food Stamps, continue to encourage the consumption of nontraditional foods. These programs were initially designed to be agricultural subsidy programs and were not focused on providing a healthful diet; however, they did help reduce undernutrition.

Because of the loss of historical lands, other natural resources, and traditional subsistence food practices, American Indians and Alaska Natives have come to rely on a cash economy to obtain food (16). In this economy, AI/AN households have increased their consumption of store-bought convenience and prepared foods, as well as fast foods. Furthermore, many AI/AN communities are in remote locations, and this limits access to healthful foods, such as fresh fruits and vegetables. As a consequence, current AI/AN diets tend to be high in calories and fat. At the same time, physical activity has decreased due to an increased reliance on motorized transportation, greater use of time-saving machinery, and more sedentary occupational and recreational activities. Thus, energy consumption has increased while energy expenditure has decreased.

The prevalence of obesity is high among AI/AN adults. According to the Centers for Disease Control and Prevention (CDC), AI/AN adults 18 years or older were more likely to be obese (38.5%) than whites (22.3%), blacks (26.6%), or Asians (6.2%) (17). As a consequence, the AI/AN population is disproportionately affected by obesity-related conditions, such as diabetes and CVD. The prevalence of obesity is greater among American Indians and Alaska Natives with diabetes than those without, and it is increasing. In 1995, 59.2 % of AI/AN adults with diabetes were obese (body mass index [BMI] ≥ 30). By 2004, 69.9% of AI/AN adults with diabetes were obese (18).

Addressing obesity and weight management may be one of the most important strategies for preventing and treating diabetes in AI/AN individuals. The risk of developing diabetes increases as BMI increases. People with a BMI equal to or greater than 35 (class II obesity) are 20 times more likely to develop diabetes than individuals with a normal BMI (19). A study was conducted among the US Pima Indians of central Arizona and the Mexican Pima Indians living in a remote region in Sonora, Mexico, to compare environmental influences on the prevalence rates of obesity and of type 2 diabetes in two genetically prone populations

(20). The Pima of the United States and Mexico have a shared genetic background but live in different environments. The US Pima Indians had much higher rates of obesity and diabetes than the Pima Indians in Mexico. The US Pima Indians consumed less fiber and more fat and expended considerably less energy in occupational and leisure-time physical activity than the Mexican Pima Indians. These findings suggest that diabetes and obesity are largely preventable conditions and that the development of diabetes and obesity is determined mostly by behavioral and lifestyle factors (20). This conclusion is further supported by the results of the Diabetes Prevention Program (DPP), a clinical trial sponsored by the NIH, which demonstrated that modest weight loss through diet, physical activity, and behavior change can often prevent type 2 diabetes in people at high risk for developing type 2 diabetes (21,22). DPP included American Indian participants, and findings for these individuals were comparable to the results for all subjects (21,22).

American Indian groups vary greatly by region, and each has its own distinct language, culture, traditions, and beliefs systems that play a significant role in food practices. Therefore, no resource can covers all groups. The rest of this chapter focuses on the food patterns of two of the largest tribal groupings in the United States, the Northern Plains Indians and the Navajo Indian tribe. With a population approaching 300,000, the Navajo Indians are among the top-10 largest American Indian tribes. They live primarily in the southwest, in parts of Arizona, Utah, and New Mexico. The Northern Plains Indians span a large geographic region (the Dakotas, Montana, Wyoming, and Nebraska) and include some of the largest tribal groupings and the most populous Indian reservations, such as the Choctaw, Chippewa, and Sioux (1). The Alaska Native population is discussed in Chapter 2.

Registered dietitians (RDs) who are interested in tribes not covered in this publication are encouraged to begin their research with government and nongovernmental organizations that focus on American Indian and Alaska Native issues, such as the IHS (http://www.ihs.gov). A good place to start is by looking up the IHS area in which the tribe resides. This will help target your research.

Northern Plains Tribes

Traditional Foods and Dishes

Northern Plains Indians lived and hunted in the area now known as North Dakota, South Dakota, Montana, Wyoming, and Nebraska. The area comprises grassy plains as well as the Black Hills and the Rocky Mountains. Historically, the people were mainly hunters and gatherers, who came to trade with other tribes for farmed items, such as corn, squash, beans, and sunflowers. These tribes considered the entire northern plains their home; they traveled and hunted during the seasons when it was possible and camped when the weather was difficult. Before a hunt they would pray for a successful and bountiful hunt. Afterward, they offered prayers for thanksgiving for a successful hunt and for the animals that gave their lives to help the people (23).

Northern Plains Indians lived in teepees, which were easy to move as the Indians followed the game animals or seasons of gathering. They ate a wide variety of meat, berries, and roots and prepared their food primarily outside. When meat was plentiful, it would be roasted over open fires, cooked in leaf-lined pits with a fire on top, or dried over a fire or in the sun. Vegetables, some fruits, and eggs were boiled or dried and mixed with fats. Many fruits were pounded raw and mixed with fat or meat to make pemmican, which was stored in containers for later use and often eaten during travel. All parts of the animals, such as tongue, brain, liver kidney, bone marrow, blood, and scrapings from the hides, were used; nothing was wasted. Bones were used to fashion weapons or fish hooks. The Plains people practiced communal food distribution, with everyone sharing in the foods from a hunt or from gathering of foods. See Boxes 1.1 and 1.2 for examples of traditional foods and dishes. Refer to Appendix A for nutrient analyses.

Box 1.1 • Foods Used in Traditional[a] Northern Plains Indian Cuisine

Starchy vegetables
- Acorns
- Corn
- Wild potatoes
- Wild rice
- Wild turnips (timpsila)
- Winter squash

Nonstarchy vegetables
- Asparagus
- Ground beans
- Hazelnuts
- Lamb's quarters (indian spinach)
- Milkweed
- Mushrooms
- Pigweed (young, tender leaves are eaten fresh or dried)
- Sunchokes (jerusalem artichokes)
- Sunflower seeds
- Wild onions
- Young dandelion leaves

Fruits
- Buffalo berries
- Cactus fruits
- Chokecherries
- Currants
- June berries
- Rose hips
- Sandcherries (ground cherries)
- Serviceberries
- Wild grapes
- Wild plums
- Wild strawberries

Meats and meat substitutes
- Antelope
- Beaver
- Bird eggs
- Buffalo
- Duck
- Elk
- Fish
- Geese
- Grouse
- Pheasant
- Porcupine
- Prairie chicken
- Prairie dog
- Rabbit
- Raccoon
- Snakes
- Squirrel
- Turtle
- Venison
- Wild turkey

[a]Pre-European, hunted, gathered, and traded foods.

Box 1.2 • Traditional Northern Plains Indian Dishes and Beverages

Dishes
- Boiled, roasted, or fried meats[a]
- Corn wasna (ground dried corn or corn meal browned and mixed with fat and raisins)
- Dried meat[a]
- Dried berries
- Meat[a] soup with timpsila (wild turnips), wild roots, vegetables
- Organs (tongue, liver, or kidney), boiled, roasted, or raw
- Pemmican/wasna (dried meat and dried berries ground together and mixed with fat)
- Taniga soup (tripe, corn, hominy, potato, timpsila, onion)

Beverages
- Juniper tea
- Leadplant tea
- Rosehip tea
- Smooth sumac tea
- Wild cherry tea
- Wild peppermint tea

[a]May be prepared with any of the meats listed in Box 1.1.

Box 1.3 • Traditional Northern Plains Indian Foods Consumed During the Christmas Holiday	
• Berry pudding	• Pemmican
• Buffalo stew	• Potato
• Corn	• Turnip
• Fry bread	• Venison roasted

Traditional Meal Patterns and Holiday Foods

Northern Plains Indians were nomadic and followed the buffalo. They also traveled where they knew plants and berries grew. They gathered berries and roots along their journey and then cooked or ate them raw during the trip or dried them for later consumption.

Traditionally, the Plains Indians did not follow the European custom of eating three meals a day. Instead, they probably ate in the morning and again later in the day. In the late 19th and early 20th centuries, however, children were sent to boarding schools, where they adapted to different foods, meal times, and holidays (24,25).

A traditional morning meal was a soup of meat and broth, which might also include *timpsila* (a starchy root vegetable) or other collected wild plants. Other meals were recently killed meat roasted in a pit or over a fire or just dried meat or jerky. A container of stew would be cooked during the day with some type of meat and vegetables and roots. It was then available when people were ready to eat. When fresh game was available, it would be roasted in an open fire and enjoyed by all. A visit from friends or relatives called for a feast, and the hosts would hunt and roast meat over the fire. The feast might also include squash and other native vegetables that the people had gathered (26).

Northern Plains Indians celebrated births, marriages, young people coming of age, and occasions when several camps came together. When children were sent to boarding schools in the 19th and 20th centuries, they learned of European holidays and celebrations, along with different types of foods and regular meal times. Refer to Box 1.3 for traditional foods served at Christmas time.

Traditional Health Beliefs

An important aspect of North Plains Indian health beliefs is the Medicine Wheel. This object includes four sacred parts, which represent north, south, east, and west; the four sacred colors; the four parts of the spiritual world and the physical world; the four values of the Lakota Oyate (respect, generosity, wisdom, and courage) that guide the lives of warriors and their families; the four stages of life; and much more. The hoop that rims the wheel represents, in totality, the circle of life (27). Northern Plains Indians also traditionally used many herbs and plants for health and medicinal purposes (see discussion of alternative and complementary medicines later in this chapter).

Historically, the Northern Plains Indians did not have a word for "diabetes" because the condition was unknown. The Sioux words for diabetes are *skuyah wahzonka* (27).

Current Food Practices

Many Northern Plains Indians still remember and enjoy what their elders ate, and older individuals in particular continue to consume game (such as deer, elk, buffalo, pheasant, and prairie chickens), berries, native vegetables, and roots—although not typically on a daily basis. Many young people have not grown up eating game, however, and do not include it in their meals.

In general, the meal practices of Northern Plains Indians have changed drastically over time, from a hunter-gather lifestyle that consisted of mostly game with limited vegetables and roots to a "meat and potatoes" diet (see Box 1.4). Fast food, fried foods, and large portions have become a part of daily life for many Northern Plains Indians. Their food choices are influenced by the use of commodity foods; the Special Supplemental Nutrition Program for

Box 1.4 • Foods Currently Consumed by Northern Plains Indians

Breads and grains

- Bagels
- Cornbread
- Fry bread
- Muffins
- Pancakes
- Pasta
- Rice
- Store-bought bread (white or wheat)
- Tortillas
- Yeast bread, home-made

Fruits

- Apples
- Bananas
- Berries
- Cantaloupe
- Cherries
- Fruit cocktail
- Fruit salad
- Grapes
- Oranges
- Peaches
- Pears
- Watermelon

Vegetables

- Broccoli
- Cabbage
- Carrots
- Cauliflower
- Commodity vegetables
- Corn, canned or fresh
- Dried beans (navy, pinto, lima)
- Green beans
- Potatoes
- Salads
- Squash
- Sweet potatoes

Meat

- Beef (all parts)
- Turkey
- Bison
- Chicken
- Crab legs
- Elk
- Jerky
- Lobster
- Lunchmeat
- Pork
- Sausage
- Tuna
- Venison

Dishes

- Beans and ham hocks
- Biscuits and gravy
- Breakfast sandwiches
- Chicken and rice
- Chili
- Goulash
- Macaroni and cheese
- Meat soup
- Popovers
- Potato soup
- Vegetable soup

Beverages

- Alcohol
- Coffee
- Juice
- Milk
- Soda pop
- Sugar-sweetened drinks
- Tea

Desserts

- Cake
- Candy
- Cookies
- Gelatin with fruit
- Ice cream
- Pastries
- Pie
- Whipped topping

Women, Infants, and Children (WIC); and Food Stamps. Typical foods include hamburgers, french fries, fried potatoes, potatoes and gravy, "all you can eat" buffets, big steaks, fried pork chops or pork steak, fried chicken, hot dogs, ring bologna, lunch meat, macaroni and cheese (sometimes fried), flavored noodles, cheese, sugary flavored drinks, large sodas, cookies, cakes, pies, ice cream, potato salad, gelatin with fruit, and fruit cocktail with whipped cream. However, with nutrition and diabetes education, many Northern Plains Indians are taking steps to live a more healthful lifestyle, such as baking, boiling, and roasting foods.

Navajos

The Navajo Nation is the largest Indian reservation in the United States. It comprises about 16 million acres (25,000 square miles) and is approximately the size of West Virginia. Navajos call themselves *Diné* (the People). Historically, the Navajo people were nomadic. They hunted game and looked for plants to feed their families and livestock, often settling near a source of water. In the past, their settlement patterns were dispersed, and they tended to live in nuclear family units that included the father, mother, and children. Some families had summer gardens and livestock. They may have had a summer, spring, fall, or winter (seasonal) home.

Today, most Navajo people live and work together in towns or cities, not villages. They may still have a summer garden and livestock, as well as a seasonal home. Traditional nuclear families still exist, but family units may also have expanded to include grandparents, grandchildren, aunts, uncles, and other relatives. Instead of dispersed settlement patterns, Navajo settlements now coalesce around government-subsidized housing on the reservation.

As a culture in transition, the Navajo people and their traditional lifestyle continue to change in response to environmental factors. For example, consumption of foods and beverages high in fat and sugar has increased; food portion sizes are larger; and their lifestyle is more sedentary.

Traditional Foods and Dishes

Navajos perceive a connection between food consumption and strength. Strength is demonstrated through eating—you eat to show that you are strong (27).

Historically, Navajos were not vegetarians, but they had a plant-based diet and ate meat only occasionally (eg, for ceremony). They believed that plant and animal foods belonged together, and each animal had a place in the universal scheme. Deer, antelope, elk, and mountain sheep had special ritualistic value.

The native dwelling of the Navajo, known as a hogan *(hoozhan)*, is a dome-shaped structure with eight corners of logs stacked together and a chimney hole at the top for the fireplace. Traditionally, cooking might take place inside the hogan, on a metal barrel cut in half (with fire inside) or on an adobe-type stove. Alternatively, an open fire could be built outdoors for roasting, boiling, and baking underground. Many families now have a regular gas or electric stove, but many people continue to bake corn, corn cakes, or parts of meat in the ground. Food preparation can involve boiling foods on top of the stove or roasting over open coals.

Corn *(Na dá)* is sacred to the Navajo people. It is a symbol of fertility and life and the basis of many Navajo dishes. In the past, the corn was dried and ground using stones and then roasted over the coals in a frying pan. It was stirred frequently to prevent from burning and then spread on a sheepskin to cool. The stones were placed in the middle of the skin and the corn was ground three times, using grass brush for sweeping the cornmeal. The meal was placed in a clean empty flour sack for later use. Refer to Box 1.5 and Table 1.1 for additional information on traditional foods and dishes (28). See Appendix A for nutrient analyses.

From the 19th century through the 1960s, the seeds of grasses and weeds were used for food. Middle-aged and elderly tribal members gathered wild plants and herbs, mostly during the spring, from their local area. Traditionally, individuals living closer to a border town or city did not eat as many plants or herbs as those who resided in more remote areas.

Box 1.5 • Foods Used in Traditional Navajo Cuisine

Starchy vegetables

- Beans
- Corn (such as blue, sweet, yellow); hominy[a]
- Wild potatoes
- Winter squash

Nonstarchy vegetables

- Pigweed[b]
- Summer squash
- Wild plants (such as celery, onion, and spinach)

Milk

- Goat milk
- Sheep milk

Fruits

- Apple
- Apricots
- Cantaloupe
- Juniper berries
- Navajo banana (wild banana)[c]
- Peaches
- Sumac berries[d]
- Watermelon

Nuts and seeds

- Piñon nuts[e]
- Squash seeds
- Tumble mustard seeds[f]

Clay, ashes, and salts

- Clay (white, gray)[h]
- Juniper ash[g]
- Rock salt
- Tumbleweed (greasewood) ash[i]

Meats

- Deer
- Horse
- Beef
- Mutton (all parts; boiled, roasted, dried, stew) and lamb[j]
- Pork
- Prairie dog
- Rabbit

[a]Hominy is kernels of dried steamed corn, which is made by steaming fresh ears of corn overnight, then drying the ears and removing the kernels. Served boiled.

[b]Common plant of the genus *Amaranthus*. The young, tender leaves are eaten fresh or dried.

[c]The fleshy fruit of the mountain yucca plant. It can be boiled, mashed, rolled flat, dried and rolled onto a stick (similar to fruit leather, which is dried fruit that has been flattened out with a stick).

[d]Small red berries that are eaten fresh, dried, or boiled with the juice strained, sweetened, and thickened to make a pudding.

[e]Nuts from the piñon pine. A popular snack roasted and sometimes salted in the shell; shelled before eating.

[f]Tiny seeds removed from the pods of dry plants. These seeds are ground and added to cornbread.

[g]Used for flavoring and coloring. Brings a distinctive taste to foods cooked with it, and people can tell when it is not used. It also has some medicinal purposes used in ceremony.

[h]Obtained from plants and used for ceremonial purposes. The body of the person for whom the ceremony is held (known as the "patient") is completely covered with the substance during traditional ceremonies for healing.

[i]The substance that remains when this plant is burned and sifted.

[j]Mutton may be dried and reheated over coals. To hydrate, it is boiled and pulverized into little pieces (muscle fibers). The pieces are grilled with onions, put in a pan and cooked with chili peppers; mostly eaten by persons living in rural areas of the reservation. Consuming the organ meats of the sheep is considered a delicacy. Other parts of the sheep eaten are the head, including the brain, heart, kidneys, skin, tongue, and eyes; the liver with the greater omentum (ie, fatty tissue or tallow that is extended over the stomach and passing inferiorly in front of the transverse colon or intestine), as well as the meat from the center of the chest area of the sheep. Navajo people traditionally did not waste in any parts of the sheep.

Table 1.1 · Traditional Navajo Breads, Dishes, Desserts, and Beverages

Food	Description
Breads	
Blue corn bread	Made from ground blue corn flour mixed with culinary ash and boiling water. Bread can be formed into round patties and cooked in a hot skillet or shaped in a loaf and baked in hot ashes.
Blue corn mush	Made from ground blue corn flour and water boiled together. It can be made with or without juniper ash.
Blue dumplings	Noodles made from blue corn flour. A dough mixture of blue corn flour, ash, and boiling water is shaped into small balls (about the size of a quarter) and boiled. A blue corn gravy forms around the dumplings.
Frozen blue corn mush	Made with blue corn four, ash and water, then frozen.
Hopi piki bread	Made of blue corn meal that is dehydrated and rolled into a long, thin bread.
Kneel-down bread	Bread made from fresh Indian corn that is ground and then wrapped in corn husks and baked. Made with or without blood of sheep.
Navajo cake (ground cake)	Bread made from ground corn flour mixed with dried, ground wheat sprouts, brown sugar, and water; sometimes raisins are added. Ground cake is baked in a cornhusk-lined pit in the ground; Navajo cake is baked in an oven. Traditionally made for a girl's puberty ceremony (*Kinaalda'*).
Navajo pancake	Pancake made of blue corn flour, white flour, and whole milk.
Tortillas and fry bread	Both of these breads are made with fat (oil, shortening, or lard). However, the amount of fat used in preparation varies. Droplets of oil, cooking spray, or a small amount of oil may be used, or breads may be deep-fried in large amount of oil. The more oil used, the more bubbles in the bread.
Dishes	
Blood sausage	Made using the intestine of the sheep and adding onions, potatoes, celery, and/or any other vegetables.
Mutton stew	A meat and vegetable stew. The most common variation includes mutton, goat, beef, or pork, as well as potatoes and onions. In the summer months, people use meat, squash or squash blossoms, corn, and onion. Other variations include carrots, potatoes, corn, green peppers, and whatever else is available. Blue dumplings can also be added.
Navajo sandwich	A meat sandwich on tortilla or fry bread. Can be made with mutton or beef, as well as lettuce, tomato, onion, roasted green chili peppers, and possibly cheese.
Navajo taco	Navajo fry bread topped with ground beef, lettuce, tomato, cheese, onions and chili beans and eaten as a meal.
Sumac berry pudding	Prepared by boiling juice of the sumac berry fruit, flour and sugar together until it forms this pudding.
Wild celery and onion soup	
Wolf berry sauce	Made with clay.
Beverages	
Goat or sheep milk	
Mormon tea	A tea (*Ephedra spp.*) introduced to the Navajos by the Mormon people.
Navajo tea	Tea made of native herbs.
Water	

Traditional Meal Patterns and Holiday Foods

Because food was scarce, the Navajo typically ate two meals a day, most often in the morning and the evening. Even when food was scarce, guests would be offered a meal upon arrival. Coffee could be considered a meal; even today, it is often offered as a meal to guests.

In traditional Navajo culture, only weddings, puberty ceremonies, and a baby's first laugh were celebrated. Presently, Navajos celebrate almost all US holidays, as well as birthdays, anniversaries, promotions, graduations, and births. Holiday foods depend on the season and food that is available at that time. Refer to Table 1.2 for more information about holiday foods and Box 1.6 for foods served at Christmas time (28).

Traditional Health Beliefs

Traditional Navajo health beliefs are complex, characterized by the seeking of harmony among human beings and between humans and the natural world. Navajo society is based on a strong clan system that traces kinship through a person's mother and her relatives. The goal is to walk in harmony or beauty *(Hozho)*. This is the guiding principal in life and health. Traditional Navajos believe that illness is due to an imbalance or disharmony between a person and nature (eg, being struck by lightning, being caught in a whirlwind or tornado, encountering a deceased human, killing a snake). Thus, there would need to be a medicine man or woman to diagnosis the illness.

Table 1.2 · Traditional Navajo Foods Consumed During Holidays

Food	Navajo Name
Blue corn mush (with ash)	*Taániil (Gad bił)*
Blue dumplings	*K'ineeshbízhii (or Naadą́ą́ ak'áán)*
Blue mush tamale	*Bé esł óní*
Cantaloupe	*Tá neesk'ání*
Fry bread	*Dah diniilghaazh*
Kneel-down bread	*Nitsidigóí*
Mutton (mutton stew, organ meats, blood sausage)	*Dibé bitsí*
Navajo banana	*Neesdoig*
Navajo cake	*Yilką́ą́d (or alką́ą́d)*
Navajo tea	*Ch'il ahwéhé nineezígíí*
Piñon nuts	*Neeshch'íí*
Roasted corn	*Naadaá ditleé sit'e*
Steamed corn coffee creamer	*Łeéshibéézh Tśáałbai*
Sumac berry pudding	*Tśiiłchin tóshchíín*
Tortilla	*Náneeskaadí*
Tumbleweed ash	*Ch'ildeeníní bileeshch'ih*
Wild rhubarb	*Chahat'inii*
Yellow squash	*Naayízí*
Yuca fruit	*Hashk'aan sit' eego (doołóhó)*
Zucchini	*Naayízí yázhí*

Box 1.6 • Traditional Navajo Foods Consumed During the Christmas Holiday	
• Blue corn bread	• Fry bread and tortillas
• Blue corn dumpling	• Mutton (all parts of the sheep)
• Blue corn tamale	• Navajo cake
• Blue mush with ash	• Navajo creamer
• Dried mutton	• Navajo tea
• Dried peaches	• Steamed corn stew with mutton
• Dried sumac berries	• Wild turkey
• Fried potatoes	• Young horse meat

Singing or prayer was thought to bring the person back into balance or harmony with nature (curing or treating the illness). Traditional treatments included herbs, roots, or plants in conjunction with a sweat bath. Many Navajos today continue to use traditional healings and participate in traditional ceremonies in addition to seeking Western medicine.

Current Food Practices

Navajo tradition is a part of an individual's history, beliefs, and culture. The substance of tradition differs from person to person and is influenced by education, religion, travel, proximity to home and/or job, income level, and geographical location on the reservation (eg, eastern, western, central). Navajo tradition shapes an individual's past experiences and memories, as well as how the individual interprets his or her own history, religion, and culture.

Current conditions, emotions, family, and friends influence the food practices of the Navajo. Meal patterns depend on the individual's preferences, work, and daily schedules. Navajos may eat one meal a day or several. Some may choose to skip a meal at home and instead purchase a meal on their way to work or a trip to town. Given the abundance of grocery stores and roadside food stands, time constraints, and limited knowledge about traditional local plants used/eaten by ancestors, very few Navajo gather, hunt or cultivate foods for consumption. Traditional cooking methods (such as underground cooking, boiling, and roasting) are still used. However, many modern-day Navajos cook with fat (frying, deep frying) and salt, and may add salt to their foods before eating. Navajos also eat commodity foods, including processed meats, cheese, powdered milk and eggs, canned vegetables and fruits, shortening and cooking oils. Many elders living in rural areas do not like spicy flavors and do not like to mix many flavors. However, the middle-aged and younger people incorporate many international flavors and foods into their meals. See Box 1.7 for more information on current food choices.

Counseling Considerations

Although there are some commonalities in values and beliefs among many American Indians and Alaska Natives, the AI/AN population is very diverse. Therefore, it is important to learn about the specific cultural and traditional practices of the AI/AN community in which you work. Poverty, lack of knowledge, and environmental changes can contribute to unhealthful lifestyle choices.

Women have historically contributed significantly to the family income and have had primary responsibility for managing the household. They must balance the needs of the individual with diabetes and those of the whole family. Therefore, schedules for counseling appointments need to be flexible—try to offer openings after work or around lunchtime.

As with many cultures in the United States, food is typically the center of many AI/AN celebrations, family gatherings, ceremonies, and special events. When a person is invited to the home of a relative and/or friend and food is offered to them, it is considered an insult to the family and/or host to refuse the food. This is why many Indian people feel compelled to eat foods, even if they are not hungry and/or do not want it. Also, the native medicine man or woman is often paid for services through food.

Box 1.7 • Foods Currently Eaten in Navajo Culture

Breads and grains

- Bagels
- Blue corn bread
- Blue corn mush
- Blue dumplings
- Hominy
- Hopi *piki* bread
- Kneel-down bread
- Muffins
- Navajo cake (ground cake)
- Pasta
- White or wheat bread[a]
- Tortillas/fry bread

Vegetables and fruits

- Apple
- Apricots
- Beans
- Cantaloupe
- Corn (steamed, roasted)
- Peaches
- Potatoes (fried, boiled)
- Squash (winter, summer)
- Sumac berry pudding
- Watermelon
- Other canned, frozen, dried, juiced and fresh fruits/vegetables[a]

Nuts and seeds

- Piñon nuts
- Other nuts/seeds (salted, shelled)[a]

Beverages

- Alcohol (beer, wine, whiskey)
- Coffee
- Energy/sport drinks
- Juice (10%, 25%, 100%)
- Milk (cow, soy, rice)
- Powdered drink mixes
- Soda pop (regular, diet)
- Tea (all varieties)

Meats[b]

- Beef
- Blood sausage
- Fish, shellfish
- Lamb (all parts)
- Mutton (all parts)
- Organ meats
- Pork
- Poultry

Desserts

- Cake
- Cookies
- Fruit gelatins
- Pastries
- Pies

Other

- Clay, ashes, rock salt[c]
- Junk food (potato chips, nachos, candy, ramen noodles)[a]

[a]Purchased at the grocery store.
[b]Can be canned, fresh, frozen or dried.
[c]Traditionally, clay and rock salt were used in ceremonial practices. At present, they both remain useful in ceremonies. For example, rock salt is used to celebrate a baby's first laugh. Ash also provides flavor in many traditional dishes (eg, blue corn mush).

Many AI/AN people are visual learners who prefer to learn by observation or by watching a video. Food models and pictures of food and portions should be used in counseling. Ask the client what he or she wants to learn and how the information can be applied or used in his or her situation. The clients are the experts in their home environment, and they are living with whatever diagnosis they are given by their health care providers. The client and the clinician should work together to create a plan.

Explain concepts in simple terms, and remember that many people do not understand grams or carbohydrates. Do not overload the client with handouts. If you give handouts, give explicit explanations.

Demonstrating Courtesy and Respect

When greeting or meeting someone, Navajos and Northern Plains Indians (especially the elderly) believe in the importance of proper introductions—shaking hands, asking what clan you are a part of, where you are from, explaining your profession, and so on. Formal greetings are customary even during routine encounters. Some handshakes are strong, and some are very light. Close friends will hug each other.

When working with the clients, sit near them, but not very close and not across from them. At the beginning of the counseling session, always ask permission before asking questions, especially about their home and /or living conditions. Speak in a friendly manner. If you are familiar with the client and his or her family, talk about common topics. This will encourage clients to listen, open up, and share.

Interpreting Clients' Nonverbal Communication

Some people may listen while sitting with their eyes closed. It is considered rude to look another person directly in the eye, so many will avoid a direct gaze. If you have been talking for a while and the person seems to close up, it is time to stop the conversation. Be observant and you will know when you have spent too much time talking.

Inquiring About Clients' Understanding of Diabetes

Northern Plains Indians know about diabetes and its devastating effects. However, they may not have an accurate understanding of the disease. For example, some mistakenly believe that insulin injections in the stomach area will lead to a need for kidney dialysis. Many people believe that they will inevitably get diabetes because their parents and grandparents had it. Ask your clients what they know about diabetes, medicines, and complications. Talk about the benefits of medicines, exercise, and preventing complications. Scare tactics are ineffective and may alienate your clients.

To encourage Navajo clients to eat more healthfully, ask them, "Which choice would work for you?" or "How does this choice fit your schedule, your family lifestyle, and/or within the limitations you have?"

Discussing Clients' Use of Complementary and Alternative Medicine

The uses of traditional medicine, healing practices, and other types of complementary and alternative medicine vary substantially among tribes and from one individual to the next. Some clients may combine traditional healing practices with the use of Western medicines and over-the-counter herbs and supplements. Clients may also use complementary or alternative medicines/remedies offered in the marketplace to heal diabetes. In a study at an Urban Indian Health center, 38% of AI/AN clients (representing 30 different tribes) reported that they saw a healer in addition to a physician. Among those who did not see a healer, 86% reported that they would consider visiting a healer in the future. Among the most commonly visited healers were spiritual healers (51%), herbalists (42%), and medicine men (28%). The most common treatments were sweat lodge ceremonies (58%), herbal remedies (55%), and spiritual healing (53%) (29).

Navajos traditionally used various herbs during ceremonies to cure many common illnesses and/or treat symptoms of illnesses (see Table 1.3 for examples). Some Navajos continue these practices.

Traditional and modern-day Navajos focus treatments on the *cause* of the illness whereas they may believe that Western medicines only treat *symptoms* (30). With regard to Western medications, elderly clients may say *aza dóó nalnish dáá* ("the medicine does not work"; "the medicine does not heal"; or "the medicine does not make well"). Clients with these beliefs may stop taking their medications. If they understand how a medication works (its mechanism of action, possible adverse effects, and food-drug interactions), they may be more likely to take it. Providers should seek their clients' cooperation to find the best care for them.

Table 1.3 • Self-Treatment Remedies Used by Navajos

Type of Remedy	Description	Usesa
• Herbal tea	A mixture of various herbs and other plants grown and/ or picked that is brewed with hot water. The ingredients vary regionally across the reservation.	• Lowering of blood glucose levels
• Juniper ash	A branch from the juniper plant is burned over hot coals with a pan underneath to collect the ashes. The whitish-gray, powder-like ashes from the plant are sifted and collected for use.	• Detoxification of the body • Relief of upset stomach • Used when mourning and/or depressed
• Pine tree sap	A clear, thick, jelly-like substance obtained from the pine tree.	• Treatment for boils

aData in this column describe *how* the remedies are used and do not reflect whether the treatments are safe or effective.

Appendix C provides general questions to assess dietary supplement use. Nutrition counselors must be sensitive to and respectful of an individual's decision to share or not share their use of traditional medicine and healing practices. These decisions are personal, and clients may not want to disclose this information. Also, some religions prohibit the sharing of specific spiritual practices, although clients may be willing to share that they are going to their holy man and receiving medicine. If you do not have an understanding of their traditions, it might be best to not broach these topics with AI/AN clients.

Considering Family Demands and Dynamics

Family and community are highly valued in AI/AN cultures. Family structures are intergenerational, and elders are highly valued for the wisdom and experience. Family, friends, and community will influence the food practices and lifestyle behaviors of AI/AN clients.

Engaging Others in Counseling Sessions

Decisions regarding food in the home are typically influenced by family, and it can be helpful to have family members accompany the person with diabetes to the counseling session. For example, many middle-aged and elderly AI/AN people rely on other family members for their food preparation and grocery shopping. Therefore, if the client consents to their presence, it can be helpful to invite those family members to participate in counseling sessions to understand the specific dietary needs of the client. As a family, they can all work together toward the individual's nutrition goals.

Community members also play a vital role in diabetes education. Role models in the community—such as spiritual leaders, local teachers, health professionals, community health representatives (CHRs), WIC counselors, health technicians, nursing aides, and Native American celebrities can serve as advocates for good nutrition and a healthful lifestyle. Also, classes (eg, a diabetes class, a native lifestyle balance program), talking circles, story-telling, and other group activities allow AI/AN people to share experiences and gain help with problem-solving. Peer educators that are members of the community can facilitate the dissemination of nutrition messages to clients and encourage them to seek nutrition services. However, it is important to provide training programs to ensure the messages are accurate and consistent across all clinicians and educators.

Nutrition Counseling

To effectively counsel clients, you must assess their readiness for change, their reasons for change, and the likelihood that they will sustain it. Many things influence a person's readiness for change. People will make a change when they can relate to it and/or find it meaningful (eg, it gives them hope).

Nutrition counseling may be more effective if you discuss how the dietary change will benefit the entire family, not just the individual client. You should promote incremental change in eating and reinforce the concept that change is a process. Acknowledge that there will be slip-ups, and this does not mean a client has failed. When clients fall off track, explore the reasons why and encourage them to start again.

Appendix B offers selected medical nutrition therapy (MNT) recommendations for individuals with diabetes and general counseling suggestions that support those recommendations. The following are culturally specific nutrition counseling strategies for AI/AN clients:

- Encourage clients to take reduced-calorie and/or low-fat potluck dishes to traditional holiday and ceremonial events.
- Explore traditional forms of physical activity, such as sheep herding, chopping wood, hunting, fishing, gathering, dancing, and engaging in traditional games.
- Encourage consumption of indigenous grains, fruits, and vegetables (either gathered or cultivated), as well as traditional foods that are good sources of protein, such as wild game, fish, and birds.
- Promote the tradition of drying foods as a low-fat method for food preparation.
- Discuss the nutrients in commodity foods and ways to make more healthful selections.

Challenges and Barriers to Dietary Adherence

There are various challenges in counseling AI/AN clients. AI/AN reservation communities are often in rural or remote locations. Some AI/AN live without electricity, running water, or modern plumbing. Many families live at or below the poverty level and therefore rely on commodity food program and other federal food assistance programs. Fast-food outlets and convenience stores are plentiful, whereas healthful foods, such as whole grains, fresh fruits, and vegetables, may be inaccessible or very expensive. Food portions are larger than necessary, which contributes to increased intake of high-fat, high-sugar, and convenience foods, and individuals often lack an understanding of recommended serving sizes. Large quantities of foods are served at holiday, traditional, and community sporting events.

AI/AN clients may lack knowledge of many nutrition-related technical terms, statistics, and concepts, such as the Dietary Guidelines for Americans. As noted previously, AI/AN people tend to be visual learners. Therefore, it is better to show or demonstrate a particular principle or idea than to tell it. For example, use food models to demonstrate the proper amounts of foods to be eaten.

When teaching clients about food labels, do not focus on just numbers and percentages. Instead, explain the components of the label and how they help the client make healthful choices. It is also helpful to quantify terms such as "low fat," "moderation," "high fat," and "portion" and provide visual props to show what you mean.

For many AI/AN elders, English may not be their first language. Some clients may not have received or completed a formal school education. Be sure to assess whether you need an interpreter who understands medical terminology to convey your thoughts to your client. Most hospitals and clinics have trained interpreters. It is best to use these personnel because medical terminology is complex and native languages often do have words for most medical terms.

Counseling Tips

The following are key objectives for the RD working with AI/AN clients:

- Establish rapport and trust.
- Be caring and show empathy.
- Inform the client that you will be asking questions and explain why.
- Ask permission before beginning an assessment.
- Have knowledge of the tribal community's cultural traditions, spiritual and religious practices, health beliefs, and food practices.

- Do not assume the extent to which the individual follows traditions, beliefs, and practices. It is important to conduct an individual assessment.
- Have knowledge of community resources, WIC, Food Stamps, commodities, tribal resources, etc.
- Determine the client's primary language, and use interpreters as needed.
- Use peer or lay health educators, preferably from the tribal community.
- Adhere to confidentiality rules and privacy laws.
- Determine the individual's preferred learning style.
- Use visual teaching aids, such as food replicas, measuring tools, and pictures, as well as hands-on teaching methods, such as cooking demonstrations and grocery store tours.
- Be knowledgeable of the foods that are available in grocery stores and other food outlets. Recommend economically available and acceptable foods. Work together on a shopping list and explore ideas for meal preparation using acceptable substitutions.
- Focus on small, incremental changes in eating and lifestyle changes. Emphasize positive messages and the benefits to the entire family.
- Reinforce the importance of eating together as a family.
- Encourage clients to incorporate traditional, indigenous foods and food acquisition practices (such as hunting, fishing, gathering, and planting and cultivating community gardens) into their lifestyle.
- Promote the cost and health benefits of breastfeeding. For every month a woman breast-feeds her baby, the child's risk for overweight, diabetes, and infant mortality decreases by 30% (31).
- Encourage clients to invite family members or caregivers that are responsible for food selection and preparation to counseling sessions.
- Ask clients to show you food labels from foods they eat at home.

Resources

Association of American Indian Physicians. http://www.aaip.org. Accessed February 9, 2009.

Association of State and Territorial Public Health Nutrition Directors. Resources and Tips for Working with American Indians and Alaskan Natives. http://www.astphnd.org/resource_read .php?resource_id=78&sid=edb35e. Accessed February 9, 2009.

Gohdes D. Diabetes in North American Indians and Alaska Natives. In: *Diabetes in America*. 2nd ed. Bethesda, MD: National Institute of Diabetes and Digestive and Kidney Diseases; 1995:683–701.

Joe JR., Young R, eds. *Diabetes as a Disease of Civilization: The Impact of Culture Change on Indigenous People*. Berlin, Germany: Mouton de Gruyter; 1993.

Kindscher K. *Edible Wild Plants of the Prairie: An Ethnobotanical Guide*. Lawrence: University Press of Kansas; 1987.

National Heart, Lung, and Blood Institute. Building Healthy Hearts for American Indians and Alaska Natives: A Background Report. Bethesda, MD: National Institutes of Health; 1998.

Office of the Assistant Secretary of Planning and Evaluation. Obesity and American Indians/Alaska Natives Report. Washington DC: Department of Health and Human Services; 2007. http://aspe.hhs.gov/hsp/07/AI-AN-obesity. Accessed February 9, 2009.

Roubideaux Y, ed. *Promises to Keep: Public Health Policy for American Indians and Alaska Natives in the 21st Century*. Washington, DC: American Public Health Association; 2001.

US Department of Agriculture. Food and Nutrition Services. Food Distribution Program on Indian Reservations. http://www.fns.usda.gov/fdd/programs/fdpir. Accessed February 9, 2009.

US Department of Health and Human Services. Indian Health Service. http://www.ihs.gov. Accessed February 9, 2009.US Department of Health and Human Services. Indian Health Service. Division of Diabetes Treatment and Prevention. http://www.ihs.gov/medicalprograms/diabetes. Accessed February 9, 2009.

Wolf WS, Weber CW, Arviso KD. Use and nutrient composition of traditional Navajo foods. *Ecol Food Nutr*. 1985;17:323–344.

References

1. US Census Bureau. The American Indian and Alaska Native Population: 2000. February 2002. http://www.census.gov/prod/2002pubs/c2kbr01-15.pdf. Accessed February 9, 2009.

2. Indian Health Service: Year 2008 Profile. http://info.ihs.gov/Profile08.asp. Accessed October 15, 2008.

3. US Department of Health and Human Services. Indian Health Service. The IHS Gold Book: Parts 1–4. http://info.ihs.gov. Accessed October 15, 2008.

4. Rimoin DL, Saiki JH. Diabetes mellitus among the Navajo: I. Clinical features. *Arch Intern Med.* 1968;122:1–5.

5. Indian Health Service. Division of Diabetes Treatment and Prevention. Fact Sheets. http://www.ihs.gov/MedicalPrograms/Diabetes/index.cfm?module=resourcesFactSheets. Accessed February 9, 2009.

6. Gohdes D. Diabetes in North American Indians and Alaska Natives. In: *Diabetes in America.* 2nd ed. Bethesda, MD: National Institute of Diabetes and Digestive and Kidney Diseases; 1995:683–701.

7. Howard BV, Lee ET, Cowan LD, Devereux JM, Go OT, Howard WJ, Rhoades ER, Robbins DC, Sievers ML, Welty TK. Rising tide of cardiovascular disease in American Indians: the Strong Heart study. *Circulation.* 1999;99:2389–2395.

8. Mokdad AH, Ford ES, Bowman BA, Nelson DE, Engelgau MM, Vinicor F, Marks JS. Diabetes trends in the U.S.: 1990-1998. *Diabetes Care.* 2000;23:1278–1283.

9. Indian Health Service. *Trends in Indian Health, 1998-99.* Rockville, MD: Department of Health and Human Services; 1999.

10. Acton KJ, Burrows, Wang J, Geiss LS. Diagnosed diabetes among American Indians and Alaska Natives ages < 35 years: United States, 1994-2004. *MMWR Morb Mortal Weekly Rep.* 2006;55:1201–1203.

11. Rios Burrows N, Geiss LS, Engelgau MM, Acton KJ. Prevalence of diabetes among Native Americans and Alaska Natives, 1990-1997: an increasing burden. *Diabetes Care.* 2000;3:1786–1790.

12. Indian Health Services. IHS National Diabetes Program Interim Report to Congress: Special Diabetes Program for Indians. December 2004:173–177.

13. Indian Health Services Division of Diabetes. Best Practice Documents. http://www.ihs.gov/MedicalPrograms/Diabetes/index.cfm?module=toolsBestPractices. Accessed May 29, 2009.

14. Burrows NR, Narva AS, Geiss LS, Engelgau MM and Acton, KJ. End-stage renal disease due to diabetes among southwest American Indians. 1990-2001. *Diabetes Care.* 2005;28:1041–1044.

15. Joe JR, Young R. Introduction. In: Joe JR, Young R, eds. *Diabetes as a Disease of Civilization: The Impact of Culture Change on Indigenous People.* Berlin, Germany: Mouton de Gruyter; 1993:1–18.

16. Conti KM. Diabetes prevention in Indian country: developing nutrition models to tell the story of food system change. *J Transcult Nurs.* 2006;17: 234–245.

17. Barnes PM, Adams PF, Powell-Griner E. *Health Characteristics of the American Indian and Alaska Native Adult Population: United States, 1999-2003.* Hyattsville, MD: National Center for Health Statistics. 2005. Advanced Data from Vital and Health Statistics no. 356.

18. Wilson C, Gilliland S, Moore K, Acton, K. The epidemic of extreme obesity among American Indian and Alaska Native adults with diabetes. *Prev Chron Dis.* 2007;4:1–8.

19. Klein S, Sheard NF, Pi-Sunyer X, Daly A, Wylie-Rosett J, Kulkarni K, Clark NG. Weight management through lifestyle modification for the prevention and management of type 2 diabetes: rationale and strategies. *Diabetes Care.* 2004;27:2067–2073.

20. Schulz LO, Bennett PH, Kidd JR, Kidd KK, Esparza J, Valencia ME. Effects of traditional and western environments on prevalence of type 2 diabetes in Pima Indians in Mexico and the U.S. *Diabetes Care.* 2006;29:1866–1871.

21. Knowler WC, Barrett-Connor E, Fowler SE, Hamman RF, Lachin JM, Walker EA, Nathan DM; Diabetes Prevention Program Research Group. Reduction in the incidence of type 2 diabetes with lifestyle intervention or metformin. *N Engl J Med.* 2002;346:393–403.

22. Hamman RF, Wing RR, Edelstein SL, Lachin JM, Bray GA, Delahanty L, Hoskin M, Kriska AM, Mayer-Davis EJ, Pi-Sunyer X, Regensteiner J, Venditti B, Wylie-Rosett J. Effect of weight loss with lifestyle intervention on risk of diabetes. *Diabetes Care.* 2006;29:2102–2107.

23. Saarita J. *The Dull Knives of Pine Ridge: A Lakota Odyssey.* Lincoln, NE: University of Nebraska Press; 2002.

24. Powers WK. *Indians of the Northern Plains.* New York, NY: Capricorn Books; 1973.

25. Kindscher K. *Edible Wild Plants of the Prairie: An Ethnobotanical Guide.* Lawrence: University Press of Kansas; 1987.

26. Walker JR. *The Sun Dance and Other Ceremonies of the Oglala.* New York, NY: American Museum of Natural History; 1917. http://sacred-texts.com/nam/pla/sdo/index.htm. Accessed May 26, 2009.

27. Satterfield DW, Shield JE, Buckley J, Taken Alive ST. So That the People May Live *(Hecel Lena Oyate Ki Nipi Kte)*: Lakota and Dakota elder women as reservoirs of life and keepers of knowledge about health protection and diabetes prevention. *J Health Dispar Res Pract.* 2007;1:1–28.

28. Bachman-Carter K, Duncan R, Pelican S. *Navajo Food Practices, Customs, and Holidays.* Chicago, IL: American Dietetic Association; 1998.

29. Marbella AM, Harris MC, Diehr S, Ignace G, Ignace G. Use of Native American healers among Native American patients in an urban Native American health center. *Arch Fam Med.* 1998;7:182–185.

30. Kim C, Kwok YS. Navajo use of native healers. *Arch Intern Med.* 1998;158: 2245–2249.

31. Shealy KR, Li R, Benton-Davis S, Grummer-Strawn LM. The CDC Guide to Breastfeeding Interventions. 2005. Atlanta, GA: Centers for Disease Control and Prevention. http://www.cdc.gov/breastfeeding/pdf/breastfeeding_interventions.pdf. Accessed February 10, 2009.

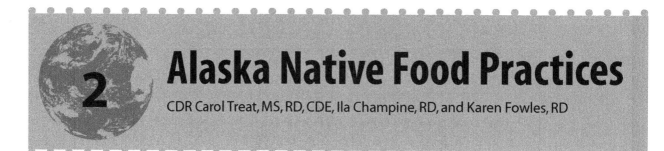

2 Alaska Native Food Practices

CDR Carol Treat, MS, RD, CDE, Ila Champine, RD, and Karen Fowles, RD

Introduction

Alaska is the largest state in terms of geographical size. Approximately one-third the size of the continental United States, Alaska has more land area than Washington, Oregon, California, Arizona, Nevada, Idaho, Utah, Wyoming, Colorado, New Mexico, and Montana combined. Alaska's land mass covers 533,000 square miles and is surrounded on three sides by water, with a total coastline of 33,000 miles. The name Alaska comes from the Aleut word for "great land."

Alaska's climate varies greatly, depending on the area. For example, winters in the southeast have mild temperatures and lots of rain, whereas winter temperatures in the north dip well below 0°F for months. Along the Aleutian and Pribilof Islands, the weather is unpredictable, but typically includes wind, mist, and gray skies. In the interior of Alaska the temperature on summer days can reach 90°F or hotter and will be as low as −50°F on winter nights, not accounting for the wind chill factor. Regardless of weather conditions, each geographic area of Alaska has its own awe-inspiring beauty—from the Brooks Range in the north to the Inside Passage along the southeast coast.

Much of Alaska does not have a highway system, and more than 200 Alaska Native villages are not accessible by road. The state ferry system (Alaska Marine Highway) operates in southeast and southwest Alaska, and the Alaska Railroad operates in the interior of the state. In the winter, people travel between villages via frozen rivers that serve as ice roads for cars, all-terrain vehicles (ATVs) or four-wheelers, and snow machines. According to the Alaska Department of Transportation, the state has only 14,788 miles of roads and 7,880 marine ferry miles. By necessity, air transportation is the primary, although most expensive, means of travel in rural Alaska. Inclement weather can delay air travel into or out of villages for days.

Alaska's natives can be divided up into five groups: the Aleut, Yupik Eskimos, Inupiat Eskimos, Athabascan Indians, and coastal Indians. According to the 2006 US Census Bureau, 88,026 individuals designated themselves as Alaska Native only; an additional 35,213 designated themselves as Alaska Native in combination with one or more other races. Approximately 55% are Eskimo, 32% are Indian (Tlingit, Haida, Tsimshian, or Athabascan), and 13% are Aleut (1).

Inupiat Eskimos mostly live in the northern and northwestern coastal regions; the Yupik Eskimos typically live in the southwestern regions. The Athabascan Indians live in the interior of the state, and the coastal Indians (Tlingit, Haida, and Tsimshian) reside in southeastern coastal Alaska. The Aleuts include residents of the Aleutian Islands, the Pribilof Islands, the western tip of the Alaska Peninsula, the Kodiak area, and the coastal regions of south-central Alaska (2).

Table 2.1 • Prevalence of Diabetes in Alaska Native Tribes, 1985–2005

Tribe	1985	2005	% Change 1985–2005
Eskimo	1%	3.2%	220%
Indian	2.4%	5.1%	113%
Aleut	4.2%	8.3%	98%

Source: Data are from reference 4.

Diabetes Prevalence

According to age-adjusted diabetes prevalence estimates from the Alaska Behavioral Risk Factor Surveillance System, 2004–2006, 6% of all adults living in Alaska have diabetes (3). Using a 3-year average, the prevalence of diabetes among Alaska Native people has steadily increased from 5.3% in 1996–1998 to 6.9% in 2003–2005 (3). Furthermore, the 3-year average of the prevalence of diabetes among Alaska Native adults (6.9%) was higher than the overall prevalence in the United States (5.6%) (3). The overall prevalence of diabetes in Alaska Natives in 2005 was 45 per 1,000, compared to 53 per 1,000 for all of United States (4). The prevalence of diabetes for all Alaska Natives combined is lower than that of non-Hispanic whites in the United States. However, prevalence of diabetes varies among the major tribes in Alaska (see Table 2.1) and prevalence rates in some Alaska Native ethnic groups exceed those of non-Hispanic whites (4). Approximately 26% of adults in Alaska have prediabetes (5). More than 95% cases of diagnosed diabetes among Alaska Natives is type 2 diabetes (4).

Risk Factors for Type 2 Diabetes

Among Alaska Natives, as in other ethnic groups, type 2 diabetes causes significant morbidity, including diabetic retinopathy, renal disease, and foot problems (6). Overweight and obesity and a sedentary lifestyle are major diabetes risk factors among Alaska Natives, who may also be genetically susceptible to type 2 diabetes (7).

Overweight and obesity seem to be increasingly prevalent in Alaska Natives. The Centers for Disease Control and Prevention Behavioral Risk Factor Surveillance System collected data on the prevalence of overweight (body mass index [BMI] 25–29.9) and obesity (BMI > 30) in Alaska from 1991 to 2007. Between 1991 and 2007, the prevalence of obesity in Alaskan adults increased from 13.4% to 28.2%, and prevalence of overweight increased from 35.3% to 36.9% (5). Thus, health care planners and providers in Alaska strongly support efforts to help the Alaska Native population achieve and maintain a healthy body weight to prevent or manage type 2 diabetes (8).

Traditional Foods and Dishes

Although Alaska is vast, there are some common cultural food practices. Whether foods come from the sea or land, most groups traditionally had a high-protein, high-fat diet. Hunting, fishing, and gathering are the traditional methods of obtaining food, so quantity and food selection change with the season. Historically, Alaska Natives would travel from place to place in search of food to feed the family and community.

The food choices of all groups in Alaska have been changing for the past 50 years. The elders of a community often maintain a subsistence lifestyle; however, the younger generations purchase more commercially prepared foods. Younger Alaska Natives are moving out of the small rural villages to more urban areas due to the high cost of living. For the many Alaska Natives who come to urban areas for work, traditional and subsistence foods are not readily available and the family must rely more on grocery stores. See Tables 2.2 and 2.3 for information about traditional foods. Refer to Appendix A for nutrient analyses.

Table 2.2 · Foods Used in Traditional Alaska Native Cuisine

	Aleut	Yupik Eskimo	Inupiat Eskimo	Athabascan Indians	Coastal Indians
Beach asparagus	X				
Beaver		X		X	
Berries	X	X	X	X	X
Birds[a]		X	X	X	
Bird eggs		X	X	X	
Blueberries	X	X	X	X	X
Broth	X	X	X	X	X
Caribou		X	X	X	
Cranberries	X	X	X	X	X
Crowberries (blackberries)	X	X	X	X	X
Deer	X				X
Dried black seaweed	X				X
Eulachon (hooligan)	X				X
Fiddlehead fern	X			X	X
Fish, freshwater[b]		X	X	X	X
Fish, saltwater[c]	X	X	X	X	X
Herring eggs	X				X
Hooligan oil	X				X
Juice	X	X	X	X	X
Moose		X	X	X	
Muktuk (whale skin and fat)		X	X		
Mush (cooked cereal)	X	X	X	X	X
Pilot bread	X	X	X	X	X
Rabbit		X	X	X	
Seal	X	X	X		X
Seal oil	X	X	X		X
Seaweed	X				X
Shellfish[d]	X				X
Walrus			X		
Whale		X	X		
Wild celery	X				
Willow leaves			X		

[a]Includes ducks, geese, and ptarmigan.
[b]Includes pike, grayling, white fish, tomcod, needlefish, and trout.
[c]Includes herring, blackfish, halibut, smelt, ling cod, and salmon.
[d]Includes clams, crab, cockles, gumboots, and mussels.

Table 2.3 · Traditional Alaska Native Dishes, Beverages, and Desserts

	Aleut	Yupik Eskimo	Inupiat Eskimo	Athabascan Indians	Coastal Indians
Boiled caribou bones		X	X	X	
Boiled meats	X	X	X	X	X
Fermented beaver tail/seal flipper	X	X	X	X	X
Fish head soup	X	X	X	X	X
Frozen fish and seal oil		X	X		
Tundra tea				X	X

Table 2.4 · Traditional Foods Consumed During Holidays

	Aleut	Yupik Eskimo	Inupiat Eskimo	Athabascan Indians	Coastal Indians
Agutuk[a]	X	X	X	X	X
Fish head soup	X	X	X	X	X
Fish pie	X	X	X	X	X
Herring eggs	X				X
Muktuk (whale skin and fat)		X	X		
Whitefish, dried		X	X	X	

[a]Dish made from berries, sugar, moose/caribou fat, or seal oil, and/or fish (exact ingredients vary by region).

Traditional Meal Patterns and Holiday Foods

Potlatches are often held to celebrate special occasions, birthdays, or holidays, or to show respect for someone who has died. A potlatch is a gathering of community members for a meal (see Table 2.4). Elders are served first by younger community members. People in attendance take the extra food home. Dancing and singing are usually part of the celebration.

Traditional Community Structure

Alaska Natives respect nature and their elders. Younger people look to elders for guidance and wisdom, and entire villages therefore take care of their elders. Traditionally, a first-time hunter will give the animal to the community to bring good luck for future hunts. Community members will share their subsistence foods, firewood, clothing and other goods with elders who are unable to provide for themselves. Those who provide for their elders believe that what is given will be returned and they will have a successful hunting/gathering season next year (9).

Current Food Practices

Many Alaska Natives live in villages and travel by boat, snow machine, and ATVs to obtain food; however, the high cost of gasoline can prohibit travel for those who live in remote villages. Many families mostly eat processed foods from the grocery store and supplement their diets with traditional foods when available. Because intake of processed foods has increased, the current Alaska Native diet is higher in carbohydrate and saturated fat than the traditional one.

The small stores in villages have limited supplies of fresh foods and large quantities of soft drinks and snack foods. Federal food programs—such as Food Stamps, the National School Lunch Program, and the Supplemental Food Program for Women, Infants, and Children (WIC)—have encouraged the use of store-bought food.

Fish consumption is high among Alaska Natives and far exceeds that of the average American diet (10). Eggs, chicken, frankfurters, ham, canned meats, and luncheon meats are other protein sources in the current diet. Popular prepared foods include frozen dinners and entrées. Dried beans and peas are not consumed frequently. Game meats are eaten more often in the winter (11).

Historically, Alaska Natives did not eat fruit and vegetables frequently. Fresh fruits and vegetables are not always available in village stores. Those that are available can be expensive, of limited variety, and poor quality. Potatoes, lettuce, onions, and carrots are among the fresh vegetables that are generally available. Many families gather wild berries, which are eaten fresh or are frozen for later use, but the short growing season in Alaska limits the availability of local edible plants. Canned fruits and vegetables are used more frequently than fresh produce (11).

Fresh milk is not always available in villages. Moreover, it is expensive—for example, a gallon of milk reportedly cost $12 in one northern Alaska village. Thus, milk, when used, is often evaporated, powdered, or in shelf-stable containers. Lactose intolerance is common among Alaska Natives.

Frequently consumed carbohydrates include sugar, bread (usually made with enriched white flour), rice, pilot bread (large, round, dense crackers), sourdough pancakes, and mush (cooked cereal). The most frequently consumed cooked cereals are oatmeal, cornmeal, and cream of wheat (11).

A dietary survey of Alaska Native adults from 13 communities described the eating practices of participants between the ages of 13 and 88 years. In all regions except coastal Indian, regular soda pop, powdered soft drinks, and fruit juice were the most frequently consumed beverages. The most frequently consumed beverage for coastal Indians was milk, followed by regular soda pop, powdered soft drinks, and fruit juice. At least 70% of Alaska Natives consumed more than 30% of their total calories from fat (12).

Mothers often pre-masticate food for their infants or young children. This custom is practiced because blenders and commercial baby foods are not readily available. However, educational efforts to discourage this practice are underway because of the risk of the transmission of bacteria and viruses to the child from the mother's saliva.

Recently, concern has mounted about the contaminants in foods caught and gathered in Alaska. Several studies (13–15) have concluded that Alaska subsistence foods are safe in moderate amounts and the benefits outweigh the harm at this time. Further studies are needed.

Health professionals, community leaders, and others should encourage the consumption of traditional foods such as fish, lean game meat, berries, greens, and seaweed for several reasons: their rich nutrient content, their ability to replace less nutritious foods, and their strong association with cultural customs. The current diet can be improved by adding more fruits and vegetables, substituting whole-grain breads for white bread, and reducing the consumption of energy-dense sweets and beverages, total fat, and cured meats.

Counseling Considerations

Counselors should keep in mind that food practices of Alaska Natives vary by region and reflect the foods that are available in the area and the season. It can be helpful to learn the client's place of origin when crafting your counseling approach.

Older clients are more likely to follow a subsistence lifestyle. In contrast, the younger generations typically eat commercially prepared foods, including store-bought foods, fast food, and food from convenience stores and restaurants.

Many Alaska Natives from small villages are shy and will not want to "burden" you with questions. They are highly appreciative of information and education on health.

You may need an interpreter to work with clients whose first language is not English. Asking open-ended questions (instead of questions that can be answered "yes" or "no") will assist you in knowing whether an interpreter is needed.

Demonstrating Courtesy and Respect

Alaska Natives typically avoid conflict and focus on building consensus in their community. They are traditionally slow to trust newcomers.

Follow your client's nonverbal cues as you seek to build rapport and individualize the counseling session. Respect is typically shown by a soft handshake and having long pauses in conversation. To improve communication, stay silent so the client can reflect and respond when ready.

Avoidance of eye contact when speaking is a traditional sign of respect. Clients who live in more urban areas may be more accustomed to direct eye contact and may benefit from motivational interviewing techniques.

Interpreting Clients' Nonverbal Communication

The proper interpretation of your clients' body language can help a counseling session to succeed. In counseling situations and when meeting someone for the first time, speak slowly and wait calmly for an answer. Observe the person to see whether eye contact is appropriate.

Inquiring About Clients' Understanding of Diabetes

You will likely want to start counseling sessions by asking clients what they know about diabetes. The following prompts may begin the conversation:

- Does any one in your family have diabetes?
- Have you ever seen a health care provider because of diabetes?
- Tell me what you know about diabetes.

Discussing Clients' Use of Complementary and Alternative Medicine

Among the complementary and alternative medicines that Alaska Natives may use for diabetes are tundra tea and devil's club. Tundra tea, also known as Hudson Bay tea *(Ledumpalustre),* is a shrub with strongly aromatic leaves that can be used to make a palatable tea. Some Alaska Natives believe this tea can help to cleanse the body of toxins. Devil's club is a plant that is purported to help manage blood glucose. The root of devil's club is boiled to make a tea. As with all complementary and alternative medicines, clients should be cautioned about the risks of using either of these teas. See Appendix C for questions to assess dietary supplement intake.

Considering Family Demands and Dynamics

Families today are more likely to work outside the home than in previous times. Such occupations may reduce the time spent hunting and gathering subsistence foods, and children may no longer learn the cultural practices of hunting and gathering.

Engaging Others in Counseling Sessions

It is always important to include caregivers, family members, and support persons in the counseling session, if the client consents to their participation. A health care condition, especially diabetes, takes team work.

Nutrition Counseling

Appendix B offers selected medical nutrition therapy (MNT) recommendations for individuals with diabetes and general counseling suggestions that support those recommendations. The following are culturally specific nutrition counseling strategies for Alaska Native clients:

- Recommend reducing the consumption of store- bought foods that are high in fat and low in nutrient density (eg, sugar-sweetened soft drinks, luncheon meats, pies, cakes, cookies, chips, and high-fat crackers).

- Help clients select healthful frozen and canned vegetables, which may be more readily available and less expensive than fresh vegetables.
- Encourage clients to gather wild greens, pick berries, and grow vegetable gardens if the climate allows.
- If fresh fruit is expensive or unavailable, recommend dried, frozen, or canned fruit with no added sugar.
- Encourage clients to use whole-wheat flour when making homemade bread.
- In social situations and on special occasions, clients may find it awkward to refuse sweets. Advise them to plan ahead before they eat a high-carbohydrate food and to exercise or eliminate a starch or fruit serving from the previous meal. Suggest self-monitoring of blood glucose to help them choose carbohydrate portions.
- Encourage the consumption of traditional fish, lean game meat, and sea mammals, chicken, turkey, and wild birds (without skin or breading) and dried fish. Educate clients about the health benefits of eating fish with n-3 fatty acids (eg, salmon, herring, trout, and whitefish) at least twice a week.
- Recommend small amounts of fish oil, seal oil, or margarine without *trans* fats instead of butter and shortening.
- Suggest the use of fresh, shelf-stable, or evaporated skim milk in coffee or tea instead of cream or nondairy creamers.
- Advise clients to restrict organ meats to one serving per month because these meats contain high levels of cholesterol.
- Discourage clients from boiling meats with added fat.

Challenges and Barriers to Dietary Adherence

People living in Alaska villages and rural areas may find it difficult to improve their food choices. Villages are often unconnected to the main road system or located on an island. When store-bought foods must be transported by ferries or planes, this makes food more expensive to buy. Furthermore, in treacherous weather conditions, grocery stores must wait long periods between shipments, and people must rely on their stock of food. In these circumstances, it is economically beneficial to purchase foods, such as canned or processed products, that have a long shelf life.

Alaska Natives do not hunt or gather as much as they once did. Individuals have jobs that limit the time they can spend collecting more healthful and natural foods from the land or sea. Clients should be encouraged to consume these more traditional foods instead of processed store-bought products.

Conclusion

Given that Alaska is such a vast region with five different cultural groups, knowing the individual's place of origin is important for tailoring therapy. The traditional subsistence lifestyle has many health benefits and sustains cultural practices. This lifestyle should be encouraged, but we must also recognize the challenges that face both the family and practitioner in today's environment. Working with the Alaska Native population offers a unique and tremendous opportunity.

Resources

Alaska Traditional Knowledge and Native Foods Database. http://www.nativeknowledge.org/start.htm. Accessed February 11, 2009.

Alaska Diabetes Prevention and Control Program. http://www.hss.state.ak.us/dph/chronic/diabetes/default.htm. Accessed February 11, 2009.

Brown TL. Meal-planning strategies: ethnic populations. *Diabetes Spectrum.* 2003;16(3):190–192. http://spectrum.diabetesjournals.org/cgi/content/full/16/3/190. Accessed February 11, 2009.

The National Diabetes Education Program. American Indian and Alaska Native Community Partnership Guide: Supplement and Activity Plans. 2004. http://www.ndep.nih.gov/diabetes/pubs/AIsupplement.pdf. Accessed February 11, 2009.

References

1. US Bureau of the Census. Alaska Quick Facts. http://quickfacts.census.gov/qfd/states/02000.html. Accessed October 4, 2008.

2. Alaska Native Heritage Center. http://www.newtradewinds.org/museums/anhc_overview.html. Accessed October 4, 2008.

3. Alaska Diabetes Prevention and Control Program. Age-adjusted diabetes prevalence among Alaska adults, AK BRFSS 2003–2005. http://www.hss.state.ak.us/dph/chronic/diabetes/default.htm. Accessed October 4, 2008.

4. Centers for Disease Control and Prevention. *Behavioral Risk Factor Surveillance System Survey Data.* Atlanta, GA: US Department of Health and Human Services, Centers for Disease Control and Prevention; 2007.

5. Cowie CC, Rust KF, Byrd-Holt DD, Eberhardt MS, et al. Prevalence of diabetes and impaired fasting glucose in adults in the U.S. Population. National Health and Nutrition Examination Survey 1999-2002. *Diabetes Care.* 2006;29:1263–1268.

6. Schumacher C, Davidson M, Ehrsam G. Cardiovascular disease among Alaska Natives: a review of the literature. *Int J Circumpolar Health.* 2003;62:343–362.

7. Risica PM, Ebbesson SOE, Schraer CD, Nobmann ED, Caballero BH. Body fat distribution in Alaskan Eskimos of the Bering Straits region: the Alaskan Siberia Project. *Int J Obesity.* 2000;24:171–179.

8. Halpern P. Obesity and American Indians/Alaskan Natives. US Department of Health and Human Services. 2007. http://aspe.hhs.gov/hsp/07/AI-AN-obesity/report.pdf. Accessed February 11, 2009.

9. Dayo D. A Gathering: Growing Strong Together, United We Make a Difference. Alaska Native Knowledge Network. University of Alaska Fairbanks, August 2006. http://www.ankn.uaf.edu/IKS/dayo.html. Accessed October 4, 2008.

10. Fish consumption advice for Alaskans: a risk management strategy to optimize the public's health. State of Alaska Epidemiology Bulletin. October 2007. http://www.epi.alaska.gov/bulletins/docs/rr2007_04.pdf. Accessed February 11, 2009.

11. Nobmann ED, Byers T, Lanier AP, Hankin HJ, Jackson MY. The diet of Alaska Native adults. *Am J Clin Nutr.* 1992;55:1024–1032.

12. Ballew C, Tzilkowski AR, Hamrick K, Nobmann ED. The contribution of subsistence foods to the total diet of Alaska Natives in 13 rural communities. *Ecol Food Nutr.* 2006;45:1–26.

13. *Alaska Native Diet. Assessing the Benefits and Risks of Diet in Rural Alaska* (DVD). Aleutian Pribilof Islands Association. 2007.

14. Use of traditional foods in a healthy diet in Alaska: risks in perspective. State of Alaska Epidemiology Bulletin. February 1998. http://www.epi.hss.state.ak.us/bulletins/docs/b1998_06.htm. Accessed February 11, 2009.

15. Contaminants in Alaska: Is America's Arctic at Risk? September 2000. http://www.akaction.org/PDFs/contaminantsinalaska.pdf. Accessed February 11, 2009.

Acknowledgments: A special thank you to Meera Ramesh, MS, RD, CDE, of the Alaska Native Diabetes Program for her assistance with the prevalence information.

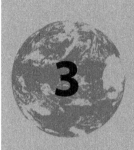

African American Food Practices

Lorraine Weatherspoon, PhD, RD, Deirdra Chester, PhD, RD, and
Tandalayo Kidd, PhD, RD

Introduction

According to the 2000 US Census, blacks/African Americans make up 12.3% of the total population in the United States of America (1). Most African Americans live in the south (55.3%), followed by the northeast (20.5%), midwest (18.1%), and west (8.6%), with 87.7% residing in metropolitan inner- and outer-city areas (1). The Census definition of African Americans refers to individuals and groups who have origins in any of the black racial groups in Africa. This includes direct descendants of captive African slaves as well as voluntary immigrants from Africa, the Caribbean, and Central and South America. The population of African Americans from sub-Saharan Africa and the Caribbean has increased substantially in the last two decades. Thus, African Americans do not share a single cultural heritage; instead, multiple cultures have evolved along a complex historical path that involves many social, political, geographic, and economic factors. The cultures of particular communities and families may include West Indian (Caribbean), African, southern US, Native American, and/or European influences. As Doris Witt notes in her book *Black Hunger* (2), this multicultural heritage is evident in the distinctive diversity of flavors, ethnic influences, and regional differences in African American cuisine.

This chapter focuses primarily on individuals whose families have a long history in the United States—ie, those with direct slave ancestry. For information on cultural food practices of Central America, the Caribbean, and South America, refer to Chapters 5, 6, and 7, respectively. In addition, Islamic dietary practices, which are covered in Chapter 15, may be of relevance when working with Muslim clients.

Data from the US Department of Agriculture's Healthy Eating Index indicate that African Americans have a lower-quality diet than other Americans (3). The prevalence of obesity and diabetes have increased in this population group. Consequently, dietary factors require special consideration both to decrease disease risk and manage health conditions.

Diabetes Prevalence

In the United States, the prevalence of diabetes and diabetes-related morbidity and mortality are disproportionately high in populations of color, especially African Americans (4–7). According to the Centers for Disease Control and Prevention (CDC), approximately 3.7 million, or 14.7% of all non-Hispanic blacks age 20 years or older have diabetes, and age-adjusted diabetes prevalence in blacks is 1.9 times greater than in non-Hispanic whites (6). In 2006, diabetes was the seventh leading cause of mortality in the United States. Compared with people without diabetes, the risk of stroke in individuals with diabetes is 2 to 4 times higher. Strokes, along with heart disease, constitute about 65% of mortality (6). Other diabetes complications include high blood pressure, blindness, kidney disease, nervous system disease, lower limb amputations, and the potential for infant birth defects in pregnant women with diabetes (6–9). African Americans have more than twice the risk of below-the-knee amputations related to diabetes than whites (8). Therefore, the high prevalence of diabetes and associated complications, especially in individuals whose diabetes is not well managed, warrants concern. Lifestyle changes, including a healthy diet and exercise, are important risk and/or modulating factors.

Risk Factors for Type 2 Diabetes

Risk factors for type 2 diabetes include overweight or obesity, a sedentary lifestyle, a strong family history of diabetes, and suboptimal blood glucose levels. Other factors, including gender, age, socioeconomic status, location of residence, education, and weight status, also affect risk. Among African Americans, females and adults between 65 and 74 years of age have the highest incidence and prevalence rates of type 2 diabetes (4–10), as well as higher complication rates. Obesity, the leading risk factor for type 2 diabetes, is widely prevalent among African Americans. Extra weight in the abdominal area (waist circumference greater than 35 inches in women and greater than 40 inches in men) is also associated with the onset of diabetes (11).

Being overweight or obese is a major risk factor for diabetes in African American women (11). Women with diabetes are at a greater risk for heart attack and stroke than those without diabetes (12). Although race/ethnicity is associated with disease incidence and prevalence (13), nongenetic factors are also predictive of disease risk in African Americans and may help explain disparities (10). In a cross-sectional study using data from the third National Health and Nutrition Examination Survey (NHANES III) to assess predictors of prevalence in African Americans compared with non-Hispanic whites, Robbins et al found that socioeconomic status was a stronger predictor than race or ethnicity of diabetes prevalence (10). Studies have also shown that the magnitude of the diabetes problem in African Americans may be greater in rural areas, where access to care, multiple chronic conditions, and cost of care are particular challenges (14,15).

Traditional Foods and Dishes

Food is an important aspect of the lifestyle of African Americans. Although they are prepared differently based on country or regional influence, four foods seem to be almost universal in the African American diet: rice, beans (typically black-eyed peas or red beans), chicken, and greens. Foods and dishes commonly eaten by African Americans are listed in Boxes 3.1, 3.2, and 3.3. Nutrient analyses are in Appendix A. Many of these foods and dishes can be classified as traditional foods or "soul food." These traditional foods, dishes, and ingredients evolved from African customs during the period of slavery in the southern United States. Influenced by American, Spanish, French, and British cuisines, African slaves modified their cooking techniques, and thus boiling, frying, and roasting became part of the African American style of cooking.

Traditional Health Beliefs

Compared with white Americans, African Americans are more likely to need health care but less likely to receive adequate care (16). Access to adequate health care remains a challenge for African Americans, especially those of low socioeconomic status. There are many reasons why health care may be inadequate. One is the lack of access to primary health care. Poverty may be a factor in some cases. However, it is important to note that even when African Americans are not poor, they may still receive inadequate or poor health care. In 1990 the Council on Ethical and Judicial Affairs of the American Medical Association acknowledged that African Americans are less likely than whites to receive the best treatment. When it comes to treating African Americans and other minorities, the report declared, some doctors tended to settle for "Band-Aid" treatment to relieve immediate symptoms (16).

Box 3.1 • Foods Traditionally Used in African American Cuisine

Grains and cereals

- Cornmeal
- Grits
- Hominy
- Oatmeal
- Pasta
- Rice
- Wheat flour

Starchy vegetables and beans

- Black-eyed peas
- Carrots
- Corn
- Dried beans (pinto, navy, lima, butter, kidney, great northern)
- Squash
- Sweet potatoes
- White potatoes

Nonstarchy vegetables

- Beets
- Cabbage
- Cucumbers
- Green/string beans
- Greens (collards, mustard, turnip)
- Kale
- Okra
- Onions
- Spinach
- Tomatoes

Fruits

- Apples
- Bananas
- Blackberries
- Cantaloupe
- Grapefruit
- Grapes
- Honeydew melon
- Oranges
- Peaches
- Pears
- Strawberries
- Watermelon

Milk and milk products

- Buttermilk
- Cheese (American, cheddar)
- Cottage cheese
- Ice cream
- Milk (whole, 2%, 1%, and nonfat)
- Yogurt

Meats and meat substitutes

- Beef
- Eggs
- Fish
- Lamb
- Pork
- Poultry

Fats and oils

- Bacon
- Butter
- Chitterlings/chitlins
- Fatback
- Hog/pork jowl
- Lard
- Pig feet
- Pork neck bones
- Salt pork

For these reasons, some African Americans think the medical system provides them care that is separate from and not equal to the care available to other Americans. Also, many African Americans still remember the Tuskegee Study of Untreated Syphilis in the Negro Male conducted between 1932 and 1972. Although clinical trials no longer use the methods employed in this controversial study, its history may contribute to some people's lack of

Box 3.2 • Traditional African American Dishes, Beverages, and Desserts

Dishes

- Baked beans
- Baked sweet potatoes
- Barbecue ribs
- Cabbage cooked with smoked meat
- Candied sweet potatoes (or yams)
- Chicken and dumplings
- Coleslaw
- Collard, turnip or mustard greens cooked with smoked meat (ham hocks, smoked turkey, smoked neckbones, salt pork, or bacon)
- Corn bread
- Corn bread dressing/stuffing
- Crab cakes
- Fried chicken
- Fried fish
- Fried green tomatoes

- Fried okra
- Glazed ham
- Green beans casserole
- Grits
- Gumbo
- Hamburgers
- Hoppin' john
- Macaroni and cheese
- Mashed potatoes
- Meatloaf
- Okra, tomato, and corn succotash
- Pork chops (baked or fried)
- Potato salad
- Red beans and rice
- Scrambled eggs
- Spaghetti with meat sauce

Beverages

- Lemonade
- Powdered fruit-flavored drink mixes
- Punch

- Sun tea
- Sweet tea

Desserts

- Apple pie
- Banana pudding
- Cherry pie
- Chocolate cake
- Ice cream
- Peach cobbler

- Pecan pie
- Pound cake
- Pumpkin pie
- Red velvet cake (especially in southern United States)
- Sweet potato pie

trust or confidence in the health care system (17). Issues and evidence related to medical trust warrant additional investigation (18). It is possible that mistrust discourages some African Americans from seeking health care, even when they need it.

Health beliefs among African Americans have evolved over time. Alternative care has been used for generations. Home remedies and self-care were important among slaves as they relied on one another or faith/spiritual or traditional healers for care when no other medical care was available (19). Slaves developed their own type of medical care, a combination of healing arts based on African practices, which combined spiritualism and herbal medicines. Many alternative medicine remedies used today were passed from "ear to ear," and from grandparent to parent to child for many generations.

Thus, traditional health beliefs among African Americans have been deeply rooted in spirituality for some time. For many individuals, health includes physical as well as emotional, intellectual, occupational, social, and spiritual components (20), and these individuals typically believe that wellness cannot be achieved without a balance in these various dimensions (21). The merging of spirituality and health can make a difference in clients' perceptions, experiences, behaviors, and outcomes in general, and affect nutrition and diabetes-related care (22,23). Recognizing the close relationship of spirituality and health, coupled

---

Box 3.3 • Traditional Holiday Foods

New Year's Day
- Banana pudding
- Barbecue ribs
- Black-eyed peas
- Collard greens (usually seasoned with smoked fatty meat such as ham hocks or fatback)

- Corn bread
- Fried catfish
- Fried chicken
- Macaroni and cheese

Easter
- Fresh turnip greens (usually seasoned with smoked fatty meat such as ham hocks or fatback)
- Seasoned green beans (usually seasoned with smoked fatty meat such as ham hocks or fatback)
- Baked ham
- Barbecue ribs

- Corn bread/dinner rolls
- Deviled eggs
- Fried corn
- Macaroni and cheese
- Roast chicken and corn bread dressing
- Sweet tea

Memorial Day, Independence Day, and Labor Day
- Baked beans
- Barbecue chicken
- Barbecue pulled pork
- Barbecue spare ribs
- Coleslaw
- Collard or turnip greens (usually seasoned with smoked fatty meat such as ham hocks or fatback)
- Corn on cob
- Dinner rolls or buns
- Fresh layer salad

- Fruit punch
- Grilled hamburgers
- Grilled hot dogs
- Lemonade
- Macaroni and cheese
- Macaroni salad
- Potato salad
- Sweet tea
- Watermelon or fresh fruit

Thanksgiving and Christmas
- Candied yams
- Corn bread
- Corn bread dressing
- Cornish hens
- Cranberry sauce
- Dinner rolls
- Giblet gravy

- Green beans
- Greens with smoked meat
- Ham
- Macaroni and cheese
- Potato salad
- Roasted turkey
- Sweet potato or pumpkin pie

---

with the central role that churches play in African American life, health promotion specialists have used community and church settings to successfully provide health interventions including diabetes education (23–30).

Current Food Practices

The dietary patterns of minority groups may differ from those of the general US population for several reasons. Factors to consider include the nature of the minority group's original diet, the ways the diet has been adapted to or supplanted by dietary patterns of the dominant US culture, the availability of preferred foods, and acculturation patterns (31,32). Among

African Americans, current food practices partially reflect the types of foods that were available to African Americans during slavery. Slaves who worked in the fields developed meals that required minimal preparation and could be prepared in large quantities. Cooks made use of cuts of pork that were inexpensive and/or undesirable to whites (eg, tail, feet, chitterlings, ears) (31,32). Today, the term "soul food" is often used to identify the foods that African Americans have consumed for years, many of which are high in salt, fat, sugar, and calories.

Compared with other Americans, African Americans consume fewer fruits and vegetables and less dietary fiber, calcium, and potassium; on the other hand, they consume excessive amounts of fatty meats, salt, and cholesterol (33–36). The eating habits and food purchasing practices of African Americans may be associated with high rates of hypertension, cardiovascular disease, and diabetes. Although there have been some marked improvements in the diet of African Americans, Healthy People 2010 recommends an increase in consumption of fruits, vegetables, and dietary fiber for this population (37). In addition, this initiative recommends that Americans reduce their intake of total fat, sugar, and saturated fat. Although this recommendation is intended for all Americans, it is especially important relative to typical African American food choices, such as fatback and bacon, that are high in fat and saturated fat. Findings of the Dietary Approaches to Stop Hypertension (DASH) study also support reduced intake of fat, sugar, and saturated fat (38). The Seventh Report of the Joint National Committee on Prevention, Detection, Evaluation and Treatment of High Blood Pressure recently recommended lifestyle modifications including weight management; consumption of more low-fat dairy foods, fruits, and vegetables; reduction in dietary salt/sodium levels; more physical activity; and limited alcohol consumption (39).

Socioeconomic status and education level have important influences on the meals consumed and hence in meal planning and nutrition education of African Americans (40). One relevant nutrition education tool is the Soul Food Pyramid, which culturally adapts traditional food choices to become healthier selections (eg, oven-fried chicken) and categorizes typical African American foods in terms of food groups and nutrient content (41).

Examples of typical traditional meals, especially in the southern United States, are as follows (32,42):

- **Breakfast:** grits often with cheese and butter/margarine; fried eggs; sausage, ham, or bacon; fried potatoes; biscuits with margarine and jelly; and coffee or tea with sugar
- **Lunch or dinner** (terms are used interchangeably to describe the main midday meal): fried chicken leg quarter; mashed potatoes; boiled dried beans or green beans seasoned with ham, ham hocks, or fatback; buttered corn on the cob, a hot buttered roll, sweetened iced tea; peach cobbler with ice cream or another baked dessert such as red velvet cake or apple pie

Currently, this type of meal pattern is reserved more for weekend/Sundays and holidays, and many "traditional fare" foods such as pig feet and chitterlings are regarded more as special occasion foods; however, greens are still prepared and eaten regularly (43).

During the work week, breakfasts and lunches are often lighter fare—eg, cereal for breakfast and sandwiches at lunch—especially in families where all adults work outside of the home. More elaborate cooked breakfasts (eg, sausage, sausage gravy, waffles, pancakes, grits, biscuits, eggs, and bacon) are prepared and consumed when more time is available. Dinner is the main meal of the day. Frying remains a popular way to prepare food, and many individuals consume convenience and fast foods (32).

Counseling Considerations

Food selection is tied to many aspects of culture and heritage. This is especially true for African Americans and other people of color. Early in life, cultural patterns are established and set. To change them is often a difficult, slow process. When diabetes or another health concern requires dietary changes, the client is more likely to comply when the counselor takes into consideration the cultural context of the foods that the client likes and values.

Counseling can be effective only if the counselor and the client truly communicate. Communication involves not only what the registered dietitian (RD) says and how she says it, but also what she implies and what the listener perceives. Key factors to keep in mind, especially when counseling an African American client, include the following: (*a*) time and cost constraints, (*b*) the possibility that the client associates health care with symptom treatment rather than with prevention or health maintenance, (*c*) the client's desire to be self-reliant, and (*d*) the possibility that the client may be uneasy working with health care providers of a different ethnicity because he or she feels patronized by them (32). The RD should adopt an engaging, nonjudgmental, conversational, and empathetic style of communication. Striking this tone will reduce the likelihood that a defensive client will think the RD is "talking down" to him or her. Be sure to listen attentively and offer support (eg, nod or say "I understand" or "That is perfectly understandable") (32,44,45). Although it is challenging in today's health care environment to find enough time to spend with clients, longer or more frequent sessions can enhance the counselor's effectiveness.

African Americans may be sensitive to any signs that suggest the counselor could be biased or racist. If clients perceive insincerity, bias, and prejudicial statements or behavior on the part of their health care providers, they may not comply with treatment. In any counseling relationship, many factors, including socioeconomic status, age, gender, educational level, or ethnicity, can shape how a client interacts with the counselor. Therefore, with all individuals, regardless of their background, health professionals should use language and mannerisms that are neutral, friendly, and culturally sensitive. Never generalize or make assumptions about clients based on their cultural background or stereotypes. Instead, phrase advice in a neutral way—for example, "Some clients have success when they do *x, y,* or *z.*"

One way to engage the client in conversation is to ask, "What does your family usually prefer to eat?" Then use that information to say, "This is great to hear because, by making some small changes, you can still enjoy your family's favorite choices while better managing your diabetes."

Counselors should have realistic expectations for all clients, regardless of their race or ethnicity. The counselor may know or perceive a certain practice to be harmful, but that does not mean that the client is ready to change his or her behavior. The client's right to determine his or her own future must be balanced against the counselor's need to promote change. Randall-David suggests that counseling recommendations should be "action- or task oriented" (46). It is more effective to help clients set realistic goals for themselves and choose their own strategies to achieve those goals than to mandate change (47). Clients who take small steps and have realistic priorities are better off than those who make no effort at all (47,48).

Self-Management Factors

Self-care is the most essential aspect of diabetes management (49), but many individuals, especially in the African American population, have not had structured, efficacious diabetes education (50). In a study of patients' priorities and needs for diabetes care interventions, urban African Americans between the ages of 35 and 75 years rated guidance on self-testing of blood glucose and taking medications as prescribed by the doctor as their top priorities and needs (51). When self-testing of blood glucose was assessed in a multi-ethnic (African American, white, and Native American) population of rural older adults, the rate of blood testing was found to be high in all the groups irrespective of their ethnicity, and the frequency of self-monitoring of blood glucose was positively associated with the recommendations of the health care providers (52).

Because spirituality is an important aspect in the lives and culture of many African Americans (53), a culturally sensitive intervention program that incorporates spiritual considerations may help African Americans better manage their diabetes. Studies indicate that church-based invention programs for African Americans with diabetes have merit, especially for those with strong church affiliations (28,29).

Demonstrating Courtesy and Respect

When providing cross-cultural counseling, counselors should not try to imitate an ethnic communication style that is not naturally their own. If a counselor who is not African American adopts African American language or speech patterns, clients may think they are being ridiculed. On the other hand, counselors should respectfully accept the client's communication style, recognizing that the "dialect" used by some African Americans is an integral part of their culture, which has been influenced by English and African languages as well as by geographical location and social factors. Some examples include one African American male greeting another with "Hey, Man," or using the term "brother" in conversation. African American females may use the term "girl" in an animated conversation with another female, especially when trying to make a point. When asked how they are doing, African Americans may automatically respond with "I'm doing good," or "I be tryin' to do good," or "I'm all right." If this is their answer, some additional probing may be needed to find out if there is in fact a problem.

In addition, the use of health terminology or jargon can confuse or mislead clients, even those who are highly educated. Therefore, it is important for counselors to speak clearly and explain terminology when discussing medical treatment with any client.

Tips for enhancing courtesy and respect toward more effective counseling include the following:

- Understand your own cultural values and biases.
- Acquire a basic knowledge of the cultural values, health beliefs, and nutrition practices of the client.
- Be respectful of, interested in, and understanding of the client without being judgmental.
- Ask how the client prefers to be addressed—do *not* assume. When addressing African Americans, use "Mr." or "Ms." or "Mrs." and their last name unless they ask you to call them by their first name.
- Avoid slang, technical jargon, and complex sentences, but recognize that a client's use of culture-specific slang or "black English" is not an indicator that they lack education or do not understand counseling messages.
- Ask open-ended questions. Asking "how" or "what" yields more informative answers than questions that require only a simple "yes" or "no" response. Consider, too, that yes/no questions can make clients feel they are admitting to some type of wrongdoing.
- Diplomatically assess the client's reading ability before introducing written materials. One way to determine literacy skills is to ask clients whether they would prefer to "discuss" all the important pieces of information in the material.

Interpreting Clients' Nonverbal Communication

The RD should use caution in interpreting clients' facial expressions or body movements. The interpretation might be quite different from the client's intent. A counselor may think a client is "noncommunicative," when the client is trying to be respectful of or testing the counselor's sincerity. The client's actions and interactions with others may provide clues about his or her nonverbal communication style. More specifically, keep the following in mind:

- Avoid body language that may be deemed offensive or misunderstood, such as a "weak" handshake. Barely touching a client's hand could be perceived as a sign of disdain, reluctance, or even prejudice. A firm handshake and smile are the expected greeting (32).
- Speak directly to the client while making eye contact, but do not stare. Also try to not break eye contact or appear to be looking away and disinterested when the client is speaking; this could be misconstrued as negative feedback or disapproval.
- Be tolerant of natural pauses or interruptions in the communication process.
- Let clients choose where they would like to sit. That will help you establish what the client views as a proper amount of personal space.
- Do not be overly judgmental of highly expressive or inexpressive individuals. African Americans often express themselves passionately (32).

Inquiring about Clients' Understanding of Diabetes

According to Fisher et al (54), both the style of the health care provider's approach and the content he or she relays should be informed by how much clients understand about diabetes. Does the client understand that the disease is serious and can lead to serious complications or death if it is not well controlled? Be sure to let the client know that "a touch of diabetes" and "sugar a little high"—phrases often used by African Americans—misrepresent the seriousness of the condition. Seek feedback on whether the client clearly understands (*a*) what diabetes self-management involves, (*b*) what to ask health care team members, and (*c*) how to seek appropriate health care.

As with clients of all races/ethnicities, make sure the client understands the importance of the following:

- Self-monitoring of blood glucose
- Self-monitoring of feet
- Eating a healthful diet
- Regular exercise
- Doctor's appointments for eye and foot checks, blood glucose and lipid tests, and general physical examinations
- Good dental care
- Avoiding risky health behaviors, such as excessive alcohol intake and smoking

Discussing Clients' Use of Complementary and Alternative Medicine

African Americans have long used complementary and alternative medicine (CAM). In 2002, 68.3% of African Americans and approximately 62% of all US adults had used some form of CAM in the previous 12 months (55). Women were more likely to use CAM than men. The therapies used most by African Americans included mind-body therapies, such as prayer specifically for health reasons (55). There is still much to be learned on the specific types of alternative therapies used by African Americans today.

Historically, African Americans used alternative therapies for many illnesses, especially when they did not have access to traditional medical care. Diseases and conditions that were treated with alternative medicine included high cholesterol, hypertension, digestive disorders, asthma, and many others. African Americans also may use herbs to treat disease. Table 3.1 lists some common remedies (19). Refer to Appendix C for questions to assess dietary supplement use.

Engaging Others in Counseling

Most African Americans are especially respectful of older relatives as well as community and church leaders. Advice and opinions of these individuals may provide a foundation for a particular belief or practice. Therefore, with the consent of the client, it may be helpful to engage them in counseling or nutrition education. As stated earlier, faith-based interventions have been shown to be successful in the African American community.

In addition, local community health workers have been shown to be successful in many programs. Some examples of successful community approaches include Diabetes Health: It's in Your Hands (56); A New DAWN (30); REACH Diabetes Program (44); Project Power (47); and Learn, Taste, and Share (28). These programs yielded improvements in diabetes knowledge, general health perceptions, lifestyle behaviors, and A1C.

Nutrition Counseling

Frequent client education is can improve self-management of diabetes (57). Despite the high prevalence of diabetes in minority groups, the cultural aspects of illness management are not sufficiently emphasized (45). Many intervention programs targeting African Americans lack cultural relevancy (58), and cultural differences between health care providers and clients can be a barrier to effective health care (59). Samuel-Hodge et al suggest an ecological approach that emphasizes family and religious factors to encourage self-management of diabetes in rural and southern African Americans (60). Davis-Mayer et al (61) documented weight loss and improved glycemic control in the POWER study, which used a culturally relevant lifestyle intervention program for African Americans with diagnosed type 2 diabetes.

Appendix B offers selected medical nutrition therapy (MNT) recommendations for individuals with diabetes and general counseling suggestions that support those recommendations. The following are culturally specific nutrition counseling strategies for African American clients:

Table 3.1 · Remedies Used by African Americans for Self-Treatment

Treatment	Uses[a]
Bearberry	Treatment for urinary tract infections
Black snakeroot or black cohosh	Treatment for rheumatism; relief of menstrual pain/discomfort
Blue cohosh or squaw vine	Relief for uterine contractions during labor
Boric acid	Douche to treat yeast infections
Catnip and wild comfrey	Treatment of seizures
Chamomile	Sleep aid; used topically to treat poison ivy
Dandelion root	Mild laxative; antidiabetic diuretic; appetite stimulant; digestive aid
Elderberry root	Treatment for bladder infections
Eyebright	Relief for watery eyes and dim vision
Flaxseed	Laxative
Juniper berry	Treatment for eczema or psoriasis
Sarsaparilla (in corn whiskey) with black cohosh	Arthritis or diabetes treatment
Shuck covering of dry corn	Treatment for influenza or colds
Virginia snakeroot	Treatment for infections, viruses, or kidney problems
Wild cherry bark	Asthma treatment
White horehound	Asthma or bronchitis treatment
Yam or sweet potato	Antispasmodic to regulate bowels; nausea relief during pregnancy

[a]Descriptions do not evaluate efficacy of these uses.
Source: Data are from reference 19.

- High-carbohydrate, sugary foods and drinks as well as bread, rice, and potatoes are abundant in the African American diet. Advise clients to substitute lower-sugar or sugar-free beverages and have smaller portions of bread, rice, and potatoes.
- Explain that sugar adds calories and increases blood glucose levels even if it is "hidden" in "healthy" foods (eg, the natural sugars in juices).
- Advise clients to sauté, bake, or "oven fry" foods instead of deep-frying them. Encourage them to choose healthier fats (such as olive or canola oil and smoked turkey) in place of fatback or ham hocks and use onions and spices to improve flavoring.
- Explain that bacon and fatback should be counted as fats, not meats, in meal plans.
- Provide a list of leaner cuts of meats that can be added to rice and vegetables (eg, smoked turkey or turkey bacon).
- African Americans do not eat enough fruits and vegetables and high-fiber grain products. To increase their fiber intake, encourage clients to have fruits instead of fruit juice and punches, eat more salads and vegetables, and choose high-fiber breads and whole-grain noodles.

Challenges and Barriers to Dietary Compliance

Challenges to diabetes self-management can include work schedules, lack of transportation, and family commitments (62). Economic factors can also be barriers to compliance. In a study of older women with type 2 diabetes, Schoenberg et al reported that 90% of the African Americans who reported financial barriers to self-management were below the poverty line (63). African Americans with less than an 8th grade education are also more likely to face barriers (63,64).

Roberts-Baptiste et al (64) found that African Americans with a family history of diabetes were more aware of the risk factors associated with the disease and were more likely to practice healthy lifestyle behaviors compared with African Americans without a family history of diabetes. For example, individuals with a family history of diabetes were more likely to participate in diabetes screening, consume healthful foods, and seek weight-loss assistance from a doctor or other health care professional.

Weight loss can be challenging for any client. In some studies (65,66), African Americans lost less weight than other participants. Setting realistic and achievable weight loss goals within a reasonable time period is important for success.

Similarly, it is important to set realistic goals for physical activity. By taking into account clients' personal physical activity preferences, counselors may help them select and achieve exercise strategies for improved glycemic control (67). If clients are not prepared to try strenuous exercise, encourage them to add more leisure-time activities, such as walking or gardening.

Counseling Tips

In conclusion, the following are some essential points to remember when counseling African American clients:

- Encourage conversation. Many clients enjoy talking. Ask them what they would like to know, instead of simply informing them about what you think they need to know.

- Build on cultural practices to reinforce positive behaviors. For example, if a client like greens, agree that this favorite food is a great choice, and then discuss preparation methods that are both healthful and acceptable to the client's tastes. Offer recommendations on modifying traditional recipes (eg, using smoked turkey in place of fatback). Ask clients if they have any recipes to share or a favorite one that you can modify together.

- Encourage positive change in harmful behaviors. Use phrases like, "It might interesting for you to challenge yourself by setting a goal to . . ." Begin with changes the individual thinks he or she can easily achieve.

- Establish rapport and show genuine concern for the client. Sometimes, it is helpful to have a general social conversation. Questions about the family and church (if the person is religious) are especially valued by African Americans. Reassure the client that your counseling interactions are confidential. This will build a level of trust that encourages more accurate responses.

- Assess the client's understanding and acceptance of recommendations. Offer to provide examples and clarification if necessary.

- Provide education materials to support desired behavior changes. Try to avoid using materials that depict other ethnic groups. Usually, the simpler the materials the better.

- Know the environment and the foods accessible to the client. If possible, plan ahead and use examples of a store or foods from the client's local area.

- Choose an age-appropriate style of interaction. If you are younger than the client, adopt a more serious, respectful attitude. Use Ms./Mrs./Mr. instead of the client's first name. If you are older than the client, try to create an informal atmosphere that allows the younger client to open up and speak more freely. Try to joke with the client and ask about school, work, hobbies, or sports. Share stories about your own children or younger relatives.

- Avoid using the word "you." For example, instead of saying "You are at an increased risk for stroke," say "People with diabetes have an increased risk of stroke."

- Be patient. Sometimes it takes years for the seeds of knowledge to take root.

Resources

American Association of Diabetes Educators. Guidelines for the Practice of Diabetes Education. http://www.diabeteseducator.org/export/sites/aade/_resources/pdf/PracticeGuidelines2009.pdf. Accessed May 16, 2009.

American Diabetes Association. http://www.diabetes.org. Accessed April 13, 2009. Search "Project Power," which has a special focus on African Americans.

American Dietetic Association. House of Delegates Backgrounder: Meeting the Challenges of a Culturally and Ethnically Diverse US Population. March 25, 2004. http://www.eatright.org/ada/files/HODBACKGROUNDERCULTURAL.pdf. Accessed May 15, 2009.

American Heart Association. Healthy Soul Food Recipes. http://www.americanheart.org/presenter.jhtml?identifier=3046994. Accessed May 26, 2009.

Centers for Disease Control and Prevention. Diabetes Public Health Resource. http://www.cdc.gov/diabetes/human_body.htm. Accessed May 16, 2009.

Centers for Disease Control and Prevention. REACH (Racial and Ethnic Approaches to Community Health). http://www.cdc.gov/reach. Accessed May 26, 2009.

Dixon B. *Good Health for African Americans.* New York, NY: Crown Publishing, 1994.

HEBNI Nutrition Consultants, Inc. http://www.soulfoodpyramid.org/web. Accessed October 20, 2007.

National Diabetes Education Program. The Diabetes Epidemic among African Americans. http://www.ndep.nih.gov/diabetes/pubs/FS_AfricanAm.pdf. Accessed May 15, 2009.

National Institute of Diabetes and Digestive and Kidney Diseases, National Diabetes Information Clearinghouse. African Americans and Diabetes. http://diabetes.niddk.nih.gov/dm/pubs/africanamerican. Accessed May 16, 2009.

Also check your state's department of community health, local hospitals, church health care ministries, and diabetes centers.

References

1. US Census Bureau. http://www.census.gov. Accessed February 10, 2009.
2. Witt D. *Black Hunger: Food and the Politics of U.S. Identity.* New York, NY: Oxford University Press;1999.
3. Basiotis PP, Lino M, Anand RS. Report card on the Diet quality of African Americans. *Fam Econ Nutr Rev.* 1999;11:61–63.
4. American Diabetes Association. Diabetes Statistics for African Americans. http://www.diabetes.org/diabetes-statistics/african-americans.jsp. Accessed April 13, 2009.
5. Carter S, Janette PA, Monterrosa A. Non-insulin-dependent diabetes mellitus in minorities in the United States. *Ann Intern Med.* 1996;125:221–232.
6. Centers for Disease Control and Prevention. National Diabetes Fact Sheet, 2007. http://www.cdc.gov/diabetes/pubs/pdf/ndfs_2007.pdf. Accessed April 13, 2009.
7. Marshall MC. Diabetes in African Americans. *Postgrad Med J.* 2005;81:734–740.
8. Resnick HE, Valsania P, Phillips CL. Diabetes mellitus and nontraumatic lower extremity amputation in black and white Americans: the National Health and Nutrition Examination Survey Epidemiologic Follow-up Study, 1971–1992. *Arch Intern Med.* 1999;159:2470–2475.
9. Leggetter S, Chaturvedi N, Fuller JH, Edmonds ME. Ethnicity and risk of diabetes-related lower extremity amputation. *Arch Intern Med.* 2002;162:73–78.
10. Robbins JM, Vaccarino V, Zhang H, Kasl SV. Excess type 2 diabetes in African-American women and men aged 40-74 and socioeconomic status: evidence from the Third National Health and Nutrition Examination Survey. *J Epidemiol Commun Health.* 2000;54:839–845.
11. Krishnan S, Rosenberg L, Djoussé L, Cupples LA, Palmer JR. Overall and central obesity and risk of type 2 diabetes in U.S. black women. *Obesity.* 2007;15:1860–1866.
12. American Heart Association . Women, Heart Disease, and Stroke. http://www.americanheart.org/presenter.jhtml?identifier=4786. Accessed April 13, 2009.
13. Winkleby AM, Kraemer CH, Ahn KD, Varady NA. Ethnic and socioeconomic differences in cardiovascular disease risk factors: findings for women from the Third National Health and Nutrition Examination Survey, 1988–1994. *JAMA.* 1998;280:356–362.
14. African American population. In: *African American Yearbook: The Resource and Referral Guide for and about African Americans.* 6th ed. McLean, VA: TIYM Publishing; 2006–2007:14–18.
15. Utz SW, Wenzel J, Hinton I, Jones R, Steeves R. Plenty of sickness": barriers and facilitators to self-management in rural African Americans with diabetes. *Diabetes Educ.* 2003;31:98–107.
16. Council on Ethical and Judicial Affairs. Black-white disparities in health care. *JAMA.* 1990; 263:2344–2346.
17. Anderson RM, Herman WH, Davis JM, Freedman RP, Funnell MM, Neighbors HW. Barriers to improving diabetes care for blacks. *Diabetes Care.* 1991;14:605–609.
18. Hall MA, Dugan E, Zheng B, Mishra AK: Trust in physicians and medical institutions: what is it, can it be measured, and does it matter? *Milbank Q.* 2001;79:613–639.
19. Sullivan SD. *A Path to Healing: A Guide to Wellness for Body, Mind, and Soul.* New York, NY: Doubleday; 1998.

20. Burkhardt MA. Spirituality: an analysis of the concept. *Holist Nurs Pract.* 1989;3:69–77.
21. Reed PG. Preferences for spiritually related nursing interventions among terminally ill and nonterminally ill hospitalized adults and well adults. *Appl Nurs Res.* 1991;4:122–128.
22. Musgrave CF, Allen CE, Allenv GJ. Spirituality and health for women of color. *Am J Public Health.* 2002;92:557–560.
23. Chester DN, Himburg SP, Weatherspoon LF. Spirituality of African-American women: correlations to health-promoting behaviors. *J Natl Black Nurses Assoc.* 2006;17:1–8.
24. Kumanyika SK, Charleston JB. Lose Weight and Win: a church-based weight loss program for blood pressure control among black women. *Patient Educ Couns.* 1992;19:19–32.
25. Melynx MG, Weinstein E. Preventing obesity in African American women by targeting adolescents: a literature review. *J Am Diet Assoc.*1994;94:536–540.
26. Pratt CA. Adolescent obesity: a call for multivariate longitudinal research on African American youth. *J Nutr Educ.* 1994;26:107–109.
27. McNabb W, Quinn M, Kerver J, Cook S, Karrison T. The PATHWAYS church-based weight loss program for urban African American women at risk for diabetes. *Diabetes Care.* 1997; 20:1518–1523.
28. Hahn MJ, Gordon HD. "Learn, taste, and share": a diabetes nutrition education program developed, marketed, and presented by the community. *Diabetes Educ.* 1998;24:153–154, 161.
29. Wisdom K, Kamilah N, Williams VH, Havstad LS, Tilley BC. Recruitment of African Americans with type 2 diabetes to a randomized controlled trial using three sources. *Ethn Health.* 2002; 7:267–278.
30. Samuel-Hodge CD, Keyserling TC, France R, Ingram AF, Johnston LF, Pullen Davis L, Davis G, Cole AS. A church based diabetes self-management education program for African Americans with type 2 diabetes. *Prev Chron Dis.* 2006;3:A93.
31. Sanjur D. *Social and Cultural Perspectives in Nutrition.* Englewood Cliffs, NJ: Prentice-Hall; 1982.
32. Kittler PG, Sucher KP. *Food and Culture.* 5th ed. Belmont, CA: Wadsworth/Thomson Learning; 2008.
33. Kumanyika SK. Diet and chronic disease issues in minority populations. *J Nutr Educ Behav.* 1990;22:89–95.
34. Fox AA, Thompson JL, Butterfield GE, Glfadottir U, Moynihan S, Spiller G. Effects of diet and exercise on common cardiovascular disease risk factors in moderately obese older women. *Am J Clin Nutr.* 1996;63:225–233.
35. Krause RM, Eckel RH, Howard B, Appel LJ, Daniels SR, Deckelbaum RJ, Erdman JW, Kris-Etherton P, Goldberg IJ, Kotchen TA, Lichtenstein AH, Mitch WE, Mullis R, Robinson K, Wylie-Rosett J, St. Jeor S, Suttie J, Tribble DL, Bazzarre TL. AHA dietary guidelines: revision 2000: a statement for healthcare professionals from the nutrition committee of the American Heart Association. *Circulation.* 2000;102:2284–2299.
36. Furumoto-Dawson AA, Pandey D, Elliott WJ, deLeon CF, Al-Hani AJ, Hollenberg S, Camba N, Wicklund R, Black HR. Hypertension in women: the Women Take Heart Project. *J Clin Hypertens.* 2003;5:38–46.
37. US Department of Health and Human Services. Heathy People 2010. http://www.healthypeople .gov. Accessed April 10, 2009.
38. Sacks FM, Svetkey LP, Vollmer WM, Appel LJ, Bray GA, Harsha D, Obarzanek E, Conlin PR, Miller ER, Simons-Morton DG, Karanja N, Lin PH. Effects on blood pressure of reduced dietary sodium and the Dietary Approaches to Stop Hypertension (DASH) diet. *N Engl J Med.* 2001;344:3–10.
39. Chobanian AV, Bakris GL, Black HR, Cushman WC, Green LA, Izzo JL, Jones DW, Materson BJ, Oparil S, Wright JT, Rocella EJ. The seventh report of the Joint National Committee on Prevention, Detection, Evaluation and Treatment of High Blood Pressure. *JAMA.* 2003;289:2560–2571.
40. Kulkarni K. Food, culture, and diabetes in the United States. *Clin Diabetes.* 2004;22:190–192.
41. HEBNI Nutrition Consultants, Inc. http://www.soulfoodpyramid.org. Accessed October 20, 2007.
42. African-American Diet. Diet.com Store Web site. http://www.diet.com/store/facts/africanamerican-diet. Accessed April 2, 2009.
43. Byars D. Traditional African American foods and African Americans. *Agric Hum Values.* 1996;13:74–78.
44. Two Feathers J, Kieffer E, Guzman R, Palmisano G, Heisler M, Anderson M, Sinco B, Wisdom K, James S. Racial and Ethnic Approaches to Community Health (REACH) Detroit partnership: improving diabetes-related outcomes among African American and Latino adults. *Am J Public Health.* 2005;95:1552–1560.

45. Becker G, Newsom E. Resilience in the face of serious illness among chronically ill African Americans in later life. *J Gerontol B Psychol Sci Soc Sci.* 2005;60:S214–S223.

46. Randall-David E. *Strategies for Working with Culturally Diverse Communities and Clients.* Bethesda, MD: Association for the Care of Children's Health; 1989.

47. Doherty Y, Robert S. Motivational interviewing in diabetes practice. *Diabet Med.* 2002;19 (suppl 3):S1–S6.

48. Clark M, Hampson SE. Implementing a psychological intervention to improve lifestyle self-management in patients with type 2 diabetes. *Patient Educ Couns.* 2001;42:247–256.

49. American Diabetes Association. Standards of medical care in diabetes—2006. *Diabetes Care.* 2006;29(Suppl 1):S4–S42.

50. Mensing C, Boucher J, Cypress M, Weinger K, Mulcahy K, Barta P, Hosey G, Kopher W, Lasichak A, Lamb B, Mangan M, Normal J, Tanja J, Yauk L, Wisdom K, Adams C. National standards for diabetes self-management education. *Diabetes Care.* 2007;30(Suppl 1):S96–S103.

51. Batts LM Gary TL, Huss K, Hill NM, Bone L, Brancati LF. Patient priorities and needs for diabetes care among urban African American adults. *Diabetes Educ.* 2001;27:405.

52. Skelly HA, Arcury AT, Snively MB, Bell AR, Smith LS, Wetmore KL, Quandt AS. Self-monitoring of blood glucose in a multiethnic population of rural older adults with diabetes. *Diabetes Educ.* 2005;31:84–90.

53. Polzer LR. African Americans and diabetes: spiritual role of the health care provider in self-management. *Res Nurs Health.* 2007;30:164–174.

54. Fisher E, Todora H, Heins J. Social support in nutrition counseling. *On the Cutting Edg*e. 2003;24:18–20.

55. Centers for Disease Control and Prevention. Complementary and alternative medicine use among adults: United States, 2002. *Adv Data.* 2004;(343):1–19.

56. Weatherspoon LJ, Saxe A. Diabetes health: it's in your hands. *On the Cutting Edge.* 2006;27:8–9.

57. Hendricks LE, Hendricks TR. The effect of diabetes self-management with frequent follow-up on the health outcomes of African American men. *Diabetes Educ.* 2000;26:995–1002.

58. Flaskerud JH. Diagnostic and treatment differences among five ethnic groups. *Psychol Rep.* 1986;58:219–235.

59. Wenzel J, Utz WS, Steeves R, Hinton I, Jones RA. Plenty of sickness: descriptions by African Americans living in rural areas with type 2 diabetes. *Diabetes Educ.* 2005;31:98–107.

60. Samuel-Hodge CD, Headen SW, Skelly AH, Ingram AF, Keyserling TC, Jackson EJ, Ammerman AS, Elasy TA. Influences on day-to-day self-management of type 2 diabetes among African-American women: spirituality, the multi-caregiver role, and other social context factors. *Diabetes Care.* 2000;23:928–933.

61. Davis-Mayer JE, D'Antonio MA, Smith MS, Kirkner G, Martin SL, Medina-Parra D, Schultz R. Pounds Off With Empowerment (POWER): a clinical trial of weight management strategies for black and white adults with diabetes who live in medically underserved rural communities. *Am J Public Health.* 2004;94:1736–1742.

62. Banister NA, Jastrow ST, Hodges V, Loop R, Gilham MB. Diabetes self-management training program in a community clinic improves patient outcomes at modest cost. *J Am Diet Assoc.* 2004;104:807–810.

63. Schoenberg NE, Drungle SC. Barriers to non-insulin dependent diabetes mellitus (NIDDM) self-care practices among older women. *J Aging Health.* 2001;13:443–466.

64. Roberts-Baptiste K, Gary TL, Beckles LA, Gregg WE, Owens M, Porterfield D, Engelgau MM. Family history of diabetes, awareness of risk factors and health behaviors among African Americans. *Am J Public Health.* 2007;97:907–912.

65. Wing RR, Hamman RF, Bray GA, Delahanty L, Edelstein SL, Hill JO, Horton ES, Hoskin MA, Kriska A, Lachin J, Mayer-Davis EJ, Pi-Sunyer X, Regensteiner JG, Venditti B, Wylie-Rosett J; Diabetes Prevention Program Research Group. Achieving weight and activity goals among diabetes prevention program lifestyle participants. *Obes Res.* 2004;12:1426–1434.

66. Kumanyika SK, Espeland AM, Bahnson LJ, Bottom BJ, Charleston BJ, Folmar S, Wilson CA, Whelton KP; TONE Cooperative Research Group. Ethnic comparison of weight loss in the Trial of Nonpharmacologic Interventions in the Elderly. *Obes Res.* 2002;10:96–106.

67. Wanko NS, Brazier CW, Young-Rogers D, Dunbar VG, Boyd B, George CD, Rhee MK, El-Kebbi IM, Cook CC. Exercise preferences and barriers in urban African Americans with type 2 diabetes. *Diabetes Educ.* 2004;30:502–513.

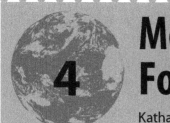

Mexican American Food Practices

Kathaleen Briggs Early, PhD, RD, CDE, and Eva Brzezinski, MS, RD

Introduction

Mexico, a Spanish-speaking country spanning from the Gulf of Mexico and Caribbean on the east to the Pacific Ocean on the west, is rich in cultural heritage and regional diversity. Internationally known foods include corn tortillas, mole sauce, fish tacos, and *ceviche*. Mexican food and culture have been influenced by a wide variety of peoples, from native Mexican Indians and South Americans to European colonists. This cultural diversity is apparent in Mexico's food practices.

Mexican cuisine has become popular throughout North America, in part due to the large influx of Mexican immigrants into the United States over the past 25 years. According the 2007 US Census Bureau, Mexican Americans comprise nearly 9% of the US population (1,2). They also account for the largest percentage (58.5%) of the US Latino/Hispanic population (1). Most Mexican Americans live in the southwest and western United States, with the largest numbers found in California, Texas, Arizona, and New Mexico (3).

Diabetes Prevalence

Prevalence of diabetes for all Hispanic Americans is 1.7 times higher than prevalence in non-Hispanic whites (4). According to the Centers for Disease Control and Prevention (CDC), in 2007, 2.5 million US Hispanics (10.4%) had diabetes (4). A comprehensive analysis of National Health and Nutrition Examination Survey (NHANES) data projects that cases of diabetes among Hispanic adults will exceed 20% by 2031—the largest diabetes caseload among any ethnic group in the United States (5).

Current data regarding rates of diabetes specifically for Mexican Americans are limited. Most data are from the San Antonio Heart Studies and the Starr County Studies, both out of Texas; the San Luis Valley Diabetes Study from Colorado; and the Hispanic Health and Nutrition Examination Survey (HHANES), based on a nationwide sample of 16,000 Hispanics from 1982 to 1984. An analysis of these data can be found in *Diabetes in America* (6), which reports that the prevalence of diabetes in Mexican Americans is two to three times higher than prevalence in non-Hispanic Americans. More recently, the CDC used NHANES data to report that the prevalence of diagnosed diabetes among Mexican Americans adults (age 20 years or older) was 11.9%, vs 10.7% for the entire US adult population (4). Smith and Barnett analyzed data from the National Vital Statistics Program and the 1990 and 2000 US Census and found that Mexican Americans had a higher diabetes-related mortality rate (251 per 100,000) than Puerto Ricans or Cuban American, whose mortality rates were 204 deaths per 100,000 and 101 deaths per 100,000, respectively (7). Fan and associates (8) examined data from NHANES III and NHANES 1999–2002. In this sample (n = 1,142), 34.5% of Mexican Americans achieved optimal glycemic control (hemoglobin A1C ≤ 7%), compared with 43.3% for non-Hispanic whites and 41.2% for blacks.

Incidence of type 1 diabetes is increasing worldwide across all ethnic groups (9). In a study of Colorado youth, Vehik et al observed that incidence was slightly higher for non-Hispanic youth compared with Hispanic youth (2.7 vs 1.6%, $P = .27$) (10).

Risk Factors for Type 2 Diabetes

Overweight and Obesity

Across the United States, prevalence of overweight (body mass index [BMI] 25–29.9) and obesity (BMI ≥ 30) has steadily increased among all groups, regardless of gender, ethnicity, or educational level (11). Among Mexican American adults and children, increases in the rates of overweight, obesity, and type 2 diabetes have been particularly dramatic, and the impact on health disparities is alarming (11). Approximately 73% of Mexican American women and 74.6% of Mexican American men are overweight or obese, compared with 57.6% of non-Hispanic white women and 71% of non-Hispanic white men (12).

Ancestry

Research is limited regarding the genetic ancestry of Mexican people and any genetic predispositions for obesity or diabetes. The prevalence of diabetes among Mexican people may be traceable to Spanish ancestry (13). Data from the Human Genome Project is expected to provide additional information regarding the risk and prevalence of diabetes among people of Mexican ancestry.

Environmental Risk Factors

Environmental risk factors for type 2 diabetes include those components in a person's surroundings that affect biology, daily habits, and decision-making in ways that will influence health status. Environmental risk factors are also thought to also be a "trigger" in the development of type 1 diabetes (14). Environmental risk factors typically include food choice options (eg, availability of fast food vs grocery stores); opportunities for physical activity (eg, availability of playgrounds); access to health care services; exposure to toxins in the water, air, and food supply; and transportation habits (eg, walking vs driving). If community surroundings are conducive to high calorie intake in combination with low physical activity levels and a reduced energy expenditure lifestyle, then people in the community have greater environmental risks for becoming overweight and developing type 2 diabetes.

Research on the role of environmental risk factors for type 2 diabetes is best illustrated by cross-border studies that compare of people living in the United States to people living in Mexico. Comparing individuals of similar ethnic backgrounds, socioeconomic status, ages, and genders from San Antonio, Texas, and Mexico City, Burke and associates found the incidence of type 2 diabetes among Mexican Americans to be higher than among Mexicans living in Mexico City (15). Most notably, San Antonio men and women between the ages of 55 and 64 years had a four-fold increased incidence of type 2 diabetes compared with Mexico City men and women in the same age range. In a study examining genetically related populations of Mexican Pima Indians (n = 224) and US Pima Indians (n = 877), Schulz and colleagues reported a significantly lower prevalence ($P < .01$) of obesity and type 2 diabetes among the Mexican Pima Indians compared with the US Pima Indians (16). These studies (15,16) suggest that environmental factors such as a more rural or physically demanding lifestyle in Mexico, compared with a more sedentary lifestyle and easier access to low-cost, high-calorie food in the United States, contribute to the higher rates of obesity and diabetes among Mexican Americans.

Traditional Foods and Dishes

Traditional Mexican cuisine has many regional variations, which can be grouped in three primary classifications: (*a*) *mestizo* foods from the central plateau and the center of Oaxaca in the south; (*b*) foods from the frontiers of the Maya in the southeast; and (*c*) the foods of the

Table 4.1 · Foods Used in Traditional Mexican American Cuisine

Food	Description
Starchy vegetables	
Beans	The most commonly used beans include pinto, red, and black. Other traditionally used beans include kidney and fava. All are good sources of fiber and protein and can be used in stews and soups. They can be served refried (fried with lard or vegetable oil) or boiled *(a la olla)* with onions, garlic, and salt. Boiled beans are served in their own broth.
Corn/*masa*	*Masa* is a type of corn flour used to make tortillas, tamales, *atole*, and *sopes*.
Nonstarchy vegetables	
Chilies, dried and fresh	Varieties include jalapeño, poblano, serrano, guajillo, chipotle, pasilla, habañero, ancho, mulato, and cascabel. Chilies are used for cooked and raw salsas (sauces), which can be added to meats, soups, and many other dishes. Chilies are a good source of vitamins A and C.
Nopales	Prickly pear cactus paddles. *Nopales* are a good source of fiber and tend to be sautéed or boiled and consumed as a vegetable. May be made into a juice or added to salsa.
Tomatoes	Essential ingredient for some Mexican salsas, such as *pico de gallo*. Tomatoes are also used in fish and beef dishes and in red rice.
Tomatillos	Small green tomatoes encased in a stiff husk. Tomatillos are tart and often used in cooked or raw green salsas. Cooked, green salsas tend to be fried.
Bread	
Tortillas	Flat breads made from corn or wheat flour. Used for tacos and enchiladas.
Milk	
Crema (cream)	Commonly used for garnish for enchiladas, tacos, eggs, and many other dishes.
Meat	
Carne asada	Thinly sliced, grilled beef.
Chorizo	Pork sausage which is spiced and used in scrambled eggs or other dishes.
Tripe	Usually fried with vegetable oil.
Fats	
Manteca (lard)	Widely used in Mexican cooking. Encourage clients to substitute heart-healthy oils.

Gulf and Pacific coast (17). Regional variations are notable, but some characteristics are common throughout Mexican food practices. The traditional Mexican meal structure consists of a succession of individual courses. For example, rice is typically eaten before the main course or the beans (17). Another characteristic common to all types of Mexican cuisine is the use of chilies, which were first domesticated in Mexico. Mexicans have the highest per capita consumption of chilies, and they are available in a great variety (17). Tables 4.1 and 4.2 summarize the commonly used traditional Mexican foods. See Appendix A for nutrient analyses.

Traditional Meal Patterns and Holiday Foods

Traditionally, Mexicans ate four to five meals per day (18–21). Today, three meals per day is a common meal pattern. The types of foods consumed vary relative to income, education, organization, geographic region, and family customs. Table 4.3 describes foods eaten during selected holidays observed in Mexican culture (22,23).

Table 4.2 • Traditional Mexican American Dishes, Beverages, and Desserts

Food	Description
Dishes	
Arroz con pollo	Rice with chicken.
Enchiladas	Usually made with corn tortillas that are fried and dipped in a chili sauce (green or red) and then filled with cheese, chicken, or beef. Usually served topped with cream cheese and shredded cheese.
Salsa	Translated as "sauce." Salsas are tomato- and chili-based garnishes use at the table. Main ingredients are tomatoes or tomatillos, onions, chilies, garlic, cilantro, and other spices.
Sopa de arroz	Rice soup. The rice tends to be fried and then cooked with or without vegetables. It can be served dry (ie, with little broth) or with broth.
Sopa de fideos	Vermicelli cooked and served with a tomato-based sauce. Other vegetables may be added.
Tacos	Corn tortillas filled with chicken, beef, pork, fish, and other ingredients.
Tamales	Steamed (cornmeal) dough filled with beef, chicken, pork, or vegetables. They can be spicy or sweet.
Beverages	
Aguas frescas	Refreshing drink made with three essential ingredients: fruit, water and sugar. Tamarind, melon, and hibiscus are popular flavors.
Alcoholic beverages	Beer, tequila, and mescal are traditional alcoholic beverages.
Atole	A porridge-like hot drink made with, cornstarch, ground rice or oats and sweetened with sugar. Flavors include chocolate, vanilla, strawberry, and fresh pineapple. It can be made with water or milk or a mixture of both. Powdered *atole* mixes can be found in US grocery stores.
Fruit juices	
Horchata	Soft drink of ground rice blended with water or juice and melon seeds. Sugar is added.
Hot chocolate	
Licuado	A cold beverage prepared with fruit and milk, blended and often sweetened with sugar. Some people add a raw egg, which may be a food safety concern.
Desserts/Sweets	
Arroz con leche	Rice cooked in milk, sweetened with sugar, and spiced with cinnamon.
Chongos zamoranos	Dessert made with curdled milk with sugar and cinnamon.
Flan	Custard.
Pan dulce	There are many varieties of *pan dulce*. These sweetened breads/pastries are usually consumed with coffee, milk, or hot chocolate for breakfast or dinner.

Table 4.3 • Traditional Foods Consumed During Holidays

Holiday	Traditional Foods
Cuaresma (Lent)	Mexican Americans commonly fast and have meatless meals on Ash Wednesday and Fridays during Lent.
Posadas (Christmas-time evening parties)	*Posadas* occur December 16–24. Dinner party foods include *buñuelos* (fried pastries with sugar), *colación* (candies), tamales, *ponche* (hot fruit punch), and *atole*.
Día de los reyes (Day of Kings)	The *Día de los reyes* celebrates the Epiphany. *Rosca* (a ring-shaped bread) is commonly shared.

Source: Data are from references 22 and 23.

Traditional Health Beliefs

Health beliefs, as defined by the Health Belief model, are the individual perceptions, modifying factors, and likelihood of taking action (24).When a patient chooses to act on a health-related issue, such as a chronic infection, or persistent hyperglycemia, these are typically referred to as "health-seeking behaviors"—ie, actions taken by patients to get medical input or medical advice regarding a health concern or condition (25).

In traditional Mexican culture, illness is sometimes understood to be a consequence of God's will or fate; it is not something individuals can personally control. In some studies, faith has been shown to take the place of professional medical care (26). In contrast, in their Arizona focus group (n = 90) and survey research (n = 132) with mostly male Hispanics (primarily Mexican Americans but exact numbers not specified), Larkey and associates found that faith in God and the seriousness of disease symptoms were both strongly related to health-seeking behaviors (27). Hence, Larkey et al concluded that faith was a support or motivator for seeking medical care. These subjects were more likely to seek prompt medical attention if they had more serious disease symptoms and a strong faith in God. Reviews of Hispanic beliefs about diabetes (28,29) concluded that Hispanics often integrate biomedical treatments with religious and folk medicine.

Herbal and folk remedies are popular in Mexican culture. In a study examining use of Mexican folk medicine in Mexican American women, Lopez (30) comprehensively reviewed folk medicine systems typically used in Mexican culture. Faith or spiritual healers, generally referred to as *señoras*, *espiritistas* or *espiritualistas*, have no specific medical training. Rather, they focus on healing the soul using séances or reading spiritual cards. Healers known as *curanderos* "may treat a full range of physical, mental, and spiritual afflictions," and sometimes perform exorcisms (30). *Yerberos* (herbalists) often dispense medicinal herbs. *Sobadores* (traditional masseuses) and *parteras* (lay midwives) perform physical treatments such as massage and manipulation.

Lopez also surveyed 70 Mexican American female university students in southern California and found the use of traditional folk medicine to be common. Seventy-one percent of respondents kept *manzanilla* (chamomile) tea and 80% kept *te de yerbabuena* (spearmint tea) at home (30). Almost 26% of the sample had used *curanderos;* almost 39% used *sobadores,* and 20% used *yerberos*. In this sample, 70% of the participants were aged 20 to 29 years, 77% were US-born, and 81% were fluent in Spanish. It is also important to note that 57% reported taking trips to Mexico in the prior 2-year period to purchase medicine; 21% obtained medical care there, and 50% brought back herbs purchased in Mexico. Findings from Lopez (30) suggest that even in groups of Mexican Americans who seem rather "acculturated" (ie, US-born, bilingual, and with high levels of education), individuals may still use a substantial amount of Mexican-based herbal and folk medicine.

In an assessment of alternative medicine use and documentation among southwestern Hispanic women, Johnson and associates (31) conducted structured interviews with a convenience sample (n = 23) of Hispanic participants. They also reviewed medical and medication charts on a group (n = 81) of randomly sampled female Hispanics (primarily Mexican Americans) who were not interviewed. The researchers found that use of herbs was very common among the interviewed participants (21 of 23 [91%] of interviewed patients). However, only 16% of the randomly selected medical charts documented herbal remedy use.

Poss and associates (32) interviewed (in Spanish) 22 Mexican Americans in El Paso, Texas, to explore use of herbal remedies for treating type 2 diabetes. Most of the interview participants reported that they use of herbal remedies to treat their diabetes in addition to prescribed Western medicine or treatments. Coronado and associates (33) reported that use of herbal remedies was common for treating type 2 diabetes based on six focus groups of 42 Mexican Americans (14 men and 28 women) in central Washington. Participants often reported use of herbal remedies as an adjunct to oral diabetes medications or insulin therapy (numbers not reported). Briggs Early and colleagues conducted in-depth interviews with 10 Mexican Americans and 8 whites with type 2 diabetes from a community health clinic (34). Nine out of 10 Mexican Americans reported herbal remedy use, whereas one white participant reported herbal remedy use. Among the more common herbal remedies used by Mexican Americans are prickly pear cactus *(nopal)* and aloe vera (31–34).

Current Food Practices

The food practices of Mexican Americans are influenced by a wide variety of issues, including the following:

- Chronic illnesses such as diabetes
- Access to health care
- Degree of acculturation
- Educational background
- Gender
- Level of food security
- Knowledge and health beliefs
- Socioeconomic status
- Self-efficacy
- Social support systems

Traditional Mexican diets are typically limited in added fat while high in fruits, vegetables, and fiber. However, current Mexican American diets are often high in fat and inadequate in fruits and vegetables (35). Surveys that assessed eating patterns in female Mexican Americans living in metro Detroit revealed use of high-fat dairy products, inadequate fruit intake, infrequent use of lean meats, and frequent consumption of fried foods (36). Questionnaire data from 1,689 Mexican Americans living in rural central Washington indicated a dietary pattern high in fat and low in fruit and vegetable consumption (35).

Counseling Considerations

Mexican Americans value family and social interactions. According to Warrix, the family unit is the single most important social unit in the life of Hispanics (22). The father is traditionally the leader of the family, and the mother runs the household, shops, and prepares the food. However, gender roles seem to be moving to a more egalitarian model with more exposure to American society. For most Mexican Americans, family responsibilities come before all other responsibilities. Therefore, during counseling sessions, it is beneficial to discuss the impact that the diabetes food plan will have on family members. A client's socioeconomic status is another important factor to consider during diabetes education.

An individual's primary language may be an indicator of success within the US health care system and is often used as a measure of acculturation (28). Compared with non-Hispanic whites, clients whose primary language is Spanish are at greater risk for developing long-term diabetes-related complications such as poorer glycemic control, blindness, end-stage renal disease or amputation (37,38). You should therefore determine the primary languages (written and oral) used in clients' homes so you can offer the most culturally appropriate education to your client.

Other essential issues for any diabetes education encounter include the following:

- How acculturated is the client? Acculturation is an independent predictor of dietary composition (39). This issue was recently and thoroughly reviewed by Ayala and colleagues (40).
- Are recommended changes in eating habits realistic and manageable for the client and his or her family?
- What is the client's lifestyle? Does the client work at night, or do seasonal schedule changes affect food habits and activity options or the client's ability to attend classes, support groups and other appointments? (For example, many Mexican American farm workers work very long hours during the spring, summer, and fall months, but fewer hours in winter months.)
- Can the client afford medications?
- Is the client willing to take the prescribed medication(s) or follow a special diet? Does the client's family support the recommended changes?
- Does the patient accept the plan of care?
- Does the client think he or she will be successful with the plan?
- Will the client's age have an impact on the educational approach used?

Demonstrating Courtesy and Respect

For a successful counseling relationship, it is essential to establish respect and trust from the start (41,42). When counseling clients, maintain their dignity by keeping a nonjudgmental attitude and accepting cultural differences. To increase credibility, understand your clients' food habits and health beliefs. Know the appropriate degree of eye contact.

Ask clients the reason for their visits—clients may have a different understanding than you regarding the reasons why their doctor made the referral for nutrition counseling. Gather information about their previous interactions with nutrition and medical personnel and ask them about their treatment expectations. According to Juckett, before providing diabetes education, the health care provider should talk with the client about their family to establish trust *(confianza)* (43).

Interpreting Clients' Nonverbal Communication

It is important to remember that clients may regard the physician, diabetes educator, or registered dietitian as a person whose authority may not be challenged. Present yourself as an approachable health care provider and frequently ask the client to summarize the main teaching concepts from the counseling session to ensure that you have conveyed the correct information in an understandable fashion. Be aware that clients may not make eye contact and may look down; also, they may nod affirmatively even when they do not understand. Asking questions may not be part of their culture.

Inquiring About Clients' Understanding of Diabetes

Some Mexican Americans may believe that diabetes is caused by the consumption of too much sugar or by God's will or punishment (44). Clients may not understand that weakness, headache, nervousness, leg pains, forgetfulness, and anger can be signs of elevated blood glucose.

Determine what your clients understand about diabetes and how it affects them. You may not be able to ask this directly. However, you can ask what they think diabetes is and if they know why they got diabetes. This line of questioning can uncover important information about the individual's beliefs and his or her receptiveness to education and treatment.

Discussing Clients' Use of Complementary and Alternative Medicine

As noted earlier in this chapter, Mexican American cultural practices sometimes include the use of herbs, teas, rituals, ointments, and various home remedies, as well as consultations with folk healers or practitioners known as *curanderos* (45). Home remedies usually take one of several forms, such as a drink, tea, poultice, or ointment. Andrade-Cetto and Heinrich have published a comprehensive review of herbal remedies used by Mexican people for diabetes and their pharmochemical properties (45). Table 4.4 lists common diabetes-related herbal remedies and how they are typically used for diabetes treatment. See Appendix C for questions to assess dietary supplement use.

Considering Family Demands and Dynamics

Health care practitioners should not underestimate the influence of family and friends on disease management among Mexican American clients (46). Many societies embrace food as part of celebration and ceremony and use it as a way for people to convey feelings to one another. Instead of focusing exclusively on the "self" part of self-management, remember to consider the social environment of the family, friends, and culture within which the client with diabetes operates (47,48). Fisher and colleagues argue that diabetes self-management education does not sufficiently emphasize the social environment of people living with diabetes (46). Family members' support and understanding is critical for clients to maintain necessary lifestyle changes (49). Intervention studies using *promotoras* (lay health-outreach education workers) obtained positive changes in family members' knowledge, attitudes, behaviors, and beliefs relative to diabetes prevention and control, thereby enhancing patient outcomes (49,50). In eight 90-minute focus groups with 45 Latino adults with type 2 diabetes, Cherrington and colleagues (51) found that patients who felt understood by their family members did better with their diabetes self-management, a finding that emphasizes the need for diabetes education to include family members in the education process.

Table 4.4 • Remedies Used by Mexican Americans for Self-Treatment

Spanish Names	Description	Methods of Use/Preparation	Health Claims[a]
Guarumbo, chancarro, hormiguillo	Cecropia obtusifolia (trumpet tree)	Leaves are boiled and steeped for tea	Hypoglycemic effect, anti-inflammatory, analgesic, muscle relaxant, antihypertensive
Maguey	Agave, century plant	Stem-macerated and consumed	Hypoglycemic effect
Nopales, nopalitos	Prickly pear cactus	Chopped in salsa, salad, boiled for tea	Hypoglycemic effect
Sábila	Aloe vera	Juice of leaves, roasted stem; mixed with nopales and eaten or drunk	Hypoglycemic effect
Uña de gato, gatuno	Cat's claw (acacia)	Leaves or bark boiled for tea	Hypoglycemic effect

[a]Data in Health Claims column do *not* evaluate whether uses are safe or effective.

There is often a pattern to the health-seeking process in Hispanic families. Usually, the mother or primary female caretaker decides when an illness is beyond her ability to treat with folk remedies and when to seek additional help. At this point, family becomes more involved in the decision-making process. Important decisions regarding health issues are made by the entire family, which may include close family friends as well as immediate and extended family members. The family serves as a strong support for the individual with diabetes, and family decisions may supersede decisions made by the health care provider. Before seeking Western health care, the family may then go to the community for help and may consult with the *curandero*. Often, the last person consulted is the Western-medicine health care provider.

Mexican Americans manage their diabetes in gender-specific ways. In the well-known intervention studies along the Texas border communities of Starr County, Brown and associates (52) used diet as a primary treatment modality and found that Hispanic men reported higher perceived control (self-perception of how well one controls one's diabetes) and more social support compared with women. Hispanic culture emphasizes cooperation rather than competition and family instead of self.

Engaging Others in Counseling Sessions

When a client does not speak or read English, the use of medically trained interpreters is necessary. Do not rely on family members to act as interpreters. They may not have sufficient knowledge of medical terminology, and confidential personal information may be revealed during counseling sessions. Written materials should be provided in English and in the clients' primary language, so that information is available to the patient and others in their support system.

Typically, male family members are not involved in grocery shopping or food preparation activities. If this is the case for your client, consider including the female head of the household in nutrition education, because she is likely responsible for shopping and cooking.

Nutrition Counseling

Depending on the client's degree of acculturation, the nutrition counseling session may be similar to any other. See Appendix B for medical nutrition therapy recommendations and general counseling suggestions. The following are culturally specific nutrition counseling strategies for Mexican American clients:

- Ask probing questions about foods currently consumed by the family. Inquire about cooking methods—especially the use of fats and oils, mayonnaise, cream, and cheese. Be sure to ask about frying methods, including what types of fat or oil the client uses, and how often the client eats fried foods.

- Encourage clients to have healthful traditional fruits and vegetables such as mangos, oranges, peaches, tomato, *nopales*, onions, garlic, peppers and chilies, salad greens, dried beans that are boiled and not fried, corn tortillas, tomatillos, and so on.
- Advise clients on lower-fat substitutions for traditional dishes and family recipes, such as heart-healthy and flavorful alternatives to lard or cream.

Challenges and Barriers to Dietary Adherence

Barriers to diabetes care for Mexican American clients may include language; financial concerns; insufficient or unsatisfactory interactions with health care providers; and the client's personal beliefs, environmental situations, and psychosocial barriers. In a retrospective cohort study of 183 Hispanic men and women (mostly Mexican Americans, ages 35 to 70 years) in Colorado, Lasater and associates found that glycemic control was not significantly better or worse in patients regardless of language spoken by the patient or the provider (53). However, Spanish speakers were much less likely than English speakers to receive written materials during diabetes education.

Depression is a barrier and comorbidity for many individuals with diabetes, and clients should be evaluated for depression at each visit. Fisher and colleagues reported that depression was a result of multiple life issues, not just diabetes alone (54). According to these researchers, focus group data indicate that people who feel understood by their family members do better with their diabetes self-management.

Physician and health care system barriers can also interfere with the quality of diabetes care. In research not specific to Mexican Americans, Freeman and Loewe found that physicians and their patients often had widely disparate notions of "diabetes control," and this greatly affected patient-physician communication (55). Using data from surveys of diabetes educators (not patients with diabetes), in the Pacific Northwest, Sprague and colleagues (56) reported that many diabetes educators believe patients do not pursue follow-up diabetes education because they seem to believe they have adequate knowledge to manage their diabetes. Patients may receive comprehensive diabetes education on diagnosis and not realize that self-management education should continue throughout their life. Although this finding was not specific to Hispanics, it is an important consideration that all patients need ongoing diabetes education. Diabetes educators, physicians, and health care organizations may therefore need to work to help clients understand that diabetes education should be a regular event, just like other medical check-ups.

Counseling Tips

Diabetes educators should make the most of counseling sessions and work with the best that Mexican culture offers. Promote consumption of traditional foods, including those that are high in vegetable protein, such as corn, beans, and *nopales*. Encourage small frequent meals as opposed to one or two very large meals. Also encourage family members to support beneficial lifestyle behaviors (57,58). Braxton suggests that health care providers acknowledge Mexican Americans' family-based lifestyle and the consumption of both traditional and contemporary foods (59). Other important points to remember when communicating with clients of Mexican heritage include the following (59,60):

- *Personalismo* (personalization): Observe courtesies such as the exchange of pleasantries and handshakes to personalize the visit. In general, it is better to ask questions about family than about work.
- *Respeto* (respect): Mexican American culture honors and respects elders and community leaders. In Spanish, elders and leaders should be addressed by the formal form of you *(usted),* not the informal *tú.*
- *Simpático* (congeniality): Polite, agreeable, and respectful interactions are the cornerstone of the Mexican American culture. During conversations, avoid confrontation and criticism.
- Nonverbal behavior: As noted earlier, nodding affirmatively does not necessarily mean agreement. Silence may indicate that a client lacks understanding and is too embarrassed to ask for clarification or disagree.

- Language comprehension: Clients may understand English better than they can speak it, especially when they are under stress.
- Modesty and privacy: Sensitive health issues should be discussed through a professional interpreter, not by using family members to translate. If client chooses to use a family member as an interpreter, it may be best to choose a family member of the same gender when personal issues are discussed. (Also, understand and observe legal regulations regarding interpreters, privacy, and patient confidentiality.)

Conclusion

It is important to understand what diabetes means to the person living with diabetes, regardless of cultural background. However, considering cultural background will allow for a more targeted and successful diabetes education encounter. Help the client become a more active participant in their own self-care. Be cognizant of the client's previous diabetes education experiences, degree of acculturation, language needs, educational background, gender roles, family structure, and socioeconomic level. Work with the client at whatever level they are at to maximize their diabetes outcomes.

Resources

American Diabetes Association Latinos and Diabetes Web page. http://www.diabetes.org/communityprograms-and-localevents/latinos.jsp. Accessed February 19, 2009.

dLife: For Your Diabetes Life. http://www.dlife.com. Accessed February 19, 2009.

Joslin Diabetes Center. http://www.joslin.org. Accessed February 19, 2009.

Latino Diabetes Association. http://www.sclda.org/Resources.htm. Accessed February 19, 2009.

Metabolic Pulse: Diabetes Education for Healthcare Professionals. http://www.metabolicpulse.org. Accessed February 19, 2009.

National Diabetes Education Program Prevengamos la diabetes tipo 2: Paso a Paso campaign. http://www.ndep.nih.gov/campaigns/PasoaPaso/Paso_a_Paso.htm. Accessed February 19, 2009.

National Diabetes Information Clearinghouse Hispanics/Latinos and Diabetes Web page. http://diabetes.niddk.nih.gov/dm/pubs/hispanicamerican/index.htm. Accessed February 19, 2009.

Sansum Diabetes Research Institute. http://www.sansum.org/index.php. Accessed February 19, 2009.

Stanford Patient Education Research Center. Tomando Control de su Salud (Spanish Chronic Disease Self-Management Program). http://patienteducation.stanford.edu/programs_spanish/tomando.html. Accessed February 19, 2009.

References

1. US Census Bureau. The Hispanic Population: 2000 Census Brief. 2001. http://www.census.gov/prod/2001pubs/c2kbr01-3.pdf. Accessed February 19, 2009.
2. US Census Bureau. Facts for Features: Cinco de Mayo. May 7, 2007. http://www.census.gov/Press-Release/www/releases/archives/facts_for_features_special_editions/009726.html. Accessed February 19, 2009.
3. Regents of the University of California and the Mexican Secretariat of Health. Mexican and Central American Immigrants in the United States: Health Care Access. 2006. http://hia.berkeley.edu/documents/hlthcareaccess2006_eng.pdf. Accessed February 19, 2009.
4. Centers for Disease Control and Prevention. National Diabetes Fact Sheet: General Information and National Estimates on Diabetes in the United States, 2007. 2008. http://www.cdc.gov/diabetes/pubs/pdf/ndfs_2007.pdf. Accessed February 19, 2009.
5. Mainous AG, Baker R, Koopman RJ, Saxena S, Diaz VA, Everett CJ, Majeed A. Impact of the population at risk of diabetes on projections of diabetes burden in the United States: an epidemic on the way. *Diabetologia.* 2007;50:934–940.
6. National Diabetes Data Group, National Institute of Diabetes and Digestive and Kidney Diseases. *Diabetes in America.* 2nd ed. Bethesda MD: National Institutes of Health; 1995. NIH publication 95-1468.
7. Smith CA, Barnett E. Diabetes-related mortality among Mexican Americans, Puerto Ricans, and Cuban Americans in the United States. *Rev Panam Salud Publica.* 2005;18:381–387.
8. Fan T, Koro CE, Fedder DO, Bowlin SJ. Ethnic disparities and trends in glycemic control among adults with type 2 diabetes in the U.S. from 1998 to 2002. *Diabetes Care.* 2006;29:1924–1925.

9. DIAMOND Project. Incidence and trends of childhood type 1 diabetes worldwide 1990–1999. *Diabet Med.* 2006;23:857–866.

10. Vehik K, Hamman RF, Lezotte D, Norris JM, Klingensmith G, Bloch C, Rewers M, Dabelea D. Increasing incidence of type 1 diabetes in 0- to 17-year-old Colorado youth. *Diabetes Care.* 2007;30:503–509.

11. Weight-control Information Network. Statistics Related to Overweight and Obesity. June 2007. http://win.niddk.nih.gov/publications/PDFs/stat904z.pdf. Accessed August 14, 2008.

12. Freedman DS, Kettel Khan L, Serdula MK, Ogden CL, Dietz WH. Racial and ethnic differences in secular trends for childhood BMI, weight, and height. *Obesity.* 2006;14:301–308.

13. Lorenzo C, Serrano-Rios M, Martinez-Larrad MT, Gabriel R, Williams K, Gonzalez-Villalpando C, Stern MP, Hazuda HP, Haffner SM. Was the historic contribution of Spain to the Mexican gene pool partially responsible for the higher prevalence of type 2 diabetes in Mexican-origin populations? The Spanish Insulin Resistance Study Group, the San Antonio Heart Study, and the Mexico City Diabetes Study. *Diabetes Care.* 2001;24:2059–2064.

14. Knip M, Veijola R, Virtanen SM, Hyöty H, Vaarala O, Akerblom HK. Environmental triggers and determinants of type 1 diabetes. *Diabetes.* 2005;54(Suppl 2):S125–S136.

15. Burke JP, Williams K, Haffner SM, Villalpando CG, Stern MP. Elevated incidence of type 2 diabetes in San Antonio, Texas, compared with that of Mexico City, Mexico. *Diabetes Care.* 2001;24:1573–1578.

16. Schulz LO, Bennett PH, Ravussin E, Kidd JR, Kidd KK, Esparza J, Valencia ME. Effects of traditional and western environments on prevalence of type 2 diabetes in Pima Indians in Mexico and the U.S. *Diabetes Care.* 2006;29:1866–1871.

17. Katz SH, Weaver WW. *Encyclopedia of Food and Culture.* New York, NY: Scribner, Gale Group; 2003:492.

18. Romero-Gwyn E, Gwynn DL, Grivetti R, McDonald R, Stanford G, Turner B, West E, Williamson E. Dietary acculturation among Latinos of Mexican descent. *Nutr Today.* 1993 July-Aug:6–11.

19. Sosa E. Ethnic Cuisine: Mexico. http://www.sallys-place.com/food/cuisines/mexico.htm. Accessed July 27, 2007.

20. Romero-Gwyn E, Gwyn D. *Dietary Patterns and Acculturation Among Latinos of Mexican Descent.* East Lansing, MI: Julian Samora Research Institute, Michigan State University; 1997. JSRI Research Report 23.

21. Hursh Graber K. Rice, the Gift of the Other Gods. January 1, 2003. http://www.mexconnect.com/en/articles/2093-rice-the-gift-of-the-other-gods. Accessed April 27, 2009.

22. Warrix M. Cultural Diversity: Eating in America: Mexican-American. Ohio State University Extension Fact Sheet. http://ohioline.osu.edu/hyg-fact/5000/5255.html. Accessed July 27, 2007.

23. Mitchell BD. Hispanics and Latinos: Diet of Characteristics of the Hispanic Diet. http://www.faqs.org/nutrition/Hea-Irr/Hispanics-and-Latinos-Diet-of.html Accessed July 30, 2007.

24. Schwab T, Meyer J, Merrell R. Measuring attitudes and health beliefs among Mexican Americans with diabetes. *Diabetes Educ.* 1994;20:221.

25. Venmans LM, Gorter KJ, Hak E, Rutten GE. Short-term effects of an educational program on health-seeking behavior for infections in patients with type 2 diabetes: a randomized controlled intervention trial in primary care. *Diabetes Care.* 2008;31:402–407.

26. Cotugna H, Subar AF, Heimendinger J, Kahle L. Nutrition and cancer prevention knowledge, beliefs, attitudes, and practices. The 1987 National Health Interview Survey. *J Am Diet Assoc.* 1992;92:963–967.

27. Larkey LK, Hecht ML, Miller K, Alatorre C. Hispanic cultural norms for health-seeking behaviors in the face of symptoms. *Health Educ Behav.* 2001;28:65–80.

28. Hunt LM, Schneider S, Comer B. Should "acculturation" be a variable in health research? A critical review of research on U.S. Hispanics. *Soc Sci Med.* 2004;59:973–986.

29. Hatcher E, Whittemore R. Hispanic adults' beliefs about type 2 diabetes: clinical implications. *J Am Acad Nurs Pract.* 2007;19:536–545.

30. Lopez RA. Use of alternative folk medicine by Mexican American women. *J Immigr Health.* 2005;7:23–31.

31. Johnson L, Strich H, Taylor A, Timmermann B, Malone D, Teufel-Shone N, Drummond R, Woosley R, Pereira E, Martinez A. Use of herbal remedies by diabetic Hispanic women in the southwestern United States. *Phytother Res.* 2006;20:250–255.

32. Poss JE, Jezewski MA, Stuart AG. Home remedies for type 2 diabetes used by Mexican Americans in El Paso, Texas. *Clin Nurs Res.* 2003;12:304–323.

33. Coronado GD, Thompson B, Tejeda S, Godina R. Attitudes and beliefs among Mexican Americans about type 2 diabetes. *J Health Care Poor Underserved.* 2004;15:576–588.

34. Briggs Early K, Armstrong Shultz J, Corbett C. Assessing diabetes dietary goals and self-management based on in-depth interviews with Latino and Caucasian clients with type 2 diabetes. *J Transcult Nurs.* April 22, 2009. [Epub ahead of print]

35. Neuhouser ML, Thompson B, Coronado GD, Solomon CC. Higher fat intake and lower fruit and vegetables intakes are associated with greater acculturation among Mexicans living in Washington State. *J Am Diet Assoc.* 2004;104:51–57.

36. Artinian NT, Schim SM, Vander Wal JS, Nies MA. Eating patterns and cardiovascular disease risk in a Detroit Mexican American population. *Public Health Nurs.* 2004;21:425–434.

37. Dagogo-Jack S, Funnell MM, Davidson J. Barriers to achieving optimal glycemic control in a multi-ethnic society: a US focus. *Curr Diabetes Rev.* 2006;2:285–293.

38. Harris MI. Racial and ethnic differences in health care access and health outcomes for adults with type 2 diabetes. *Diabetes Care.* 2001;24:454–459.

39. Sarkar U, Fisher L, Schillinger D. Is self-efficacy associated with diabetes self-management across race/ethnicity and health literacy? *Diabetes Care.* 2006;29:823–829.

40. Ayala GX, Baquero B, Klinger S. A systematic review of the relationship between acculturation and diet among Latinos in the United States: implications for future research. *J Am Diet Assoc.* 2008;108:1330–44.

41. Brown S. Diabetes interventions for minority populations: We're really not that different, You and I!" *Diabetes Spectrum.* 1998;11:145–149.

42. Whittemore R. Culturally competent interventions for Hispanic adults with type 2 diabetes: a systematic review. *J Transcult Nurs.* 2007;18:157–166.

43. Juckett G. Cross-cultural health beliefs and folk remedies. *Am Fam Physician.* 2005;72:2267–2274.

44. Tripp-Reimer T, Choi E, Kelley S, Enslein JC. Cultural barriers to care: inverting the problem. *Diabetes Spectrum.* 2001;14:13–22.

45. Andrade-Cetto A, Heinrich M. Mexican plants with hypoglycaemic effect used in the treatment of diabetes. *J Ethnopharmacol.* 2005;99:325–348.

46. Fisher EB, Brownson CA, O'Toole ML, Shetty G, Anwuri VV, Glasgow RE. Ecological approaches to self-management: the case of diabetes. *Am J Public Health.* 2005;95:1523–1535.

47. Norris SL, Engelgau MM, Narayan KM. Effectiveness of self-management training in type 2 diabetes: a systematic review of randomized controlled trials. *Diabetes Care.* 2001;24:561–587.

48. Vincent D, Clark L, Zimmer LM, Sanchez J. Using focus groups to develop a culturally competent diabetes self-management program for Mexican Americans. *Diabetes Educ.* 2006;32:89–97.

49. Teufel-Shone NI, Drummond R, Rawiel U. Developing and adapting a family-based diabetes program at the U.S.-Mexico border. *Prev Chronic Dis.* 2005;2:A20.

50. Lorig KR, Ritter PL, Jacquez A. Outcomes of border health Spanish/English chronic disease self-management programs. *Diabetes Educ.* 2005;31:401–409.

51. Cherrington A, Ayala GX, Sleath B, Corbie-Smith G. Examining knowledge, attitudes, and beliefs about depression among Latino adults with type 2 diabetes. *Diabetes Educ.* 2006;32:603–613.

52. Brown SA, Harrist RB, Villagomez ET, Segura M, Barton SA, Hanis CL. Gender and treatment differences in knowledge, health beliefs, and metabolic control in Mexican Americans with type 2 diabetes. *Diabetes Educ.* 2000;26.

53. Lasater LM, Davidson AJ, Steiner JF, Mehler PS. Glycemic control in English- vs Spanish-speaking Hispanic patients with type 2 diabetes mellitus. *Arch Intern Med.* 2001;161:77–82.

54. Fisher L, Chesla CA, Mullan JT, Skaff MM, Kanter RA. Contributors to depression in Latino and European-American patients with type 2 diabetes. *Diabetes Care.* 2001;24:1751–1757.

55. Freeman J, Loewe R. Barriers to communication about diabetes mellitus. Patients' and physicians' different view of the disease. *J Fam Pract.* 2000;49:507–512.

56. Sprague MA, Shultz JA, Branen LJ, Lambeth S, Hillers VN. Diabetes educators' perspectives on barriers for patients and educators in diabetes. *Diabetes Educ.* 1999;25:907–916.

57. Kittler PG, Sucher KP. Accent on taste: an applied approach to multicultural competency. *Diabetes Spectrum.* 2004;17:200–204.

58. Hispanic American Influences on the U.S. Food Industry. Selected References prepared in commemoration of the USDA Hispanic Heritage Month Celebration. September 15–October 15, 2002. http://www.nal.usda.gov/outreach/HFood.html. Accessed September 21, 2007.

59. Braxton DM. Hispanics and Latinos, Diet of. http://findarticles.com/p/articles/mi_gx5200/is_2004/ai_n19120863/pg_1. Accessed July 27, 2007.

60. Rhode Island Department of Health. Latino/Hispanic Culture & Health. http://www.health.state.ri.us/chic/minority/lat_cul.php#diet. Accessed July 30, 2007.

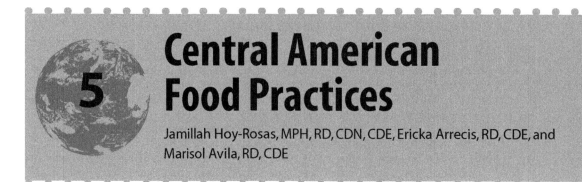

Central American Food Practices

Jamillah Hoy-Rosas, MPH, RD, CDN, CDE, Ericka Arrecis, RD, CDE, and Marisol Avila, RD, CDE

Introduction

Central America is a tropical isthmus that connects North America to South America. It includes seven nations: Belize, Costa Rica, El Salvador, Guatemala, Honduras, Nicaragua, and Panama. These nations are bordered by the Pacific Ocean to the southwest, the Caribbean Sea to the northeast, and the Gulf of Mexico to the north. Spanish is the primary language in all Central American countries except Belize, where English is the official language (1). Central Americans, even within the same country, can be of diverse ancestry, including indigenous, *mestizo*, African, and European roots. They represent an array of distinct and diverse cultures, languages, and socioeconomic and educational backgrounds (1). Table 5.1 compares the population size in the seven countries in 2006 (2). The US Census recognizes Central Americans in the United States as part of the Hispanic ethnic group and does not distinguish them by race (3).

Most Central American immigrants have moved to the United States since 1980, when political and economic instability erupted in the region. Between 1980 and 2000, the rate of US immigration from Central America increased from 2.7% to 6.3% (4). In 2005, 2.7 million foreign-born Central Americans lived in the United States, accounting for 7.3% of the foreign population. In the same year, the US population included approximately 1.3 million US-born descendants of Central American immigrants (5).

Many Central Americans living in the United States reside on the west coast and are primarily from El Salvador, Guatemala, Honduras, and Nicaragua. Recent immigrants from Central America have mostly been undocumented. In 2000, an estimated 57% of Guatemalan, 58% of Honduran, and 47% of Salvadorian immigrants were undocumented (4). Living illegally in the United States limits job and education opportunities. Illegal immigrants often live in poverty, lack health insurance, and work in positions with few or no benefits and low annual wages (4).

Diabetes Prevalence

Diabetes is a serious concern among Central Americans living in the United States and a growing public health problem in their native countries. Table 5.2 lists the 2003 prevalence of diabetes in absolute numbers for the seven countries of Central America and provides projections for 2030 from the World Health Organization (WHO) (6). The financial burden of diabetes on the health care infrastructure of some of these nations is expected to more than double. Compared with the WHO projections, the International Diabetes Foundation suggests an even greater rise in diabetes prevalence to more than 10% in 2025 in countries like Costa Rica and Panama (7).

Table 5.1 • Central American Population (2006) by Country

Country	Population
Belize	282,000
Costa Rica	4.4 million
El Salvador	6.76 million
Guatemala	13 million
Honduras	7.0 million
Nicaragua	5.5 million
Panama	3.2 million

Source: Data are from reference 2.

Table 5.2 • Diabetes Prevalence in Central America

Country	Diabetes Prevalence, 2000	Projected Diabetes Prevalence, 2030
Belize	5,000	15,000
Costa Rica	76,000	237,000
El Salvador	103,000	320,000
Guatemala	139,000	447,000
Honduras	81,000	269,000
Nicaragua	68,000	246,000
Panama	59,000	155,000

Source: Data are from reference 6.

Hispanics represent the largest minority population in the United States and will comprise almost 24.4% of the US population by 2050 (8). There is a lack of data examining health outcomes for Central Americans in the United States. However, if the prevalence of diabetes among Mexican Americans were generalized to the Hispanic population older than 20 years, approximately 2.5 million Hispanic Americans (9.5%) would have diabetes (9). These numbers would be expected to increase as the population grows older. Hispanic adults also tend to have higher rates of undiagnosed diabetes and greater morbidity and mortality associated with diabetes than other ethnic groups (9).

Risk Factors for Type 2 Diabetes

Overweight and Obesity

Obesity rates are on the rise in Central America and have become a public health issue as countries transition from problems of underweight and malnutrition to overweight and chronic disease (10). Much of the "nutrition transition" has occurred as a result of populations moving from rural to urban areas. Some of the risk factors for overweight associated with urbanization of the population include decreased breastfeeding rates and duration, increased poverty, increased cigarette smoking, greater exposure to environmental pollutants, and changes in diet and physical activity patterns (11). Rural or traditional diets typically include high intake of fruits, vegetables, and grains. Urbanization is associated with the adoption of a more Western-style diet characterized by high levels of fat and refined sugars and low fiber intake. Combined with increasingly sedentary lifestyles, this dietary pattern contributes to obesity and the rise of associated chronic diseases, including diabetes (12). In response to the increasing prevalence of obesity and diabetes in Central America, the Pan American Health Organization has started the Central American Diabetes Initiative (CAMDI), which is intended to address surveillance and intervention to halt the progression of diabetes in Costa Rica, El Salvador, Guatemala, Honduras, and Nicaragua (13). According to preliminary data, 8% of participants in Guatemala had diabetes and the most common risk factor was the combination of being overweight (body mass index [BMI] ≥ 25) and having low levels of physical activity (defined as less than 150 minutes per week). Researchers also found that the prevalence of diabetes was greatly increased among individuals 40 years of age and older, compared with those between the ages of 20 and 39 (14).

Differences in Risk Factors for Central Americans vs Mexican Americans

Research suggests that diabetes risk factors among Central Americans living in the United States may vary from those established for Mexican Americans. More research in this area is warranted. In a study using data from the 2001 California Health Interview Survey, the prevalence of overweight and obesity in Mexican Americans and Central Americans residing in California were similar: 36.8% of the 8,304 Mexican Americans in the survey were overweight and 26.2% were obese, whereas 39.2% of the 1,019 Central Americans surveyed were overweight and 22.2% were obese. However, the factors associated with being overweight or obese differed notably between these two populations. Among Central American men, those with more than a college education were more likely than those with less than a high school education to be overweight. In addition, Central American men with no health insurance were more likely to be overweight compared with those with health insurance. Among Mexican American men, however, a high school education and having health insurance were each associated with higher prevalence of overweight. Among Central American women, those with three children were more likely to be overweight than women with no children, whereas having four or more children was associated with obesity in Mexican American, but not Central American, women (15).

Kieffer and associates used national data to examine the impact of birthplace on prevalence of diabetes during pregnancy. In general, US women born in other countries were significantly more likely to have diabetes during pregnancy than those born in the United States. This finding was true for US women of Central American descent, even after data were adjusted to account for increased maternal age among immigrant mothers. However, among Mexican American women, rates of diabetes during pregnancy were higher for women born in the United States (16).

Acculturation

Acculturation describes how immigrants adopt the behaviors, knowledge, attitudes, values, and beliefs of their new culture, and it may play a factor in health outcomes among Central Americans in the United States. In a 2007 review, Perez-Escamilla and Putnik argue that research on acculturation and health issues in Latino ethnic subgroups must take into account complex factors, including diet and lifestyle choices in the country of origin, movement from rural to urban settings, social support, and family structure (17). In one study, acculturation (indicated by United States residency of 15 years or more) was a strong correlate of obesity for Central American men but not women. In addition, fair-to-poor self-reported health status was consistently associated with an increased risk of being overweight or obese (15).

Socioeconomic Factors and Language Barriers

Socioeconomic factors influence health outcomes among Central Americans with diabetes. People from economically disadvantaged backgrounds are less likely to have insurance or access to health care. Cost is also a factor for patients reducing or discontinuing their diabetes medications (18). Compared with 28% of non-Hispanic whites with diabetes, 60% of Hispanic adults with diabetes have an annual income below $20,000 (18). The Institute of Medicine has found that ethnic minorities tend to receive a lower quality of health care than whites, even after controlling for confounding factors such as insurance status and income. Reasons for this disparity include bias, stereotyping, discrimination, prejudice, and discomfort by health care providers when treating patients from unfamiliar cultural or ethnic backgrounds (19).

Campos found that Spanish-speaking Hispanic patients were significantly less likely than non-Hispanic whites to use insulin or have diabetes specialists as their primary care provider. Spanish-speaking Hispanics also had lower rates of self-monitoring blood glucose and had worse glycemic control (18). Low health literacy may make it difficult for patients to understand written medication instructions or educational materials. In Campos's study, low health literacy in patients with type 2 diabetes was correlated with poor outcomes, lower likelihood of tight glycemic control, and greater likelihood of developing retinopathy (18).

In the Translating Research into Action for Diabetes (TRIAD) Study, a multicenter study of diabetes care in managed care settings, 23% of Spanish-speaking Hispanic patients reported language as a barrier in communication with the provider. After controlling for ethnicity and other variables, individuals with low language acculturation were significantly more likely to have diabetes than those with the highest level of language acculturation (20).

Genetics

Genetic factors may play a role in the development of diabetes in Central Americans, but it is difficult to generalize because the ancestry of Central Americans is diverse and the interaction between genetic and environmental factors is complex. Most Central Americans are of mixed indigenous and European lineage *(mestizos)*. El Salvador, Honduras, Guatemala and Belize have the largest *mestizo* populations. Some Central Americans include African slaves among their ancestors—for example, the Creoles and Garifuna in Belize and populations in Nicaragua, Panama, and Costa Rica. Among Central American countries, Guatemala has the largest percentage of indigenous groups (21).

Traditional Foods and Dishes

The diets of people from the various countries in Central America share several commonalities, although there can be great differences in preparations and ingredients used. The staples of the traditional diet are corn (maize), rice, and beans *(frijoles)*. Maize is often treated with lime and ground into flour *(masa)*, which is pressed into tortillas or used in other preparations, including tacos, tamales, enchiladas, and a thin porridge called *atole*. White rice is more typical than brown. The most popular type of beans varies from country to country: black beans are common in Guatemala and most of Costa Rica, and red or pinto beans are typical elsewhere in the region (22). Beans may be served stewed with onions, spices, and tomato; fried; or ground and eaten with white rice. These staples are supplemented with meat, animal products, and local fruits and vegetables.

Flavor principles vary among regions. Common seasonings in main dishes include onions, garlic, peppers, orange, lemon, mint, and cilantro. Wheat flour is used in white or sweet rolls. Noodles *(fideos)* served in soups or mixed with vegetables are also popular (22).

Central Americans often drink coffee at breakfast time and as an after-meal or afternoon snack. With their coffee, they may eat *pan dulce/conchas* (lightly-sweetened bread made with lard or vegetable shortening) or *pan de manteca* (thin-crust loaf bread made with lard). Other beverages include hot chocolate, *refrescos* (cold drinks made from tropical fruit with milk or water), and *horchata* (rice flour mixed with sugar and milk and/or water). In Nicaragua, *triste* (a cold drink made from roasted corn, cocoa powder, and sugar) is popular. Central American desserts *(dulces)* include *nogadas* (sweetened baked plantains), rice puddings, custards, and sweet fried fritters (22).

In Belize, coconut is a popular ingredient in Garifuna food. Offerings include coconut candy, *pan de coco* (coconut bread), coconut water, *leche de coco* (coconut milk), and coconut soup. *Sere* is a stew of fish cooked with herbs in coconut cream. A popular dessert is grated banana cooked in sweetened coconut milk. Sweet potatoes and yuca (cassava, a starchy root) are common vegetables in the Garifuna diet.

Common foods in Panama include fish and seafood. Popular dishes include breaded, fried fish balls made from conger or *corvina,* Panama's most common fish. *Ceviche* (fish and shellfish marinated and cooked in lemon or vinegar with herbs and spices) is also eaten. Stews made with seafood *(sancocho de mariscos),* chicken *(sancocho de gallina),* or red meat *(sancocho de carne)* are local favorites. Other typical dishes include friend pork rinds *(chicharrones)*, rice with chicken *(arroz con pollo),* ground corn balls *(pelotitas de maiz),* and *empanadas* (pies filled with meat and vegetables). Many of these dishes are also common in other Central American countries. See Box 5.1 and Table 5.3 for more information on traditional cuisine. Refer to Appendix A for nutrient analyses.

Box 5.1 • Foods Used in Traditional Central American Cuisine

Starchy vegetables

- Corn
- Chayote
- Dried beans (black, red, pinto, garbanzo, kidney)
- *Guineos* (small, green unripe bananas)
- Malanga (taro)
- Plantains
- Pumpkin
- Sweet potato
- Squash
- Yams
- Yuca (cassava)

Nonstarchy vegetables

- Avocados
- Beets
- Broccoli
- Cabbage
- Carrots
- Collard greens
- Cucumbers
- Date palm (*pacaya* or *palmito*)
- Hearts of palm
- Lettuce
- Onions
- Peppers
- Radishes
- Spinach
- String beans
- Tomatoes
- Tomatillos
- Watercress
- Yuca flowers (*flores de Izote*)

Fruits

- Apples
- Bananas
- Blackberries
- Breadfruit
- Cashew nuts, yellow or red
- Cherries
- Chirimoya (custard apple)
- Coconut
- Figs
- *Guanabana* (soursop)
- Guava
- *Jobos* (sweet fruit with an almond-like nut inside)
- *Jocote* (Spanish plum)
- Loquat/*sapodilla* (known as *níspero* in Colombia, Nicaragua, and El Salvador; apple-like fruit with high acid, sugar)
- *Mamey sapote* (meaty-textured, bright salmon-colored, round or oval, sweet fruit with a black shiny pit)
- Mango
- *Nance* (cherry sized, yellow fruit)
- Oranges
- Passion fruit
- Papaya
- Pawpaw (edible berry)
- Peaches
- *Pejibaye* (a palm fruit)
- Pineapple
- *Pitaya* (dragon fruit)
- Plums
- Pomegranate
- Quince
- Starfruit
- Strawberries
- Tamarind
- Tangerines
- Watermelon
- White sapote

Milk and milk products

- *Crema* (creamy, sour cream similar to crème fraiche)
- Evaporated milk
- Milk (mostly consumed mixed with cocoa, barley, rice, or corn)
- *Pupusa* (Chihuahua-style cheese)
- *Quesillo* or *queso fresco* (soft, fresh cheese)
- *Queso crema* (cream cheese)
- *Queso duro* (hard cheese)

(continued)

Box 5.1   *(continued)*

Meats and meat substitutes

- Beef (including tongue, oxtail, short ribs, liver, rib eye steak, sweetbreads, and cow foot)
- Chicken
- Eggs
- *Embutidos* (cold meats and sausages, including chorizo, *morcilla, longaniza, salchicha,* and *salchichón*)

- Fish and shellfish
- Fried pork rinds
- Pork
- Tripe (usually made into a soup or stew with root vegetables or beans)

Herbs and seasonings

- Achiote (annato seeds)
- Allspice
- Anise
- Chiles
- *Chipilin* (plant leaves used in soup; can be boiled and served green, dried and used as an herb, or added to tamale dough for color and flavor)
- Cilantro
- Cinnamon
- Garlic

- *Loroco* (an edible flower with pungent taste)
- Mint
- Nutmeg
- Oregano
- *Panela/tapa de dulce* (block of dark brown sugar)
- Parsley
- Seeds *(semillas;* eg, sesame, squash)
- Vanilla

Table 5.3 · Traditional Central American Dishes, Breads, Beverages, and Desserts

Food	Description
Dishes	
Baleadas	Handmade tortillas filled with beans and sour cream then folded like a taco
Casamiento/gallo pinto	Rice and beans
Ceviche	Raw fish marinated in coconut milk and/or lime juice
Chiles rellenos	Stuffed peppers, usually filled with cheese, meats, and spices
Curtido Salvadoreño	Pickled cabbage mixed with chilies, carrots, and vinegar; eaten with *pupusas*
Empanadas	Pastry filled with any combination of chicken, beef, cheese, or beans
Empanadas de plátano	Fried plantain filled with meat
Enchiladas catrachas	Crispy tortilla filled with ground beef, chile sauce, lettuce, and tomato; very similar to a tostada
Espaguetis	Spaghetti
Garnaches	Belizean dish consisting of refried beans served on a tortilla topped with cheese and pickled cabbage and carrots
Guacamole	Avocado mixed with lime or lemon juice, salt, and sometimes tomatoes
Hilachas	Guatemalan shredded beef in a tomato sauce, eaten with rice or tortillas
Huevos rancheros	Eggs and salsa served with tortillas
Mariscada	Mixed seafood dish
Nacatamales	Small, tamale-like dish made from corn dough, vegetables, and mint; cooked in banana leaves
Pasteles	Corn dough stuffed with meat
Pasteles de chucho	Fried yuca and beef patties

(continued)

Table 5.3   (continued)

Food	Description
Pepian de pollo	Guatemalan dish of boiled chicken in a spicy tomato-based sauce, served with rice or tortillas
Pupusas	El Salvador's national food—fritters made of two corn tortillas filled with meat and seasoned with chilies, onion, garlic, and cheese
Revolcado de panza	Tomato-based curry dish with cow's intestines
Rondon	Dish prepared with turtle meat, fish, and red meat or pork
Salpicón	Cold, chopped roast beef seasoned with lemon juice, minced onions, radishes, mint, and salt
Sopa de albóndiga	Meatball soup
Sopa de caracol/sopa de jaibas	Coconut-based soup with conch meat
Sopa de mondongo	Heavy stew made with tripe, root vegetables, beans, and spices
Tacos	Hard- or soft-shell corn tortillas filled with ground meat, sauce, and cheese
Tamales/*montucas*	Corn dough stuffed with meat, rice, seasoning, potato, olives, and garbanzo beans. The tamale is wrapped with a banana leaf.
Torta de papa	Potato omelet, usually served with salsa
Vaho/baho	Nicaraguan dish of meat, green plantains, and yuca (cassava)
Vigoron	Nicaraguan and Costa Rican dish of pickled cabbage, tomatoes, and onions, served with *yuca con chicharron*
Yuca con chicharrón	Cassava and crispy pork rind
Breads	
Pan de coco	Coconut bread
Pan de guineo	Banana bread
Pan de mantequilla	Buttered bread
Beverages	
Agua de Jamaica	Hibiscus tea
Agua de tamarindo	Tamarind drink
Agua dulce	*Panela* or *tapa de dulce* mixed with water or milk
Beer	
Cebada	Barley drink with cinnamon
Chicha	A fruit drink, or a fermented beverage made of maize or pineapple peel and cashew or cassava
Chicheme	Fruit drink with sugar, milk, and vanilla
Chocolate caliente	Hot chocolate, often prepared with whole milk
Coconut water	
Coffee	Often served with whole milk and sugar
Fruit nectars	Fruit pulp mixed with water and sugar
Ginger beer	Belizean drink
Horchata	Roasted rice flour mixed with cinnamon, sugar, and milk or water
Leche poleada	Beverage that contains, milk, cornstarch, egg yolk, cinnamon and sugar
Liquados	Beverages made with tropical fruit (eg, papaya, mango, banana, blackberries) mixed with milk or water
Palm wine	
Pinolillo	Sweet cornmeal and cacao-based drink in Nicaragua
Resbaladera	Costa Rican chilled barley drink made with rice, barley, sugar, spices, milk and vanilla

(continued)

Table 5.3 *(continued)*

Food	Description
Rompope	Eggnog
Rum	
Serase wine	Belizean drink
Sorrel wine	Belizean drink
Shuco	Hot beverage made with purple corn, powered pumpkin seeds, beans and chile
Desserts	
Arroz con leche	Rice pudding
Buñuelos	Bread fritters with cinnamon and sugar
Coconut bread	
Flan	Soft custard dessert topped with a layer of soft caramel
Hojaldras	Panamanian deep-fried doughnut, covered with sugar
Manjar blanco	Dessert similar to *dulce de leche* (sweetened milk dessert)
Mousse de frutilla	Fruit mousse
Pastel de tres leches	Cake made with homogenized, evaporated, and condensed milk
Pastelitos	Baked turnovers filled with custard or fruit preserves
Plátanos fritos	Fried ripe plantains
Plátanos en mole	Plantains in chocolate-chipotle sauce
Semita	Coffe cake-type pastry filled with jams/preserves
Sopa borracha	Pound cake with sugar, spices, raisins, run or brandy
Rellenitos de platano	Guatemalan dish consisting of plantains that are first boiled, mashed, then stuffed with refried beans and deep fried into balls, sprinkled with sugar
Rice with coconut or mango	
Torrejas	French toast-like dessert filled with custard

Traditional Meal Patterns and Holiday Foods

Most Central Americans eat three meals a day and sometimes may have a snack after lunch. Breakfast may simply be coffee and bread. More substantial breakfasts typically include beans, eggs, coffee, and corn tortillas or bread. The beans can be served *parados* (whole), *revueltos* (refried), or *licuados* (a runny paste). Other common breakfast options may include oatmeal, bread *(pan dulce),* and Incaparina, a low-cost, high-nutrient, protein-fortified hot cereal made from cottonseed, corn, sorghum flours, and yeast—this cereal was developed by the Institute of Nutrition in Central America and Panama (INCAP) to prevent protein-deficiency. Some Central Americans have fried plantains, sour cream, and cheese for breakfast. Guatemalans may also eat *longaniza* (sausage) and *chirmol* sauce (grilled whole plum tomatoes crushed to a salsa-consistency sauce and seasoned with lemon juice, salt, cilantro, and scallions).

For lunch, Central Americans typically eat chicken or beef with rice, vegetables, and tortillas. Beverages include fresh-squeezed lemonades or regional sweetened drinks. Dinner may include leftover food from lunch as well as beans, plantains, and tortillas or bread.

The most important celebrations for Central Americans are those that focus on Catholic holidays such as Christmas, Easter, Lent, and All Saints Day (November 1). On the days that people attend Mass, they usually have larger, holiday-type meals as well. Each country has its own popular holiday dishes. In Guatemala, plantains in chocolate sauce may be served around Easter. See Table 5.4 for traditional Christmas foods.

Table 5.4 · Traditional Foods Consumed During the Christmas Holiday

Country	Foods
Belize	• *Kriol* rice and beans
	• Spiced potato salad with turkey and ham
	• Black fruitcake laced with rum or brandy
	• *Pebre* (roast pork with gravy served with hot corn tortillas)
	• Tamales
	• Turkey or pork
Costa Rica	• *Tamal de cerdo* (pork-filled tamale)
	• *Pierna de cerdo asada* (roasted leg of pork)
	• *Ensalada de papa* (potato salad)
	• *Arroz con pollo*
	• *Pancitos de amor* (spongy baked cakes with a sugary glaze)
	• *Flan de coco al caramelo* (coconut flan with caramel glaze)
El Salvador	• *Pupusas*
	• *Hojuelas* (fried puffs served with honey or sugar)
	• *Torrejas*
	• Roast turkey with olives and capers
	• Tamales
	• *Gallo en chicha* (meat from a rooster seasoned with fruits)
Guatemala	• Tamales
	• *Torrejas*
	• Turkey
	• Pork leg
	• *Ponche* (hot fruit punch)
Honduras	• *Ayote en miel* (boiled pumpkin and honey)
	• *Sopa de caracol* (conch soup)
	• *Nacatamales* (tamales wrapped in banana leaves)
	• *Torrejas*
Nicaragua	• *Gallina rellena navidena* (hen stuffed with fruit and vegetables)
	• *Marquesote* (cinnamon-flavored dessert)
	• *Sopa borracha* (sponge cake soaked in syrup and rum)
	• *Manjar* (dulce de leche)
	• *Rompope* (eggnog; traditional beverage for Christmas)
	• *Pinol* (traditional Nicaraguan cocoa drink)
Panama	• *Carimanolas* (yuca fritters stuffed with eggs and meat)
	• *Flan de caraemelo* (caramel custard)
	• *Tres leches* (cake made with three kinds of milk)
	• *Delicia de coco* (coconut delight)
	• *Arroz dulce* and tamales
	• *Pavo* (turkey) and *relleno* (stuffing)

Traditional Health Beliefs

Commonly held beliefs regarding illness and disease may include the following (23):

- Evil eye *(mal de ojo)*—the belief that diseases may occur in small children if they receive compliments without also receiving God's blessing. An adult who wishes to compliment a child would say, for example, "Melissa has beautiful eyes and may God bless her," instead of "Melissa has beautiful eyes."
- Fright *(susto)*—the belief that physical conditions such as diabetes have emotional causes and traumatic events can lead to illness.
- Spasm *(pasmo)*—the belief that exposure to cold air or *sereno* (morning or evening dew) can cause temporary paralysis of the face or legs.
- Bile *(bilis)*—the belief that a strong emotional occurrence causes bile to pour into the bloodstream, leading to livid rage and worsening health conditions, such as high blood pressure or elevated blood glucose levels.

Current Food Practices

As in other parts of the world, Central American diets are expanding to include more processed foods, and the consumption of processed foods is contributing to the increasing prevalence of obesity and diet-related chronic diseases such as diabetes. For example, in Guatemala, obesity is becoming more prevalent, especially in urban areas, as incomes in low-income groups rise and members of those groups consume more high-fat and/or high-carbohydrate, energy-dense foods (10).

Information on food habits of Central Americans in the United States is scarce. Low rates of assimilation among many Central American immigrants may preserve many traditional food habits.

Central Americans in the United States may adapt their diets in healthy and unhealthy ways. A focus group study of women from Honduras living in New Orleans found them to have both positive and negative diet changes since immigrating to the United States. Healthful changes included eating more fruit, frying less often, baking more, and using vegetable oil instead of pork or coconut fat. However, these women also reported skipping meals and not having enough time to cook and therefore eating more fast foods (24).

Counseling Considerations

When counseling Central American clients with diabetes, practitioners should ask them in-depth questions about their diet and lifestyle factors. This information will be useful to determine which topics to address during counseling and education. When recommending lifestyle changes, practitioners should discuss practical concerns, such as transportation and financial issues.

Use of trained interpreters is essential when the clinician and client do not speak the same language. Do not use family members or acquaintances as interpreters unless the patient requests this.

The health care provider must properly assess the literacy level of clients and adjust the level of health information that is given. Practitioners should emphasize basic self-management skills, such as home glucose monitoring, as well as the importance of a healthy diet, stress management, and physical activity.

Demonstrating Courtesy and Respect

Central American clients value signs of courtesy such as kindness, politeness, pleasantness, and avoidance of hostile confrontation. Neutral attitudes may be perceived as negative, resulting in decreased satisfaction with care and poor follow-up (25). When interacting with clients, show interest in their lives (eg, start the visit with a brief conversation about family, work, or school). Clients interpret these gestures as signs that the provider cares about them, and this encourages them to share crucial details about their health status.

Interpreting Clients' Nonverbal Communication

Nonverbal cues may indicate that the client does not understand the health information provided or has limited literacy. Failure to make eye contact may indicate lack of understanding, or it could be a sign of deference and respect. Often, if a client is living in the United States illegally, he or she may avoid in-depth conversations, for fear of deportation. In such circumstances, small group sessions may lead to a more relaxed atmosphere and better communication (23). In addition, try asking open-ended questions that allow for detailed explanations and information sharing.

Inquiring About Clients' Understanding of Diabetes

Most studies of Hispanic health beliefs have focused on Mexican Americans, and information about other Hispanic subgroups is lacking. Therefore, the practitioner should make an effort to explore each Central American client's personal knowledge, beliefs, and attitudes about diabetes. Clients often try to connect their illnesses in a direct and specific way to personal history. They may perceive diabetes as being linked to specific events in their life history and seek treatment that is consistent with their personal and cultural beliefs. Their perceptions may be incorrect or distorted, which can lead to difficulty with adherence to treatment (26).

Hispanic culture strongly emphasizes religious beliefs and spirituality, but few studies have evaluated how religious beliefs affect approaches to diabetes self-management. Hatcher and Whittemore note that Hispanic clients may believe that diabetes is caused and controlled by God, often as a punishment. Clients may also pray to God for support in diabetes management. Some people derive strength, hope, and respect for their bodies from their religious beliefs (26).

The following questions can help practitioners explore clients' understanding of diabetes:

- In your own words, what can you tell me about your diabetes?
- What caused your illness?
- Why do you think it started when it did?
- What have you noticed since you became diagnosed with diabetes? How does diabetes work?
- How severe is diabetes? Will it last a short time or a long time?
- What has your experience been with your care?
- How has diabetes changed your life?
- How do you describe the treatment for diabetes?
- What would you say about living with diabetes to another person who has just been diagnosed?

Discussing Clients' Use of Complementary and Alternative Medicine

In Central America, individuals commonly use herbal remedies as an adjunct to their diet. However, research about these practices as related to diabetes care is limited. To address diabetes, clients may use cinnamon, bitter melon, *nopal* (prickly pear), aloe, or stevia as ingredients or supplements. They may also seek the advice of herbalists or folk healers to manage their symptoms. Practitioners should inquire about the use of supplements, herbs, teas, and salves and be prepared to provide information about safety and efficacy. See Appendix C for questions to assess use of dietary supplements.

Considering Family Dynamics

Central Americans are often bound by strong familial and cultural ties. *Familismo* (a collective loyalty to the extended family that is greater than the needs of the individual) may make it difficult for clients to make with lifestyle changes or adhere to medication schedules that inconvenience other family members. To overcome this barrier, practitioners should encourage clients to invite family members to visits. Family should be educated about the importance of treatment adherence and the need to support the client's treatment efforts. Encourage them to join the client in making relevant diet and lifestyle changes, and give them tools, such as culturally appropriate recipes, that support these efforts.

Engaging Others in Counseling Sessions

Practitioners should provide sufficient time and opportunity for extended family to discuss important medical decisions during counseling sessions. Home health aides, caregivers, and others in the client's support network may also help increase treatment success. Lay health professionals who share linguistic or cultural characteristics with the client are another possible resource, particularly if they are successfully managing their own chronic illness and can serve as role models.

Nutrition Counseling

Appendix B offers selected medical nutrition therapy recommendations for individuals with diabetes and general counseling suggestions that support those recommendations. The following are culturally specific nutrition counseling strategies for Central American clients:

- Rice and starchy vegetables are abundant in the Central American diet. Encourage clients to replace some portions with nutritious nonstarchy vegetables.
- Advise clients to have only one small (6-inch diameter) tortilla per meal. Ask clients if they are willing to have corn or whole wheat tortillas instead of tortillas made from white flour.
- Discuss ways to cook beans without added fats. Suggest the use of canola or olive oil instead of pork fat (lard) and provide options for seasoning beans.
- Encourage clients to freeze stews and soups so they can scrape fat from the surface of the frozen dishes.
- Provide alternatives to high-fat meat products. For example, instead of pork skin, sausage, or lard, suggest clients use smoked turkey meat, turkey bacon, or liquid smoke for flavoring.

Challenges and Barriers to Dietary Compliance

Barriers to dietary compliance may include limited literacy and lack of support. Low-income clients and those who live in neighborhoods that lack access to healthful foods such as fruits and vegetables may have worse diets and health outcomes.

Counseling Tips

Counseling should involve understanding the client's thoughts and preferences, reaching a shared understanding of the problem, and including the client in the decision-making process. The following LEARN model is a well-established mnemonic device that providers can use to improve cross-cultural communication with clients, thereby improving compliance and outcomes (27):

- Listen with sympathy and understanding to the client's perception of the problem.
- Explain your perception to the problem.
- Acknowledge and discuss the differences and similarities in your perceptions.
- Recommend treatment.
- Negotiate agreement.

Resources

American Diabetes Association ADA Latino Initiatives: Por tu familia: http://www.portufamilia.org. Accessed May 20, 2009.

The Cross Cultural Health Care Program: http://www.xculture.org. Accessed May 20, 2009.

EthnoMed—Hispanic: http://ethnomed.org/ethnomed/cultures/hispanic/hispanic.html. Accessed May 20, 2009.

National Alliance for Hispanic Health: http://www.hispanichealth.org. Accessed March 18, 2009.

National Center for Chronic Disease Prevention and Health Promotion. Controle Su Diabetes (Control Your Diabetes): http://www.cdc.gov/diabetes/pubs/controle/index.htm. Accessed May 20, 2009.

National Center for Cultural Competence: http://www11.georgetown.edu/research/gucchd/nccc. Accessed May 20, 2009.

National Diabetes Education Program Diabetes Prevention for Latinos and Hispanics: http://www.ndep .nih.gov/campaigns/Tipo2/Tipo2_index.htm. Accessed May 20, 2009.

References

1. US Central Intelligence Agency. The World Factbook 2007. https://www.cia.gov/library/publications/the-world-factbook/geos/bh.html. Accessed September 1, 2007.

2. World Health Organization. Countries. http://www.who.int/countries/en. Accessed May 1, 2009.

3. US Census Bureau. Population Division. Hispanic Population of the United States. http://www.census.gov/population/www/socdemo/hispanic/hispdef.html. Accessed August 7, 2007.

4. Zúñiga E, Castañeda X, Averbach A, Wallace SP. *Mexican and Central American Immigrants in the United States: Health Care Access*. Los Angeles, CA: Regents of the University of California and Mexican Secretariat of Health; 2006.

5. Pew Hispanic Center. A Statistical Portrait of Hispanics at Mid-Decade. http://pewhispanic.org/reports/middecade. Accessed September 1, 2007.

6. World Health Organization. Prevalence of Diabetes in the WHO Region of the Americas. http://www.who.int/diabetes/facts/world_figures/en/index3.html. Accessed September 1, 2007.

7. International Diabetes Foundation. Diabetes Atlas. http://www.eatlas.idf.org/Prevalence. Accessed August 18, 2007.

8. US Census Bureau. Projected population of the United States, by race and Hispanic origin: 2000 to 2050. http://www.census.gov/population/www/projections/usinterimproj. Accessed August 13, 2007.

9. Centers for Disease Control and Prevention. National Diabetes Fact Sheet: General Information and National Estimates on Diabetes in the United States, 2005. http://www.cdc.gov/diabetes/pubs/pdf/ndfs_2005.pdf. Accessed August 18, 2007.

10. Uauy R, Albala C, Kain J. Obesity trends in Latin America: transiting from under- to overweight. *J Nutr*. 2001;131(suppl):893S–899S.

11. Valdes-Ramos R, Solomons N. Preventive nutrition: its changing context in MesoAmerica. *Nutr Research*. 2002;22:145–152.

12. Kain J, Vio F, Albala C. Obesity trends and determinant factors in Latin America. *Cad Saude Publica*. 2003;19(Suppl 1):S77–S86.

13. Pan American Health Organization. The Central America Diabetes Initiative. http://www.paho.org/English/ad/dpc/nc/camdi.htm. Accessed September 3, 2007.

14. Pan American Health Organization. The Central America Diabetes Initiative, Preliminary Results: Prevalence of Diabetes, Hypertension and Their Risk Factors in the Municipality of Villa Nueva, Guatemala. http://www.paho.org/English/ad/dpc/nc/dia-camdi-gut-2003-result.pdf. Accessed September 3, 2007.

15. Bowie JV, Juon HS, Cho J, Rodriguez EM. Factors associated with overweight and obesity among Mexican Americans and Central Americans: results from the 2001 California Health Interview Survey. *Prev Chron Dis*. 2007;4:1–17. http://www.cdc.gov/pcd/issues/2007/jan/06_0036.htm. Accessed August 12, 2007.

16. Kieffer EC, Martin JA, Herman WH. Impact of maternal nativity on the prevalence of diabetes during pregnancy among US ethnic groups. *Diabetes Care*. 1999;22:729–735.

17. Perez-Escamilla R, Putnik P. The role of acculturation in nutrition, lifestyle, and incidence of type 2 diabetes among Latinos. *J Nutr*. 2007;137:860–870.

18. Campos C. Addressing cultural barriers to the successful use of insulin in Hispanics with type 2 diabetes. *South Med J*. 2007;100:812–820.

19. Geiger J. Racial and ethnic disparities in diagnosis and treatment: a review of the evidence and a consideration of causes. In: *Unequal Treatment Confronting Racial and Ethnic Disparities in Healthcare*. Washington DC: Institute of Medicine; 2003.

20. Brown AF, Gerzoff RB, Karter AJ; for the TRIAD Study Group. Health behaviors and quality of care among Latinos with diabetes in managed care. *Am J Public Health*. 2003;93:1694–1698.

21. US Central Intelligence Agency. The World Factbook 2007. Field Listing—Ethnic Groups. https://www.cia.gov/library/publications/the-world-factbook/fields/2075.html. Accessed September 3, 2007.

22. Kittler P, Sucher K. *Food and Culture*. 4th ed. Belmont, CA: Thomson Wadsworth; 2004.

23. Juckett G. Cross-cultural medicine. *Am Fam Physician*. 2005;72:2267–2274.

24. Edmonds VM. The nutritional patterns of recently immigrated Honduran women. *J Transcult Nurs*. 2005;16:226–235.

25. Diaz VA. Cultural factors in preventive care: Latinos. *Prim Care*. 2002;29:503-517.

26. Hatcher E, Whittemore R. Hispanic adults' beliefs about type 2 diabetes: clinical implications. *J Am Acad Nurs Pract*. 2007;19:536–545.

27. Berlin EA, Fowkes WC. A teaching framework for cross-cultural health care—application in family practice. *West J Med*. 1983;139:193–198.

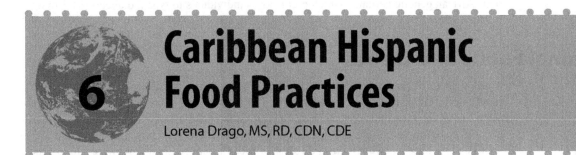

Caribbean Hispanic Food Practices

Lorena Drago, MS, RD, CDN, CDE

Introduction

The Caribbean islands are located southeast of North America, east of Central America, and to the north and west of South America. There are more than 7,000 islands, islets, reefs, and cayes in the region. This chapter focuses on the Spanish-speaking Caribbean region: Puerto Rico, an unincorporated US territory with Commonwealth status; Cuba; and the Dominican Republic.

The US Census Bureau defines a Hispanic/Latino as "a person of Cuban, Mexican, Puerto Rican, South or Central American, or other Spanish culture or origin regardless of race" (1). According to the 2000 US Census, Puerto Ricans, Dominicans, and Cubans represent 15.3% of the total US Hispanic population. The largest population of Caribbean Hispanics is in the eastern United States, particularly in New York, New Jersey, and Florida (2).

Diabetes Prevalence

According to the National Institute of Diabetes and Digestive and Kidney Diseases, the age-adjusted prevalence of type 2 diabetes for US Hispanic adults age 20 years or older is 13.7% (3). Data are not sufficient to estimate the prevalence of type 2 diabetes in Hispanic groups other than Mexican Americans. Most Hispanic Americans with diabetes (approximately 90% to 95%) have type 2 diabetes. A small number of Hispanic Americans (approximately 5% to 10%) have type 1 diabetes. The prevalence of type 1 diabetes in Hispanics is the same or lower than in non-Hispanic whites, whereas the prevalence of type 2 diabetes in Hispanics is twice the rate for non-Hispanic whites (4).

Type 2 diabetes is most common among middle-aged and older Hispanics. Approximately 25% to 30% of Hispanics older than age 50 have diabetes (5). In a cross-sectional study of 656 subjects ages 60 to 96 years, type 2 diabetes was more prevalent in Puerto Ricans (38%) and Dominicans (35%) compared with non-Hispanic whites (23%) (6). Also compared with non-Hispanic whites, Puerto Ricans were two times more likely and Dominicans were three times more likely to have A1C equal to or greater than 7%, which may increase the risk of diabetes complications (6).

Risk Factors for Type 2 Diabetes

Overweight

Adults who are overweight (body mass index [BMI] ≥ 25) and of Hispanic/Latino origin are at increased risk of developing type 2 diabetes (7). Among Hispanic Americans (as well as Asians, African Americans, Native Americans, and Pacific Islanders), increased visceral adiposity is associated with risk for type 2 diabetes (8).

Ancestry and Environmental Factors

Genetic factors contribute to the development of type 2 diabetes in this population. The principal ancestral background of Caribbean Hispanics includes Spanish, American Indian, and African ancestry. In particular, type 2 diabetes in Puerto Ricans may possibly be traced to their African genetic heritage, which predisposes individuals to type 2 diabetes (9). Environmental factors (eg, exercise, diet, and smoking) are also risk factors for type 2 diabetes (9).

Traditional Foods and Dishes

Traditional Caribbean foods began with the Taíno Indians, the natives Columbus encountered during his discovery of the New World (10). When Columbus arrived in 1492, there were five Taíno kingdoms or territories on Hispaniola. By the 18th century, foreign diseases and forced assimilation into the Spanish colonial plantation economy had decimated Taíno society (11). Cassava (yuca), *casabe* (cassava bread), peppers, and corn were Taíno foods. The names of certain plants and fruits, such as *guayaba* (guava), *guanábana* (soursop), and *cajuil* (cashew nut fruit) have Taíno origins.

Africans also influenced Caribbean foods, introducing plantains, coconuts, okra, and taro, a starchy vegetable also known as *yautía*. Many of these foods serve as the basis for Caribbean cuisine today (see Table 6.1) (12). Refer to Appendix A for nutrient analyses.

Table 6.1 · Foods Used in Traditional Caribbean Hispanic Cuisine

Food	Spanish Name(s)/Description
Starchy vegetables	
Beans	*Habichuelas* (Puerto Rico and Dominican Republic), *frijoles* (Cuba), *judías* (Cuba), *alubias, porotos, caraotas*
Cassava	*Yuca*
Chayote squash	*Chayote* (Puerto Rico), *tayota* (Dominican Republic)
Corn	*Maíz*
Green bananas	*Guineos verdes*
Green peas	*Petit pois* (Dominican Republic), *arvejas, chícharos*
Peppers	*Pimientos, ajís*
Pigeon peas	*Guandules, gandules*
Plantain	*Plátano* (resembling large, thick-skinned green bananas; when ripe, the outer skin turns yellow with black pigmentation and the fruit is sweet)
Pumpkin	*Calabaza* (Puerto Rico), *ahuyama* (Dominican Republic)
Sweet potato	*Batata* (Puerto Rico and Dominican Republic), *boniato* (Cuba)
Taro	*Yautía/tannier* (a starchy root vegetable; white, yellow, or pale pink when raw; turns mauve-gray or violet when cooked; tastes like a combination of chestnuts and artichoke hearts)
Yam	*Ñame*
Nonstarchy vegetables	
Broccoli	*Brocoli, brecól*
Cabbage	*Repollo*
Cucumber	*Pepino*
Eggplant	*Berenjena*
Lettuce	*Lechuga*
Okra	*Quimbobó*
Onion	*Cebolla*
String beans	*Vainitas, habichuelas tiernas, habichuelas*
Watercress	*Berro*

(continued)

Table 6.1   (continued)

Food	Spanish Name(s)/Description
Milk and milk products	
Cheddar cheese	*Queso de papa, queso cheddar*
Gouda cheese	*Queso amarillo guda*
Milk	*Leche*
White cheese	*Queso blanco, queso para freir* (this is a firm cheese that doesn't melt when fried)
Whole milk	*Leche entera*
Fruits	
Avocado	*Aguacate*
Banana	*Banana, guineo*
Breadfruit	*Pana, panapén* (a large, round green fruit with a rough rind and pale flesh)
Cashew nut fruit	*Cajuil*
Cherimoya	*Cherimoya* (a heart-shaped or oval fruit with white flesh that has a sweet-sour flavor)
Chico zapote	*Chico zapote, nispero* (a sweet fruit with a flavor similar to maple sugar)
Coconut	*Coco*
Grapefruit	*Toronja, pomelo*
Guava	*Guava, guayaba*
Mamey	*Mamey, mamey sapote* (large, football-shaped fruit)
Mango	*Mango*
Orange	*China* (Puerto Rico and Dominican Republic), *naranja* (Cuba)
Papaya	*Papaya, lechoza* (Cuba and Dominican Republic), *fruta bomba* (Cuba and Dominican Republic)
Parcha (yellow passion fruit)	*Parcha, maracuyá* (a round, green fruit with orange pulp)
Passionfruit	*Parcha, chinola, ceibey* (round or oval fruits with green-orange pulp and sour-sweet flavor)
Pineapple	*Piña*
Quenepas (Spanish limes)	*Quenepas, limoncillos, mamoncillos* (this fruit grows in clusters, similar to green grapes; the sweet yellow flesh is surrounded by a large inedible pit)
Soursop	*Guanábana* (deep-green, heart-shaped fruit with white juicy flesh and a tangy, acidic flavor)
Star fruit	*Carambola* (star-shaped fruit with golden yellow skin and crisp juicy flesh)
Tamarind	*Tamarindo* (cinnamon-brown pods that contain sticky and tart brown pulp and inedible large brown seeds)
Meats	
Beef	*Carne de res*
Blood sausage	*Morcilla*
Chicken	*Pollo*
Codfish	*Bacalao*
Eggs	*Huevos*
Goat	*Cabra*
Oxtail	*Rabo, cola*
Pork rind, fried	*Chicharrón* (crunchy piece of fat-back pork that is sold in Puerto Rico; small pieces of *chicharrón* are used to season rice dishes, especially rice with pigeon peas)
Salami	*Salchichón*
Shredded beef	*Carne ripiada, ropa vieja*
Tripe	*Mondongo, tripas, panza, menudo*

(continued)

Table 6.1   *(continued)*

Food	Spanish Name(s)/Description
Seasonings	
Adobo	*Adobo* (mixture of crushed peppercorns, oregano, garlic, and salt, with olive oil and lime juice or vinegar)
Annatto seeds	*Achiote* (used to impart a yellowish color to rice dishes)
Bay leaves	*Hojas de laurel* (used in fricassee and other stews)
Coriander/cilantro	*Cilantro*
—	*Alcaparrado* (capers and olives in brine that are added to rice dishes and stews)
—	*Sofrito* (made of tomatoes, garlic, cilantro, peppers and *recao* (a green leafy vegetable with a pungent, peppery taste); the principal condiment used to season stews, beans, and meats)

Source: Data are from reference 12.

The staple dish of the Caribbean is rice and beans (10). Puerto Ricans and Dominicans refer to the traditional rice and beans dish as *arroz y habichuelas.* Dominicans refer to a dish of rice, beans, and meat as *la bandera* (the flag). In Cuba, *moros y cristianos* is a traditional dish of black beans and white rice whose name refers to the war between the Moors (black) and the Spanish Christians (white). Long-grain and converted rices are commonly used. Typically, one part rice is cooked with two parts water plus vegetable oil and salt. Rice is often cooked in a *caldero* (aluminum pot), and the sticky, crusty portion that sticks to the bottom is a favorite part of the meal. The sticky crusty rice is called *pegao* in Puerto Rico, *con-con* or *raspa* in the Dominican Republic, and *raspa* in Cuba. For the traditional dish of rice and beans, Puerto Ricans enjoy pink and red kidney beans, Dominicans prefer Roman beans, and Cubans use black beans. See Table 6.2 for additional traditional Caribbean dishes, beverages, and desserts (10,12–14). Refer to Appendix A for nutrient analyses.

Traditional Meal Patterns and Holiday Foods

Despite the common ingredients used throughout the region, traditional meal patterns differ from country to country.

Puerto Rico

In Puerto Rico, meals consist of breakfast *(desayuno)*, lunch *(almuerzo),* dinner *(cena),* and one or more snacks *(meriendas).* Breakfast may include juice, eggs, white bread, and *café con leche* (hot steamed milk and espresso). Oatmeal *(avena)* with cinnamon is another breakfast option. Lunch is often the most substantial meal in Puerto Rico and may include root vegetables *(viandas),* rice, beans, and fish, chicken, or beef. In the US mainland, Puerto Ricans may select a sandwich with processed meats such as bologna or ham, along with a beverage or fruit. They may also eat dinner leftovers or fast foods (10). A typical dinner dish is rice and stewed beans seasoned with *sofrito,* a mixture of tomatoes, garlic, cilantro, peppers, and *recaoa* (a green leafy vegetable with a pungent, peppery taste). Salads made of lettuce and tomatoes with avocados are commonplace in the US mainland; avocado is also often served on its own in the island. Soft drinks, water, and other beverages may accompany dinner.

Starchy root vegetables such as green or yellow plantains, *tannier/yautia* (taro), yuca/cassava, and green bananas may be a side dish at dinner. A snack often consists of *café con leche* with saltine (soda) crackers. Saltine crackers may be eaten with cheddar cheese *(queso de papa)* and salami.

Dominican Republic

A traditional Dominican breakfast consists of mashed boiled green plantains *(mangús)* served with fried white cheese, salami, eggs, and *café con leche.* Boiled cassava or boiled green bananas with sliced onions is a breakfast alternative to *mangús.* A popular breakfast beverage called *morirsoñando* ("to die dreaming") is made with orange juice, milk, and often sugar.

Table 6.2 · Traditional Caribbean Dishes, Beverages, and Desserts

Spanish Name	Description
Dishes	
Arroz con camarones	Rice with shrimp
Arroz con pollo	Rice with chicken
Arroz y habichuelas	Rice and beans (Puerto Rico, Dominican Republic)
Asopaos	A soupy rice, vegetable and protein mixture
Bandera, la	Rice and beans (Dominican Republic)
Casabe	Cassava bread
Empanadas	Chicken or meat turnovers wrapped in flour dough
Guineitos en escabeche	Green bananas in a vinegar/oil dressing
Kipe	Fried meat patty made of ground beef, bulgur wheat, and spices
Locrio	A dish of mixed rice, beans, and meat
Maduros	Sweet fried plantains
Mangú	A Dominican dish of green plantains that are boiled and mashed and used in place of bread or cereal for breakfast
Mariquitas, maraquitas	Thinly sliced, fried plantain chips
Media noche	Cuban-style panini sandwich with ham, sliced pork, and cheese
Mofongo	Mashed green plantains with added meats such as pork
Moros y cristianos	Black beans and white rice (Cuba)
Pan con bistec	Bread with steak (Cuba)
Pastelón	A Hispanic variation of lasagna that uses slices of fried sweet plantains instead of pasta
Pernil	Pork chops and roasted pork shoulder
Picadillo	Chopped ground beef seasoned with *sofrito* (Cuba)
Ropa vieja	Seasoned shredded beef
Serenata	Puerto Rican dish that mixes codfish *(bacalao)* with root vegetables
Tortilla española	Egg omelet with potatoes
Tostada	Toasted *pan cubano* with butter
Tostones	Twice-fried green plantains
Beverages	
Café	Coffee
Café con leche	Coffee with steamed milk
Café cubano	Espresso-style black coffee
Ron	Rum
Malta	Nonalcoholic beverage made of barley and hops; often perceived as highly nutritious and iron-rich
Morirsoñando	Literally, "to die dreaming"; beverage made with orange juice, milk, and often sugar (Dominican Republic)
Té de hierbas	Herbal tea (such as chamomile, passiflora, cinnamon, peppermint, ginger, and aloe; considered to have medicinal properties, especially among Dominicans)
Desserts	
Dulce de leche, flan, majarete, tembleque	Types of dairy desserts
Piraguas	Shaved ice cones with syrup flavors such as tamarind, raspberry, pineapple and coconut

Source: Data are from references 10 and 12–14.

A traditional Dominican lunch may consist of *la bandera dominicana,* which includes rice, beans, and a meat (such as beef, seafood, or chicken). Dinner is similar in composition to lunch, with choices such as rice, beans, and starchy root vegetables. Meat choices at dinner may range from stewed goat or oxtail to beef and chicken. Dominicans often have two starches for either lunch or dinner. For example, dinner might include Dominican-style spaghetti (cooked softer than al dente, the dish contains vinegar, salami, and chopped onions and peppers) as well as rice.

Rum and beer are popular alcoholic beverages. Beer is colloquially referred to as a *fría* ("cold one").

Cuba

A traditional Cuban breakfast is *tostada* (a Cuban bread made with lard, spread with butter, and pressed in a panini machine) and *café con leche*. Egg omelets are called *tortilla española* (Spanish tortilla) and should not be confused with the Mexican tortilla, which is a flat corn or wheat bread.

Lunch may consist of *empanadas* (chicken or meat turnovers wrapped in flour dough) or Cuban sandwiches. A typical Cuban sandwich is called *media noche* (midnight sandwich) and includes ham, pork, and cheese, grilled panini-style, and topped with pickles and mustard. *Pan con bistec* (bread with steak) is a thin slice of *palomilla* steak (boneless round or sirloin steak) on Cuban bread garnished with lettuce and tomatoes and accompanied by potato sticks or thinly sliced, fried plantain chips (*mariquitas* or *maraquitas*).

A typical dinner consists of a meat, chicken, or fish entrée accompanied by white rice, black beans, and sweet fried plantains *(maduros)*. Typical meat dishes are *picadillo,* chopped ground beef seasoned with *sofrito* and *ropa vieja* (literally "old clothes"), which is seasoned shredded beef. *Café con leche* and *café cubano* (espresso-style coffee served in a small cup) are traditional after-dinner beverages.

Holiday Foods

The most important Caribbean Hispanic celebrations focus on Christian holidays and include the feast of the Epiphany on January 6 (also known as *Día de los Reyes* or Three Kings Day), Easter, and Christmas (15). For a list of foods consumed during the Christmas holiday, see Table 6.3 (15,16).

Holidays honoring patron saints and virgins are important celebratory occasions, especially in the islands. Traditional Caribbean holiday meals include various turkey, pork, bean, and rice dishes, and alcoholic beverages.

Between Ash Wednesday and Easter (Lent), most Caribbean Catholics abstain from eating red meat on Fridays and consume fish instead. Dominicans prepare *habichuelas con dulce* (sweet beans) and *casabe,* a dish made of beans, coconut milk, and cassava bread. On Palm Sunday, Puerto Ricans serve a marinated fish dish called *escabeche.*

Traditional Health Beliefs

Caribbean Hispanics traditionally believe that health exists only when the body, mind, and spirit are in balance. Commonly held beliefs regarding illness and disease include the following (17):

- Evil eye *(mal de ojo)*—the belief that diseases may occur in small children if they receive compliments without also receiving God's blessing. An adult who wishes to compliment a child might say, for example, "Melissa has beautiful eyes and may God bless her," instead of "Melissa has beautiful eyes."
- Fright *(susto)*—the belief that physical conditions such as diabetes have emotional causes and traumatic events can lead to illness.
- Spasm *(pasmo)*—the belief that exposure to cold air or *sereno* (morning or evening dew) can cause temporary paralysis of the face or legs.
- Bile *(bilis)*—the belief that a strong emotional occurrence causes bile to pour into the bloodstream, which causes livid rage and worsens health conditions such as high blood pressure or elevated blood glucose levels.

Table 6.3 · Traditional Christmas Foods

Spanish Name	Description
Puerto Rico	
Arroz con gandules	Rice and pigeon peas
Coquito	Eggnog made with rum, sweetened condensed milk, evaporated milk, egg yolks, coconut milk, and sugar
Pasteles	Ground root vegetables with meat filling wrapped in plantain leaves or wax paper and then boiled
Pernil	Roast pork
Cuba	
Arroz con leche	Rice pudding
Boniatillo	Sweet potato pudding
Buñuelos	A fritter made with cassava and Caribbean sweet potato *(boniato)*
Congrí	Bean and rice casserole
Lechón asado	Roasted pig made with bitter orange marinade
Pan cubano	Cuban bread, traditionally prepared with lard
Tostones	Fried green plantains
Turrón	Nougat
Yuca con mojo	Cassava with garlic sauce
Dominican Republic	
Arroz	Rice
Arroz con dulce	Rice pudding with coconut milk
Jamón	Baked ham
Pavo asado	Roast turkey
Perni	Roast pork
Pasteles	Ground root vegetables with meat filling wrapped in plantain leaves or wax paper and then boiled

Source: Data are from references 15 and 16.

Current Food Practices

The food practices and meal patterns of Caribbean Hispanics living in the United States are strongly influenced by the following:

- Degree of acculturation
- Socioeconomic status
- Place of origin
- Daily exposure to food advertising
- Food availability
- Access to places to buy and/or prepare food
- Health beliefs
- Participation in government food programs

Counseling Considerations

Demonstrating Courtesy and Respect

When counseling clients, ask them, "How are you feeling today?" Smile and shake hands or place your hand on the client's shoulder. If you have an established relationship with a client, it is proper to ask about the client's spouse or family members—"How is your husband? Your children?" Look directly at your clients during counseling. Address older adults in a formal manner. For example, use the terms, *señor* (sir/mister) and *señora* (ma'am/missus).

Interpreting Clients' Nonverbal Communication

Caribbean Hispanic clients with limited English proficiency and/or low health literacy may not verbalize their lack of comprehension about the treatment modality, particularly if they have high respect for health care providers. Clients may respond with "yes" or "no" even when they do not clearly understand the content of the counseling session (18). Whenever possible, ask open-ended questions. For example, instead of asking the yes-or-no question, "Do you understand which foods you need to eat?" ask, "Can you tell me three foods you will now include in your diet?"

Inquiring About Clients' Understanding of Diabetes

Health care professionals should ask clients about their understanding of their illness and its consequences. For example, when counseling patients, ask the following questions:

- What do you think caused your diabetes?
- How do you take care of your diabetes?"

As you listen to their responses, be aware that clients may believe diabetes is caused by divine punishment or feel ashamed, out of control, or depressed when they are diagnosed.

Discussing Clients' Use of Complementary and Alternative Medicine

Caribbean Hispanics may seek folk treatments, use home remedies, and/or try traditional procedures. Sources of folk treatment may include the following:

- *Botanicas*—herbalist stores
- *Yerberos*—herbalists
- *Curanderos*—healers who use prayer, massage, and herbs to treat physical, spiritual, and emotional conditions
- *Espiritistas/santeros*—practitioners believed to have spiritual or psychic abilities

Caribbean Hispanics may use multiple folk remedies as well as herbals and dietary supplements to treat and manage diabetes and other conditions. Refer to Appendix C for questions to assess dietary supplement use. Health care providers may also use the following questions to initiate conversations with clients about complementary and alternative medicine:

- Have you seen other practitioners for the treatment of diabetes and its related conditions?
- If yes, what treatments or remedies are you taking?
- We all have favorite remedies that we use when we are sick. Which home remedies do you use?

Considering Family Demands and Dynamics

Family dynamics are an important counseling consideration. In a series of focus groups, Anderson and colleagues found that Caribbean Hispanic women placed their family's needs above their own and believed that playing the role of wife and caretaker should take precedence over their own health (19).

Engaging Others in Counseling Sessions

With the client's consent, health care providers should include clients' support systems in counseling. For example, a client may invite friends and relatives to be part of the goal-setting process. Family members can aid in successful outcomes if they understand the importance of the treatment, and their participation may keep them from undermining the client's efforts. Health care providers may also want to engage the use of community health workers, if they are available.

Nutrition Counseling

Appendix B offers selected medical nutrition therapy recommendations for individuals with diabetes and general counseling suggestions that support those recommendations. The following are culturally specific nutrition counseling strategies for Caribbean Hispanic clients:

- Rice and starchy vegetables are abundant in the Caribbean Hispanic diet. Suggest that clients eat more nonstarchy vegetables and smaller portions of rice.
- Rice and bean dishes traditionally have more rice than beans. Encourage clients to increase the amount of beans and reduce the amount of rice.
- Clients may refer to low-fat milk and whole-wheat bread as "diet milk" and "diet bread," respectively. Emphasize that "diet" foods are neither calorie- nor carbohydrate-free.
- Encourage clients to choose codfish and other lower-fat protein choices.
- Suggest lower-fat substitutes to season rice dishes, such as using lean ham instead of pork fat.
- Provide a list of leaner cuts of meats that can be added to traditional stews and soups.
- Discuss lower-fat alternatives for holiday beverages (eg, using fat-free evaporated milk or low-fat coconut milk in drink recipes).

Challenges and Barriers Affecting Dietary Compliance

Dietary interventions can be difficult because the behavioral goals are multifaceted. For example, a client who aims to eat less fat would need to change food selections, purchasing patterns, preparation techniques, and condiment use. The following are some of the issues that may affect a Caribbean Hispanic client's ability to follow a meal plan and comply with other recommendations (19–31):

- Portion control.
- An external or internal locus of control: Some clients are fatalistic or believe that external, divine powers control destiny; others believe in self-efficacy.
- Income levels and food budgets: For example, low-income clients may rely on Food Stamps and/or Meals on Wheels, and other clients, too, may be concerned about the cost of foods included in their meal plans.
- Food availability: In some geographic areas, clients do not have easy access to well-stocked grocery stores or may not be able to buy the traditional foods they enjoy.
- Time constraints and other limitations on meal preparation: Clients may perceive new cooking methods to be too time-consuming (eg, they may think frying is quicker and easier than baking). Some clients, such as the elderly, may rely on others to prepare their meals.
- Limited understanding of the role of food in disease management: For example, clients may assume that certain "healthy" foods, such as oatmeal, grapefruit, and yogurt, do not affect blood glucose levels, or they may avoid other foods that they perceive to be too sweet (eg, mango) or unhealthy (pork).
- Dental health, general health status, and health insurance status.
- Language issues: the client's ability to read, write, and understand English and/or Spanish.

Counseling Tips

The following tips can help in counseling Caribbean Hispanic clients with diabetes:

- Assess the client's beliefs about the role of religion in health outcomes. Seek advice and insight from religious leaders in the client's community.
- Recommend economically available and acceptable foods. Provide a shopping list and ideas for meal preparation that use foods the client finds acceptable.
- Focus on changes that are feasible, sensible, and practical for the client and his or her family.
- Whenever possible, use visual tools rather than written examples and handouts. For example, teach portion control using food replicas, pictures, and measuring cups, spoons, and devices. In particular, clients with low literacy levels want simple, practical, and relevant information on what foods to eat and how to prepare them and express a preference for hands-on activities that are enjoyable and allow them to share ideas and experiences (32).
- Become familiar with cultural beliefs about health and be prepared to demonstrate the difference between myths and facts.
- Encourage clients to bring food labels from foods they eat at home to counseling sessions.

- Ask patients to bring supermarket fliers that contain ethnic foods to counseling sessions.
- Encourage patients who own cameras to take pictures of their meals and use these photos to evaluate portion sizes.

Resources

Epicurious.com. http://www.epicurious.com. Accessed March 30, 2009. Includes database of more than 4,000 food terms.

Latino Health Beliefs. A Guide for Health Care Professionals. Washington, DC: National Council of La Raza; 1998.

National Diabetes Information Clearing House – Hispanics/Latinos and Diabetes. http://diabetes.niddk .nih.gov/dm/pubs/hispanicamerican/index.htm. Accessed May 20, 2009.

US Department of Agriculture. National Agriculture Library. Ethnic and Cultural Resources. http://grande.nal.usda.gov/nal_display/index.php?info_center=4&tax_level=2&tax_subject= 270&topic_id=1339. Accessed March 31, 2009.

References

1. US Census Bureau. The American FactFinder Glossary: Hispanic or Latino origin. http://factfinder.census.gov/home/en/epss/glossary_h.html. Accessed March 20, 2009.
2. US Census Bureau. The American FactFinder. http://factfinder.census.gov. Accessed March 20, 2009.
3. National Institute of Diabetes and Digestive and Kidney Diseases. *National Diabetes Statistics Fact Sheet: General Information and National Estimates on Diabetes in the United States.* Bethesda, MD: National Institutes of Health; 2005.
4. Centers for Disease Control and Prevention: Prevalence of diabetes among Hispanics—selected areas, 1998–2002. *MMWR Morb Mortal Wkly Rep.* 2004;53:941–944. http://www.cdc.gov/ mmwr/preview/mmwrhtml/mm5340a3.htm. Accessed March 30, 2009.
5. US Department of Health and Human Services. Office of Minority Health. HHS Fact Sheet: Minority Health Disparities at a Glance. http://www.omhrc.gov/templates/content.aspx?ID=2139. Accessed March 30, 2009.
6. Tucker K, Bermudez O, Castaneda C. Type 2 diabetes is prevalent and poorly controlled among Hispanic elders of Caribbean origin. *Am J Public Health.* 2000;90:1288–1293.
7. American Diabetes Association. Standards of medical care in diabetes—2006. *Diabetes Care.* 2006;29(Suppl 1):S4–S42.
8. Jovanovic L, Harrison RW. Advances in diabetes for the millennium: diabetes in minorities. *Med Gen Med.* 2004;6(3 Suppl):3.
9. Hanis CL, Hewett-Emmett D, Bertin TK, Schull WJ. Origins of U.S. Hispanics. implications for diabetes. *Diabetes Care.* 1991;14:618–627.
10. Sanjur D. *Hispanic Foodways, Nutrition and Health.* Needham Heights, MA: Allyn & Bacon; 1995.
11. Guitar L. Criollos: the birth of a dynamic new Indo-Afro-European people and culture on Hispaniola. *J Carib Amerindian Hist Anthropol.* 2000;1:1–17.
12. Drago L. *Beyond Rice and Beans: The Caribbean Latino Guide to Eating Healthy with Diabetes.* Alexandria, VA: American Diabetes Association; 2006.
13. Kittler PG, Sucher KP. *Food and Culture.* 5th ed. Belmont, CA: Wadsworth/Thomson Learning; 2008.
14. Aunt Clara's Kitchen Dominican Cooking. http://www.dominicancooking.com. Accessed March 30, 2009.
15. Menard V. *The Latino Holiday Book.* New York, NY: Marlowe; 2000.
16. Three Guys from Miami. A Cuban Christmas: A Traditional Celebration. http://cuban-christmas .com/christmas_menu.html. Accessed March 20, 2009.
17. Juckett G. Cross-cultural medicine. *Am Fam Physician.* 2005;72:2267–2274.
18. Diaz VA. Cultural factors in preventive care: Latinos. *Prim Care.* 2002;29:503–517.
19. Anderson RM, Goddard CE, Garcia R, Guzman JR, Vazquez F. Using focus groups to identify diabetes care and education issues for Latinos with diabetes. *Diabetes Educ.* 1998;24:618–625.
20. Walker E, Caban A. A systematic review of research on culturally relevant issues for Hispanics with diabetes. *Diabetes Educ.* 2006;32:584–595.
21. Chavez N, Telleen S, Kim YO. Food insufficiency in urban Latino families. *J Immigr Minor Health.* 2007;9:197–204.
22. Kristal AR, White E, Shattuck AL, Curry S, Anderson GL, Fowler A, Urban N. Long-term maintenance of a low-fat diet: durability of fat-related dietary habits in the Women's Health Trial. *J Am Diet Assoc.* 1992;92:553–559.

23. Gans KM, Burkholder GJ, Risica PM, Lasater TM. Baseline fat-related dietary behaviors of white, Hispanic, and black participants in a cholesterol and education project in New England. *J Am Diet Assoc*. 2003;103:699–706.

24. Karliner S, Crewe SE, Pacheco H, Gonzalez YC. *Latino Health Beliefs: A Guide for Health Care Professionals*. Washington DC: National Council of La Raza; 1998.

25. Melnik TA, Spence MM, Hosler AS. Fat-related dietary behaviors of adult Puerto Ricans, with and without diabetes, in New York City. *J Am Diet Assoc*. 2006;106:1419–1425.

26. Horowitz, CR, Colson KA, Hebert PL, Lancaster K. Barriers to buying healthy foods for people with diabetes: evidence of environmental disparities. *Am J Public Health*. 2004;94:1549–1554.

27. Lin H, Bermudez OI, Tucker KL. Dietary patterns of Hispanic elders are associated with acculturation and obesity. *J Nutr*. 2003;133:3651–3657.

28. Dotty M, Ives BL. Quality of Health Care for Hispanic Populations. Findings from the Commonwealth Fund 2001 Health Care Quality Survey. March 2002. http://www .commonwealthfund.org/usr_doc/doty_factsheethisp.pdf. Accessed March 30, 2009.

29. Centers for Disease Control and Prevention. A Demographic and Health Snapshot of the U.S. Hispanic/Latino Population. 2002. http://www.cdc.gov/NCHS/data/hpdata2010/chcsummit.pdf. Accessed March 30, 2009.

30. National Institute for Literacy. Current Population Survey. http://www.nifl.gov/nifl/facts/CPS.html. Accessed March 30, 2009.

31. Gettleman L, Winkleby MA. Using focus groups to develop a heart disease prevention program for ethnically diverse, low-income women. *J Commun Health*. 2000;25:439–453.

32. Hartman TJ, McCarthy PR, Park RJ, Schuster E, Kushi LH. Focus group responses of potential participants in a nutrition education program for individuals with limited literacy skills. *J Am Diet Assoc*. 1994;94:744–748.

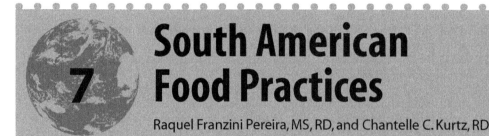

South American Food Practices

Raquel Franzini Pereira, MS, RD, and Chantelle C. Kurtz, RD

Introduction

Approximately 37 million people live in South America, with its population distributed among the French province of French Guiana, the British Falkland Islands, and 12 countries: Argentina, Bolivia, Brazil, Chile, Colombia, Ecuador, Guyana, Paraguay, Peru, Suriname, Uruguay, and Venezuela. Spanish is spoken in all countries except Brazil, where Portuguese is the main language. Other languages spoken in the region include French, Quechua, Aymara, Guaraní, Italian, English, German, Dutch, and Japanese.

Historically and culturally, South America has connections with both the European nations that colonized it and, more recently, the United States. South American culture and cuisine also reflect African, Asian, and indigenous influences (1).

Most South Americans are Catholics (more than 90% in Peru, 84% in Brazil, and 91% in Argentina) (2); others are Muslims, Jews, Protestants, Jehovah's Witnesses, Mormons, Buddhists, agnostics, or atheists. Some South Americans practice African-influenced religions such as Candomblé and Umbanda, and some people may practice more than one religion (3,4).

The 2000 US Census defines "Hispanic" or "Latino" as follows (5):

> Those who classify themselves in one of the specific Hispanic or Latino categories listed on the Census 2000 or ACS questionnaire—"Mexican," "Puerto Rican," or "Cuban"—as well as those who indicate that they are "other Spanish, Hispanic, or Latino. Origin can be viewed as the heritage, nationality group, lineage, or country of birth of the person or the person's parents or ancestors before their arrival in the United States. People who identify their origin as Spanish, Hispanic, or Latino may be of any race.

According to these criteria, in 2000 the US Latino population was approximately 35 million (12.5% of the total US population) (6). Approximately 1.35 million US residents (3.8% of all Latinos) were from South America (6).

Diabetes Prevalence

Diabetes prevalence is greater in Hispanics in the United States than in the non-Hispanic white US population. Diabetes tends to occur in Hispanics at younger ages—between 35 and 64 years (7)—compared with the non-Hispanic white population in developed countries, where most people with diabetes are older than the age of retirement. Among Hispanics, type 2 diabetes is more prevalent among women and people in urban areas (8). Diabetes is the fifth leading cause of death among Hispanics in the United States. Diabetes rates are more than doubled for obese Hispanics compared with other obese Americans (9).

In 2003, the prevalence of diabetes in South America was 5.9% (8). In Latin American countries, diabetes prevalence ranges from 3.1% to 8.2% of the population. Prevalence in Latin America is predicted to double by 2025, to 32.7 million people (10). Type 2 diabetes is most prevalent, whereas the prevalence of type 1 diabetes in Latin America is generally lower than in the United States (11).

Risk Factors for Type 2 Diabetes

South Americans are at higher risk for type 2 diabetes than ever before. Urbanization, globalization, and economic factors all contribute to increased rates of chronic diseases such as diabetes. Whereas overweight and obesity were once considered more characteristic of high-income people, individuals from all income levels are now affected. In some South American communities, being overweight or obese is regarded as a sign of prosperity and health, a sedentary lifestyle is idealized, and physical labor is unattractive (10). The media promotes contradictory messages—on the one hand, idealizing thinness; on the other hand, selling high-calorie convenience and fast foods (12,13).

In developing countries, nutrition transitions are accelerating (10). The problem of dietary deficit is shifting to one of dietary excess, with increased prevalence of physical inactivity, dietary fat consumption, and weight gain ultimately contributing to an increased prevalence of diabetes (14,15). In Latin American countries, these nutrition transitions seem to be greater among lower-income people (16), vary among countries from 22% to 26%, and are higher among females (17).

The combination of factors such as excess of food consumption, weight gain, physical inactivity, and the entry of women into the workforce (which increases the likelihood of physical inactivity and consumption of unhealthful convenience foods) has contributed to the development of diabetes in countries like Brazil (18). Although fruits and vegetables are abundant in Latin American countries, daily consumption of these foods is low in Brazil—41% of adults report daily intake of fruits, and 30% report eating vegetables daily (19,20).

Traditional Foods and Dishes

South American cuisine includes many regional variations. Climate, geography, religion, and culture influence which foods are cultivated and served, and the cuisines of natives and colonizers have mingled to create different regional styles. Selected popular foods and dishes are listed in Tables 7.1 (1,21–23) and 7.2 (21–27). Refer to Appendix A for nutrient analyses.

Traditional Meal Patterns and Holiday Foods

Meal patterns and holidays vary among South American countries. Many follow the European custom of three meals a day (breakfast, lunch, and dinner) plus a few snacks. The time allocated for meals is usually sufficient for a sit-down meal with multiple courses. Some, but not all, South Americans customarily take a siesta (nap after lunch). Dinner may be eaten in the late evening. This meal can be a large social gathering, either at home or in a restaurant, rather than a quick, "convenient" meal.

Traditional meals include beans; rice; meat, chicken, pork, or seafood; vegetables; fruits; and desserts. Pasta dishes and pizza are common in the regions influenced by Italians, such as southeastern Brazil, Argentina, and Uruguay (1). Home-cooked meals are not as common as they once were, and people now consume more processed food items (28).

During holidays, meals are abundant, include a variety of food choices, and are sometimes associated with superstitions. Important holidays include Easter, Christmas, and New Year's Eve. Box 7.1 lists holiday foods (21).

Table 7.1 · Foods Used in Traditional South American Cuisine

English Name	Spanish Name	Portuguese Name
Grains		
Amaranth	*Amaranto*	*Amaranto*
Bread crumbs	*Pan rallado*	*Farinha de rosca*
Pasta	*Pasta*	*Massa*
Quinoa	*Quínoa*	*Quínoa*
Rice	*Arroz*	*Arroz*
Tortillas	*Tortillas*	N/A
Starchy vegetables		
Arracacia (Andean root vegetable)	N/A	*Mandioquinha*
Beans	*Frijoles/porotos*	*Feijão*
Chickpeas/garbanzo beans	*Garbanzo*	*Grão de bico*
Corn/maize	*Maíz*	*Milho*
Jicama	*Jicama*	N/A
Peas	*Arvejas*	*Ervilha*
Potato	*Papa/patata*	*Batata*
Sweet potato	*Papa dulce*	*Batata doce*
Tapioca/cassava/manioc/yuca	*Yuca*	*Mandioca*
Taro	*Taro/malanga*	N/A
Water yam (root vegetable)	N/A	*Inhame*
Nonstarchy vegetables		
Broccoli	*Brécol/brócoli*	*Brócolis*
Cabbage	*Repollo*	*Repolho*
Carrot	*Zanahoria*	*Cenoura*
Cauliflower	*Coliflor*	*Couve flor*
Garlic	*Ajo*	*Alho*
Heart of palm	*Chonta/palmito*	*Palmito*
Kale	*Col rizada*	*Couve*
Lettuce	*Lechuga*	*Alface*
Mushroom	*Seta/champiñon*	*Cogumelo/champignon*
Okra	*Okra*	*Quiabo*
Onion	*Cebolla*	*Cebola*
Pepper	*Chiles (ají, amarillo, malagueta, pimiento)*	*Pimenta*
Spinach	*Espinaca*	*Espinafre*
Tomato	*Tomate*	*Tomate*
Fruits		
Açai	N/A	*Açaí*
Acerola/barbados cherry	*Acerola*	*Acerola*
Avocado	*Aguacate/palta*	*Abacate*
Banana	*Banana/plátano*	*Banana*
Breadfruit	*Fruta de pan/pana*	*Fruta pão*
Cashew	*Caja*	*Caju*
Cherimoya/sugar apple	*Chirimoya*	*Fruta do conde*
Citrus juices	*Jugos cítricos*	*Sucos cítricos*

(continued)

Table 7.1   *(continued)*

English Name	Spanish Name	Portuguese Name
Coconut	*Coco*	*Côco*
Cupuaçu/nicaragua chocolate	N/A	*Cupuaçu*
Grapes	*Uvas*	*Uvas*
Guava	*Guayaba*	*Goiaba*
Jaboticaba	*Jabuticaba*	*Jabuticaba*
Jackfruit/durian	*Jaca*	*Jaca*
Kiwi fruit	*Kivi/kiwi*	*Kiwi*
Lemon	*Limón*	*Limão*
Mango	*Mango*	*Manga*
Orange	*Naranja*	*Laranja*
Papaya	*Papaya*	*Mamão papaia*
Passionfruit/granadilla	*Maracuyá*	*Maracujá*
Peach	*Durazno*	*Pêssego*
Pear	*Pera*	*Pêra*
Persimmon/kaki	*Caqui*	*Caqui*
Pineapple	*Piña*	*Abacaxi*
Plum	*Ciruela*	*Ameixa*
Pomegranate	*Granada*	*Romã*
Prune	*Ciruela pasa*	*Ameixa seca*
Quince	*Membrillo*	*Marmelo*
Soursop/guanabana	*Guanábana*	*Graviola*
Starfruit	*Carambola*	*Carambola*
Surinam cherry/pitanga	*Pitanga*	*Pitanga*
Watermelon	*Sandía*	*Melancia*
Dairy		
Cottage cheese	*Queso blanco grumoso*	*Queijo cottage*
Cream cheese/cheese curd	*Requesón*	*Requeijão*
Creamy cheese	N/A	*Queijo catupiry*
Farmer's (fresh) cheese	*Queso fresco*	*Queijo fresco de minas*
Ricotta	*Ricota*	*Queijo ricota*
Sour cream	*Cuajada*	*Coalhada*
Yogurt	*Yogur*	*Iogurte*
Meats and meat alternatives		
Barbecue	*Parillada/barbacoa*	*Churrasco*
Beef jerky	*Carne seca*	*Carne seca*
Beef steak	*Asado/parilla*	*Bife*
Blood sausage/chorizo	*Chorizo*	*Chouriço*
Chicken/hen	*Pollo/gallina*	*Frango/galinha*
Codfish/dried cod	*Bacalao*	*Bacalhau*
Eggs	*Huevos*	*Ovos*
Guinea pig	*Cuy/cuye/conejillo de india*	N/A
Llama	*Llama*	N/A
Lobster	*Langosta*	*Lagosta*

(continued)

Table 7.1   *(continued)*

English Name	Spanish Name	Portuguese Name
Mutton/sheep	*Carnero*	*Carneiro*
Oyster	*Ostra*	*Ostra*
Pork	*Cerdo*	*Porco*
Salami	*Salchichón*	*Salame*
Salmon	*Salmón*	*Salmão*
Shredded beef	*Carne ripiada*	*Carne desfiada*
Shrimp	*Camarón*	*Camarão*
Squid/calamari	*Calamar*	*Lula*
Spices, seasonings, and herbs		
Chili	*Chiles (ají, amarillo, malagueta, pimiento)*	*Pimenta*
Basil	*Albahaca*	*Manjericão*
Cilantro	*Cilantro*	*Coentro*
Cinnamon/canella	*Canela*	*Canela*
Oregano/origan/sweet Marjoram	*Orégano*	*Orégano*
Parsley	*Perejil*	*Cheiro verde/salsa*
Rosemary	*Romero*	*Alecrim*
Salt	*Sal*	*Sal*
Vanilla	*Vainilla*	*Baunilha*

N/A = not applicable. Used for foods that are not commonly eaten by speakers of that language.
Source: Data are from references 1, 21, 22, and 23.

Table 7.2 • Traditional South American Dishes, Beverages, and Desserts

Name (Language)	Description
Combination dishes	
Acarajé (Portuguese)	Deep-fried black-eyed peas little cake
Ajiaco colombiano (Spanish)	Colombian chicken and vegetable stew
Albóndigas (Spanish)/*Almôndegas* (Portuguese)	Meatballs
Anticuchos (Spanish)	Peruvian beef kebabs
Arepas (Spanish)	Flat cornmeal cakes or fritters
Arroz con frijoles (Spanish)/ *Arroz com feijão* (Portuguese)	Rice and beans
Asado (Spanish)	Grilled beef, lamb, or pork
Bife à milanesa (Portuguese)	Thin-cut beef or pork that is battered and fried; usually served with wide-cut French fries
Biscoito de polvilho (Portuguese)	Crunchy snack made with tapioca starch
Bolinho de arroz (Portuguese)	Deep-fried rice cake made with milk and parsley
Bolinho de bacalhau (Portuguese)	Small, deep-fried codfish cake
Caldo marino (Spanish)	Chilean seafood stew
Ceviche (Spanish)	Raw fish marinated in lemon or lime juices, garlic, and onion; served at room temperature
Choclo (Spanish)	Toasted corn
Churrasco (Spanish or Portuguese)	Various grilled meats served on skewers and carved onto your plate
Coxinha (Portuguese)	Appetizer made from deep-fried dough filled with chicken

(continued)

Table 7.2   (continued)

Name (Language)	Description
Croquete de carne, de milho, de miolo (Portuguese)	Croquettes/deep-fried cakes filled with meat or other ingredients
Empadinha (de frango, de palmito) (Portuguese)	Small pies filled with chicken, hearts of palm, among other ingredients
Empanadas (Spanish)	Stuffed flaked pastry with meats and cheeses
Ensaladas mixtas a la vinagreta (Spanish)	Mixed greens salad with vinaigrette
Esfiha (Portuguese)	Small pie filled with meat, cheese or vegetables
Farofa (Portuguese)	Flour of tapioca with oil
Feijoada completa (Portuguese)	Black beans with pork meat dish served with white rice, kale and oranges
Fiambres (Spanish)/*Frios* (Portuguese)	Coldcut meats
Humitas (Spanish)	Cornmeal tamales stuffed with meats and cheeses
Kibe (Spanish)/*Quibe* (Portuguese)	Ground beef and wheat bulgur dish, fried or baked
Massas (Portuguese)	Pasta with red or white sauces, vegetables, meats/seafoods
Matambre (Spanish)	Literally translates as "hunger killer," a stuffed, rolled, grilled flank steak flavored with peppers and vegetables
Milanesa (Spanish)	Thin-cut beef, chicken or pork that is battered and fried; usually served with wide-cut French fries *(papas fritas)*
Misto quente (Portuguese)	Ham and cheese sandwich, served hot
Pamplona de pollo (Spanish)	Stuffed, rolled and grilled chicken breast
Pan de queso (Spanish)/*Pão de queijo* (Portuguese)	Bread or roll made with tapioca flour and cheese; served plain or filled with cream cheese or jelly
Panquecas (Portuguese)	Savory crepes filled with ground beef, creamed spinach, or cheese and ham
Parrillada (Spanish)	Grilled steak; various types of meat or chicken
Pastas (Spanish)	Pasta with red or white sauces, vegetables, meats/seafoods
Pastel de queijo, carne moída, or *palmito* (Portuguese)	Deep-fried or baked dough filled with cheese, or ground meat, hearts of palm, or other filling
Patacón (Spanish)	Fried and smashed green plantains
Pizza (Spanish and Portuguese)	Pizza made with meats and cheeses and/or vegetables
Rissolis (Portuguese)	Deep-fried dough filled with cheese, meat, and/or hearts of palm
Salada mista acom vinagrette (Portuguese)	Mixed vegetable salad with vinaigrette
Sándwich de jamón y queso (Spanish)	Ham and cheese sandwich, served hot
Sopas (Spanish and Portuguese)/*Sancochos* (Spanish)	Soups made with various ingredients such as vegetables, meats, spices; can be in broth or creamy base
Vatapá (Portuguese)	Shrimp and coconut milk based side dish
Beverages	
Agua de coco (Spanish)/*Água de coco* (Portuguese)	Coconut water
Café con leche (Spanish)/*Café com leite* (Portuguese)	Coffee with milk
Café pintado (Spanish)	Coffee with hot water
Café tinto or *café negro* (Spanish)/*Café preto* (Portuguese)	Very strong black coffee; usually the espresso size
Caipirinha (Portuguese)	Alcoholic drink made with *pinga* (sugar-cane liquor), sugar, ice and limes
Cerveza (Spanish)/*Cerveja* (Portuguese	Beer, malt liquor
Chá de ervas (Portuguese)	Herbal tea
Chá pretomate (Portuguese)	Black tea
Chá verde (Portuguese)	Green tea

(continued)

Table 7.2   *(continued)*

Name (Language)	Description
Chicha (Spanish)	Fermented drink made from maize, rice, or yucca
Chocolate caliente (Spanish)/*Chocolate quente* (Portuguese)	Hot chocolate/cocoa
Guaraná (Portuguese)	Soft drink made with guaraná fruit; available in regular and diet versions
Hervidas (Spanish)	Hot drinks made with *trago,* honey, and orange or blackberry juice
Jugo de frutas (Spanish)	Fruit juice
Laranjada (Portuguese)	Orange juice diluted in water
Licuado de frutas (Spanish)	Blended yogurt or milk and fruit
Limonada (Spanish or Portuguese)	Lemonade
Pinga or *aguardente* (Portguese)	Distilled sugar-cane liquor
Suco de frutas (Portuguese)	Fruit juice
Té de herbario or *agua aromáticas* or *yerbas* (Spanish)	Herbal tea
Té negro (Spanish)	Black tea
Té verde (Spanish)	Green tea
Trago (Spanish)	Distilled sugar-cane liquor
Vino blanco (Spanish)/*Vinho branco* (Portuguese)	White wine
Vino tinto (Spanish)/*Vinho tinto* (Portuguese)	Red wine
Vitamina (Portuguese)	Blended yogurt or milk and fruit
Desserts and sweets	
Abóbora com côco (Portuguese)	Pumpkin dessert with coconut
Alfajor (Spanish or Portuguese)	Crackers filled with condensed milk and covered in chocolate
Arroz dulce (Spanish)/*Arroz doce* (Portuguese)	Sweet rice pudding
Bocadillo, pasta de guayaba (Spanish)	Guava dessert (guava and sugar)
Bomba de chocolate/creme (Portuguese)	Chocolate or cream eclair/puff
Brigadeiro (Portuguese)	Chocolate fudge candy chocolate and condensed milk dessert
Budín de pan (Spanish)	Bread pudding usually served with dulce de leche
Cajuzinho (Portuguese)	Cashew nuts based dessert and condensed milk dessert
Churros con dulce de leche (Spanish)/ *Churros com doce de leite* (Portuguese)	Deep-fried dough (similar to a doughnut) with sweetened condensed milk filling
Dulce de leche or *cajeta* (Spanish)/*Doce de leite* (Portuguese)	Milk caramel syrup (made from cooking sweetened condensed milk)
Ensalada de frutas con helado (Spanish)	Fruit salad with ice cream or cream
Flan (Spanish or Portugese)	Flan, pudding, or custard made with milk and eggs; served with dulce de leche, fruit, and chocolate
Flan de coco (Spanish)	Coconut flan
Flan de leche (Spanish)	Pudding made from sweetened condensed milk with caramel sauce
Goiabada (Portuguese)	Guava dessert (guava and sugar)
Helado (Spanish)	Ice-cream
Helado en paleta (Spanish)	Fruit bar or popsicle
Manjar branco (Portuguese)	Coconut flan
Olho de sogra (Portuguese)	Prune, coconut, and condensed milk dessert
Pão de mel (Portuguese)	Honey cake
Pé de moleque (Portuguese)	Peanuts and sugar candy

(continued)

Table 7.2 *(continued)*

Name (Language)	Description
Picolé (Portuguese)	Fruit bar or popsicle
Pudim (Portuguese)	Pudding or custard made with milk and eggs
Pudim de leite (Portuguese)	Pudding made from sweetened condensed milk with caramel sauce
Pudim de pão (Portuguese)	Bread pudding usually served with dulce de leche
Quindim (Portuguese)	Egg-based dessert
Romeu e Julieta (Portuguese)	Guava dessert with fresh cheese
Salada de frutas com sorvete ou creme (Portuguese)	Fruit salad served with ice cream or cream
Sorvete (Portuguese)	Ice-cream
Tortas (Spanish or Portuguese)	Pies, cakes, or pastries with dulce de leche or fruit purees

Source: Data are from references 21–27.

Box 7.1 • Traditional Foods Consumed During Holidays

- Chocolate Easter eggs
- Codfish
- Cookies
- *Cuy* (guinea pig)
- Desserts, pies, cakes
- Fresh and dried fruits
- Ham
- *Hervidas* (hot drinks with *trago*, honey, and orange or blackberry juice)
- Nuts
- Panettone/*pan de pascua* (Christmas cake filled with candied fruits and raisins)
- *Parrilladas/asados/churrasco* (barbecue)
- Pork
- Rice
- Salads
- Seafood
- Turkey
- Wine

Source: Data are from reference 21.

Traditional Health Beliefs

Traditional South American health beliefs are rich and varied, and it is important to understand their specific role in each client's life. Many South Americans believe that certain foods, herbs, plants, or natural medications can cure chronic diseases. The use of Western medicine in combination with alternative/indigenous medicine is common (29–32).

Current Food Practices

South Americans in both the United States and their countries of origin are increasingly choosing processed foods. Many South American countries are experiencing a significant cultural "switch": individuals consume fewer staple foods (such rice and beans), and consumption of chicken, milk, eggs, vegetable oils, and processed foods is increasing (33). Snacking and the adaptation of traditional recipes are also becoming more common (1). In larger US cities, imported traditional foods are available in specialty shops and grocery stores, but individuals may choose to eat fast food for convenience.

Counseling Considerations

People of South American origin are not a uniform group, and they do not take a uniform path to acculturation in the United States. This diversity can present a challenge to counselors (34). Proper assessment of and respect for each client's culture is essential (35). Educational materials need to be culturally appropriate for the target audience. Factors to consider include the client's race/ethnicity, gender, age, education, income, and stage of readiness to change. Above all, you should focus on factors such as family structure, financial concerns, and eating habits that influence health behaviors (36). To identify these factors, prompt clients to elaborate on the context and circumstances of their relevant health behaviors. For example, ask how other people's behaviors or expectations affect the client or how certain changes in the meal plan may change the client's role and image in his or her family. To succeed in counseling, you should assess the barriers that could keep a client from achieving his or her goals, demonstrate respect for the client, and evaluate his or her learning style and reading level. The use of cultural metaphors and examples to deliver nutrition messages can also help you to reach your clients (37).

Language barriers can be a challenge. In many cases, a client who does not fully comprehend English will seem to agree and understand. If a client feels intimidated, he or she may become passive and not ask questions. A trained interpreter should be used if the counselor and client do not speak the same language.

Demonstrating Courtesy and Respect

Clients will look for verbal and nonverbal cues of your respect for them. It is difficult to generalize about South Americans' expectations in this regard, but the counseling relationship will benefit if you are courteous and take time to get to know each client on a personal level.

Interpreting Clients' Nonverbal Communication

When working with South American clients, observe how members of the community interact with each other, instead of relying on stereotypes or generalizations (38). For example, try observing how a client greets other people from his or her social circle. This can shed some light on what is expected and appropriate behavior in this specific group. South Americans tend to make eye contact and will typically face each other when they speak; they may also touch each other while talking (39).

Clients may be more satisfied with care received when nutrition educators express emotions through their body language (40). Most clients prefer that nutrition educators shake their hands, but you should observe the client for signs that such contact is welcome (41).

Inquiring About Clients' Understanding of Diabetes

It is important to assess each client's specific level of understanding of diabetes because there are substantial cultural and socioeconomic variations. In your evaluation, take into account the client's socioeconomic, literacy, education, and acculturation levels, as well as the depth of his or her connection with a community or country of origin.

Asking the client the right questions will help you determine his or her understanding of diabetes. For example, ask the client to summarize information covered in current or previous sessions, or ask what the client's family knows about diabetes and its treatment. Developing a personal relationship with client is essential to create open communication.

Discussing Clients' Use of Complementary and Alternative Medicine

Evidence is inconsistent and varied, but it has been suggested that more than half of people with diabetes are inclined to use complementary and alternative therapies in conjunction with conventional health care services (42,43). It is therefore important to evaluate the client's use of alternative medications and treatments or folk healers, as well as any fatalistic beliefs that little can be done to manage or prevent diabetes (44).

There are hundreds of South American herbal remedies (45). Hispanics have one of the highest rates of herbal use, but they may also be unlikely to disclose their use to health

Table 7.3 • Selected Remedies Used by South Americans for Self-Treatment of Diabetes

Spanish/Portuguese Name	English Name	Description/Preparation
Ajo/Alho	Garlic	Fresh garlic mashed and diluted in water
Alcachofa/Alcachofra	Artichoke	Herbal tea from base leaves of artichoke
Berenjena/Berinjela	Eggplant	Eggplant juice with lemon and water
Carqueja	Carqueja	Herbal tea from leaves of carqueja plant
Cebolla/Cebola	Onion	Onion juice diluted with water
Dente-de-leão/Amor-de-homen	Dandelion	Juice from dandelion leaves
Erva de passarinho		Tea from Struthanthus flexicaulis leaves
Eucalipto	Eucalyptus	Tea from eucalyptus leaves
Graviola	Graviola tree	Tea from leaves of graviola tree
Ipê-roxo/Ipê-Amarelo/Pau-d'Arco	Pau d'arco	Tea from inner bark of pau d'arco tree
Limón/Limão	Lemon	Lemon juice; the number of lemons used each day increases progressively
Manzana verde/Maçã verde	Green apples	Whole fresh green apples are believed to help with gastrointestinal problems, lower cholesterol and blood glucose
Pata-de-vaca/unha-de-vaca	Pata-de-vaca tree	Herbal tea from leaves of pata-de-vaca tree
Picão preto/amor-de-mulher/Pico-pico	Picão preto herb (a tropical plant)	Juice from leaves of picão preto herb
Chanca-piedra/Quebra-pedra	Breakstone (chanca piedra)	Herbal tea from leaves of chanca piedra (breakstone) herb
Salva/Salvia	Sage	Tea made from sage leaves; sage may also be burned to create smoke, which is believed to help to purify the spiritual energy around people and of the environment
Stevia/Estévia	Stevia	Natural sweetener

Source: Data are from references 1, 47, 48, and 49.

care professionals (46). Table 7.3 lists some of the many natural remedies used for treatment of diabetes and other conditions and diseases (1,47–49). Refer to Appendix C for questions to assess dietary supplement use.

Considering Family Demands and Dynamics

Family dynamics in South America may vary by region, economic status, culture, and education level. Women who are married and have children are less likely to work outside the home than women who are single (50). In traditional South American families, women may be primarily responsible for taking care of the house and the family, and therefore they will take the lead on meal planning and preparation. However, these women may be guided by their husbands' and children's food preferences when making food choices. To help clients succeed in diabetes management, counselors should consider the significance of gender roles in household labor and support (51).

Engaging Others in Counseling Sessions

South Americans are family-oriented and social people, whose health behaviors are greatly influenced by the people with whom they live and interact. Clients often indicate that meal planning choices depend in part on the food preferences of family members and friends.

Clients can benefit from a community-based, family-oriented intervention that provides social support to promote healthful lifestyles (52). In addition to one-on-one counseling, group interventions, such as culinary demonstrations, games, interactive activities, and presentations, may succeed because they combine education with social elements.

Nutrition Counseling

Today's nutrition educator facilitates behavior changes. The counselor partners with clients, motivating them to make choices among options; and helping them address their thoughts, feelings, and behaviors. This counseling approach promotes the client's independence, and its success is measured subjectively (53).

The nutrition assessment should cover the specific foods consumed, as well as food preparation methods, the timing and frequency of meals, and usual portion sizes (37). Be sure to assess each client's potential barriers to dietary adherence, such as socioeconomic limitations, literacy skills, education level, and learning style (35). Appendix B offers selected medical nutrition therapy recommendations for individuals with diabetes and general counseling suggestions that support those recommendations.

Challenges and Barriers to Dietary Compliance

Culture, poverty, and acculturation levels can greatly affect dietary compliance and consequent health outcomes (54). Although poverty rates are higher among Hispanics in the United States than non-Hispanic whites, the all-cause mortality rate is lower for Hispanics—this is known as the Latino mortality paradox (55). Among Hispanics in general, higher levels of acculturation are associated with the following: lower intake of fruits and vegetables; higher consumption of fats, alcohol, and drinks with refined sugar; smoking; and higher BMI; however, the likelihood of exercise increases with acculturation (55,56). On the other hand, lower levels of acculturation are related to healthier diets (57–59), lower blood pressure and cholesterol values, and lower rates of smoking and type 2 diabetes (60).

Counseling Tips

Consider the following key strategies for the nutrition education sessions:

- Use visual aids to illustrate nutrition concepts.
- Choose individualized and interactive (hands-on) activities, such as games and demonstrations, to provide knowledge and increase self-efficacy and skills.
- Look for opportunities to include the whole family.
- Use written or videotaped testimonials from other similar clients (preferably told by these clients themselves) and culturally appropriate materials.
- In written materials, include spaces for the client to make notes.
- Provide samples of foods and demonstrate culinary techniques when you introduce new foods and nutrition concepts to clients.

Resources

US Resources in Spanish

American Diabetes Association Spanish Web site. http://www.diabetes.org/espanol. Accessed February 23, 2009.

Centers for Disease Control and Prevention Web site in Spanish. http://www.cdc.gov/spanish. Accessed February 23, 2009.

Latino Nutrition Coalition. http://www.latinonutrition.org. Accessed February 23, 2009.

National Diabetes Education Program. Diabetes Education Materials in Spanish. http://www.ndep.nih.gov/diabetes/pubs/catalog.htm. Accessed February 23, 2009.

National Diabetes Information Clearinghouse. Information in Spanish. http://diabetes.niddk.nih.gov/spanish/index.asp. Accessed February 23, 2009.

South American Resources

Tabela Brasileira de Composição de Alimentos—TACO. Versão 2—Segunda Edição [Nutrition Information of Brazilian Foods from the University of Campinas in Brazil; document is in Portuguese]. http://www.unicamp.br/nepa/taco/contar/taco_versao2.pdf. Accessed February 23, 2009.

Asociacion Latinoamericana de Diabetes (ALAD) [Latin American Diabetes Association; site available in Spanish or Portuguese only]. http://www.pitt.edu/~iml1/diabetes/ALAD.html. Accessed February 23, 2009.

Sociedade Brasileira de Diabetes [Brazilian Diabetes Society; site available in Portuguese only]. http://www.diabetes.org.br. Accessed February 23, 2009.

Sociedad Argentina de Diabetes [Argentinean Diabetes Society; site available in Spanish only]. http://www.diabetes.org.ar. Accessed February 23, 2009.

References

1. Kittler P, Sucher K. Caribbean Islanders and South Americans. In: Bahlinger L, Boyd J, Craig S, Keough S, Larson L, eds. *Food and Culture*. 3rd ed. Belmont, CA: Wadsworth/Thomson Learning; 2001:227–254.

2. Vlahou A. Vaticano: Católicos são 17.3% da população mundial. BBC Brazil. http://www.bbc.co.uk/portuguese/reporterbbc/story/2007/04/070424_vaticano_estatisticasrg.shtml. Accessed August 26, 2007.

3. Religion and Theology—Regional Resources. Latin American Network Information Center (LANIC). http://lanic.utexas.edu/la/region/religion. Accessed August 16, 2007.

4. Fernandes RC. Religião [Religion]. Ministério das Relações Exteriores [Brazilian Ministry of Foreign Relations]. http://www.mre.gov.br/cdbrasil/itamaraty/web/port/artecult/religiao/apresent/index.htm. Accessed August 16, 2007.

5. US Census Bureau. Glossary—Spanish/Hispanic/Latino. http://factfinder.census.gov/home/en/epss/glossary_s.html#spanish_hispanic_latino. Accessed July 23, 2007.

6. US Census Bureau. QT-P9. Hispanic or Latino by Type: 2000. http://factfinder.census.gov/servlet/QTTable?_bm=y&-geo_id=01000US&-qr_name=DEC_2000_SF1_U_QTP9&-ds_name=DEC_2000_SF1_U. Accessed July 23, 2007.

7. Boutayeb A, Boutayeb S. The burden of non communicable diseases in developing countries. *Int J Equity Health*. 2005;14:4:2.

8. International Diabetes Federation. *Diabetes Atlas*. 2nd ed. Brussels, Belgium: International Diabetes Federation; 2003.

9. Centers for Disease Control and Prevention. Fact Sheet: Prevalence of Diabetes Among Hispanics in Six U.S. Geographic Locations from 1998 to 2002. http://www.cdc.gov/diabetes/pubs/pdf/hispanic.pdf. Accessed July 25 2007.

10. World Diabetes Foundation. Annual Review. 2006. http://www.worlddiabetesfoundation.org/media(3466,1033)/WDFAR06Singlepages.pdf.pdf. Accessed July 23, 2007.

11. Moore PA, Zgibor JC, Dasanayake AP. Diabetes: a growing epidemic of all ages. *J Am Diet Assoc*. 2003;134(suppl):11S–15S.

12. Almeida GAN, Santos JE, Pasian SR, Loureiro SR. Percepção de tamanho e forma corporal de mulheres: estudo exploratório [Perceptions of body shape and size in women: an exploratory study]. *Psicol Estud*. 2005;10:27–35. http://www.scielo.br/pdf/pe/v10n1/v10n1a04.pdf. Accessed Aug 31, 2008.

13. Serra GMA, Santos EM. Saúde e mídia na construção da obesidade e do corpo perfeito [Health and media in the construction of obesity and perfect body]. *Ciênc Saúde Coletiva*. 2003; 8:691–701. http://www.scielo.br/pdf/csc/v8n3/17450.pdf. Accessed Aug 31, 2008.

14. Rewers M, Hamman RF. Risk factors for non-insulin-dependent diabetes. In: *Diabetes in America*. 2nd ed. http://diabetes.niddk.nih.gov/dm/pubs/america/pdf/chapter9.pdf. Accessed July 15, 2007.

15. Monteiro CA, Mondini L, de Souza AL, Popkin BM. The nutrition transition in Brazil. *Eur J Clin Nutr*. 1995;49:105–113.

16. Monteiro CA, Benicio MH, Conde WL, Popkin BM. Shifting obesity trends in Brazil. *Eur J Clin Nutr*. 2000;54:342–346.

17. Braguinsky J. Prevalencia de obesidad en America Latina [Obesity prevalence in Latin America]. *ANALES SIS San Navarra*. 2002;25(Suppl 1):S109-S115. http://www.cfnavarra.es/salud/anales/textos/vol25/sup1/pdf/25s110.pdf. Accessed August 6, 2007.

18. Philippi ST. Brazilian Food Pyramid. *Nutrition Today*. 2005;40(2):1–5.

19. Castillo C, Atalah E, Benavides X, Urteaga C. Food patterns in Chilean adults from the metropolitan region. *Rev Med Chil*. 1997;125:283–289.

20. Jaime PC, Monteiro CA. Fruit and vegetable intake by Brazilian adults. 2003. *Cad Saúde Pública*. 2005;21:S19–S24.

21. Philippi ST. *Tabela de Composição de Alimentos: Suporte para Decisão Nutricional*. Sao Paulo, Brazil: Anvisa, Finatect/Nut-UnB; Brasília, DF; 2001.

22. Latino Nutrition Coalition. Latino ingredients, A to Z. Available at: http://www.latinonutrition.org/LatinoFoodsAtoZ.html. Accessed July 10, 2007.

23. Philippi ST. *Nutrição e Técnica Dietética*. 2nd ed. São Paulo, Brazil: Manole; 2008.

24. American Heart Association. *Around the World: Healthy Recipes with International Flavor Cookbook.* New York, NY: Random House; 1996.

25. Discovery Channel. *Insight Guide: Ecuador and Galápagos.* Maspeth, NY. Apa Puplications; 2000.

26. National Cancer Institute. *Celebre la Cocina Hispana: Healthy Hispanic Recipes.* Bethesda, MD: National Institutes of Health; 2000.

27. Núcleo de Estudos e Pesquisas em Alimentação—NEPA. Universidade Estadual de Campinas—UNICAMP. Tabela Brasileira de Composição de Alimentos. 2nd ed. 2006. http://www.unicamp .br/nepa/taco/contar/taco_versao2.pdf. Accessed July 7, 2007.

28. Bleil SI. O Padrão Alimentar Ocidental: considerações sobre a mudança de hábitos no Brasil. *Cadernos de Debate.* 1998;1–25. http://www.unicamp.br/nepa/arquivo_san/O_Padrao_ Alimentar_Ocidental.pdf. Accessed Aug 31, 2008.

29. Reyes-García V, Godoy R, Vadez V, Apaza L, Byron E, Huanca, Leonard WR, Pérez E, Wilkie D. Ethnobotanical knowledge shared widely among Tsimane' Amerindians, Bolivia. *Science.* 2003;299:1707.

30. Miranda JJ, Nuñez H, Alca A. Traditional healers, still part of the community health systems in the Andes. *J Epidemiol Coummun Health.* 2002;56:733.

31. Miller MJ, MacNaughton WK, Zhang XJ, Thompson JH, Charbonnet RM, Bobrowski P, Lao J, Trentacosti AM, Sandoval M. Treatment of gastric ulcers and diarrhea with Amazonian herbal medicine sangre de grado *Am J Physiol Gastrointest Liver Physiol.* 2000;279:G192–G200.

32. Kitajima M, Hashimoto K, Sandoval M, Aimi N, Takayama H. New oleanan-type triterpene and cincholic acid glycosides from Peruvian "Uña de Gato" *(Uncaria tomentosa). Chem Pharm Bull.* 2004;52:1258-1261.

33. de Oliveira SP. Changes in food consumption in Brazil. *Arch Latinoam Nutr.* 1997;47 (2 Suppl 1):22–24.

34. Aguirre-Molina M, Molina C. Latino population: who are they? In: Molina C, Aguirre-Molina M, eds. *Latino Health in the United States: A Growing Challenge.* Washington, DC: American Public Health Association; 1994:3–22.

35. Brown T. Meal planning strategies: ethnic populations. *Diabetes Spectrum.* 2003;16:190-192.

36. Gehling E. The next step: stage-matching your patient education materials. *Diabetes Care and Education Newsflash.* 2002;23:24–26.

37. Tripp-Reimer T, Choi E, Kelly LS, Enslein JC. Cultural barriers to care: inverting the problem. *Diabetes Spectrum.* 2001:14:13–22.

38. Encina GB. Cultural Differences? Or, Are We Really That Different? http://www.cnr.berkeley.edu/ ucce50/ag-labor/7article/article01.htm. Accessed August 26, 2007.

39. Argyle M. *Bodily Communication.* 2nd ed. London, England: Methuen; 1988.

40. DiMatteo MR, Taranta A, Friedman HS, Prince LM,. Predicting patient satisfaction from physicians' nonverbal communication skills. *Med Care.* 1980;18:376–387.

41. Makoul G, Zick A, Green M. An evidence-based perspective on greetings in medical encounters. *Arch Intern Med.* 2007;167:1172-1176.

42. Teixeira ER, de Nogueira JF. Uso popular das ervas terapêuticas no cuidado com o corpo [The popular use of therapeutic herbs in body care]. *Rev Gaúcha Enferm.* 2005;26:231–241.

43. Chang HY, Wallis M, Tiralongo E. Use of complementary and alternative medicine among people living with diabetes: literature review. *J Adv Nurs.* 2007;58:307–319.

44. Walker E, Caban A. A systematic review of research on culturally relevant issues for Hispanics with diabetes. *Diabetes Educ.* 2006;32:584–595.

45. Di Stasi LC, Oliveira GP, Carvalhaes MA, Queiroz M Jr, Tien OS, Kakinami SH, Reis MS. Medicinal plants popularly used in the Brazilian tropical Atlantic forest. *Fitoterapia.* 2002;73:69–91.

46. Kuo GM, Hawley ST, Weiss LT, Balkrishnan R, Volk RJ. Factors associated with herbal use among urban multiethnic primary care patients: a cross-sectional survey. *BMC Complement Altern Med.* 2004;4:18.

47. Spethmann CN. *Medicina Alternativa de A a Z* [Alternative Medicine from A to Z]. 6th ed. Uberlandia, Brazil: Ed. Natureza;. 2000.

48. Coutinho V. Projeto Sementinha—Nossos Chás—2000. http://www.cpcd.org.br/livro/ervas.pdf. Accessed Aug 27, 2007.

49. Casas Pedro. Enciclopédia das Plantas e Ervas. http://www.casaspedro.com.br/Plantaservas.htm. Accessed Aug 27, 2007.

50. Psaharopoulos G, Tzannatos Z. Economic and demographic effects on working women in Latin America. *J Popul Econ.* 1993;6:293–315.

51. Wong M, Gucciardi E, Li L, Grace SL. Gender and nutrition management in type 2 diabetes. *Can J Diet Pract Res.* 2005;66:215–220.

52. Thornton PL, Kieffer EC, Salabarría-Peña Y, Odoms-Young A, Willis SK, Kim H, Salinas MA. Weight, diet, and physical activity-related beliefs and practices among pregnant and postpartum Latino women: the role of social support. *Matern Child Health J.* 2006;10:95–104.

53. Mendonça DRB. A importância da Educação Nutricional [The importance of nutrition education]. Sociedade Brasileira de Diabetes [Brazilian Diabetes Society]. http://www.diabetes.org.br/ Colunistas/Nutricao_e_Ciencia/index.php?id=1005. Accessed Aug 26, 2007.

54. Balcazar H, Castro FG, Krull JL. Cancer risk reduction in Mexican American women: the role of acculturation, education, and health risk factors. *Health Educ Q.* 1995;22:61–84.

55. Abraído-Lanza AF, Chao MT, Flórez KR. Do healthy behaviors decline with greater acculturation? Implications for the Latino mortality paradox. *Soc Sci Med.* 2005;61:1243–1255.

56. Prez-Escamilla R, Putnik P. The role of acculturation in nutrition, lifestyle, and incidence of type 2 diabetes among Latinos. *J Nutr.* 2007;137:860–870.

57. Dixon LB, Sundquist J, Winkleby M. Differences in energy, nutrient, and food intakes in a US sample of Mexican-American women and men: findings from the Third National Health and Nutrition Examination Survey, 1988–1994. *Am J Epidemiol.* 2000;152:548–557.

58. Marks G, Garcia M, Solis JM. Health risk behaviors of Hispanics in the United States: findings from NHANES, 1982–84. *Am J Public Health.* 1990;80:20–26.

59. Guendelman S, Abrams B. Dietary intake among Mexican-American women: generational differences and a comparison with white non-Hispanic women. *Am J Public Health.* 1995;85:202–205.

60. Sundquist J, Winkleby MA. Cardiovascular risk factors in Mexican American adults: a transcultural analysis of NHANES III, 1988–1994. *Am J Public Health.* 1999;89:723–730.

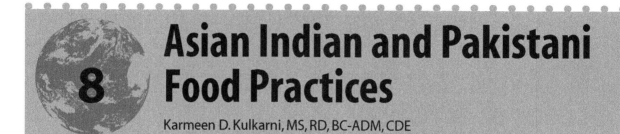

8 Asian Indian and Pakistani Food Practices

Karmeen D. Kulkarni, MS, RD, BC-ADM, CDE

Introduction

Pakistan and India are located in South Asia. Known collectively as India during the British Empire, they were separated and established as independent nations in 1947. (At that time, Bangladesh was part of Pakistan; it became independent in 1971.) Although Indians and Pakistanis share some common food practices (1), the cuisines of South Asia are diverse, in part because of the wide variety of religions practiced in this region.

Hindus comprise 80.4% of India's population. Religious minorities include Muslims (13.4%), Christians (2.3%), Sikhs (1.9%), Buddhists (1.1%), Jains (0.4%), and Parsis, Jews, and others (0.5%) (2). India's official language is Hindi, but because of British influence before 1947, English is spoken nationwide. In addition, approximately 850 other languages and dialects are spoken.

In Pakistan, Urdu is the official language. English is also widely spoken, and there are numerous other languages and dialects. Most Pakistanis are Muslim. In addition, Pakistan has Christian, Parsi, and Hindu minorities (1).

In 1980 the US Census Bureau first designated the terms "Pakistani" and "Asian Indian" to describe immigrants from the Asian subcontinent (3). Together, these ethnic groups are one of the fastest-growing populations in the United States. In the 2000 Census, Indians comprised 15% of the US Asian population, making them the third largest group of Asian Americans (after Chinese and Filipino Americans) (2). The Pakistani community in the United States is smaller, but growing in size.

Diabetes Prevalence

Environmental factors affect the prevalence of diabetes in various ethnic groups, including Asian Indians (4). In rural India, prevalence is between 2% and 6%, whereas prevalence in urban India is 12% (5). Diabetes prevalence in Asian Indians living in Western nations is approximately 4 times greater than overall rates for individuals living in India (4). This data suggest that urbanization and Westernization increase diabetes prevalence in Asian Indians. However, lifestyle and environmental factors are not the only diabetes risk factors—as Abate and Chandalia have noted, diabetes is more prevalent in Asian Indian populations than in people of European descent living in the same environmental conditions (4).

Risk Factors for Type 2 Diabetes

Compared with whites in the United States or other Western countries, Asian Indians in the United States have lower rates of obesity. However, the risk for insulin resistance and diabetes increases at a lower body mass index (BMI) in Indians and other Asians than in people of European descent—the BMI cut-off is 23 for Asian Indians, compared with 25 for whites (4,6). The World Health Organization defines the normal BMI for Asians as between 18.5 and 22 (4).

Traditional Foods and Dishes

Eating and social life are intertwined in India and Pakistan, as they are elsewhere in the world. Traditional dishes include grains cooked with vegetables; legumes cooked with vegetables; milk products combined with vegetables or fruits; and grains combined with meat, poultry, or seafood. Meals are traditionally served on *thalis* (brass, stainless steel, or silver plates) or on fresh banana leaves and *katoris* (small bowls). Indian and Pakistani cuisines include a wide variety of snacks and desserts for social occasions. Many traditional snacks are high in fat, sugar, and/or salt. Milk desserts predominate in these cuisines and are made by gently evaporating whole milk with sugar and butter to varying degrees of sweetness, color, and consistency, and adding nuts, lentils, grains, and/or flavorings (7).

Alcoholic beverages are forbidden in Islam, so observant Muslims from India and Pakistan do not consume alcohol. (See Chapter 15 for more information on Islamic food practices.) However, among the Asian Indian and Pakistani populations in the United States, alcohol consumption may be understood as a personal choice.

With a few regional differences (discussed in the next section), traditional Asian Indian and Pakistani meals include variations of the following:

- Homemade bread
- Rice
- *Dal* (legume-based dishes)
- Sautéed vegetables
- Meats, poultry, fish, and eggs for nonvegetarians
- Roasted or fried wafers, chutneys, pickle salads, and other condiments and flavors to enhance the meal
- Plain yogurt, buttermilk, or *raita* (yogurt with cucumber or tomatoes)
- Desserts
- Spiced tea or coffee
- Mouth fresheners, such as betel leaves, nuts, or fennel seeds
- Water (usually filtered or boiled in India), which is usually the preferred beverage with a meal

The meaning of the term "curry" in this cuisine is different from the typical Western definition. To Indians and Pakistanis, curry can refer to any spicy stir-fried vegetable dish or gravy dishes with meat or vegetables. South Asians do not use a single type of curry powder. Instead, they mix various spices and condiments in different proportions for particular dishes; many curries have regional variations (1,7). Dishes are seasoned with salt to taste. See Box 8.1 and Table 8.1 for additional information about traditional foods. Refer to Appendix A for nutrient analyses.

Traditional Meal Patterns and Holiday Foods

As mentioned previously, most South Asian meals feature some variation of rice, *dal*, meat or eggs, condiments, and desserts. Beverages include spiced tea, coffee, and water. However, food practices vary according to each region's agricultural production, and these variations affect the nutrition profile of the foods consumed. For example, all regions of India eat rice and wheat; however, wheat is the staple grain of the north, and rice is the staple grain of the south. Spiced and sweetened tea with milk is favored in the north, spiced tea is enjoyed in the west, and coffee is preferred in the south.

Box 8.1 • Foods Used in Traditional Asian Indian and Pakistani Cuisine

Grains
- Rice, including basmati rice
- Wheat

Legumes
- Black-eyed peas
- Chickpeas
- Lentils
- Pink beans (valore)

Starchy vegetables
- Corn
- Peas
- Plantains
- Potatoes
- Pumpkin
- Squash, green, yellow, acorn, or butternut
- Sweet potatoes
- Yams

Nonstarchy vegetables
- Bean sprouts, mung
- Beets (chukander)
- Bitter melon (karela)
- Bottle gourd (lauki)
- Brussels sprouts
- Cabbage
- Carrots (gajar)
- Cauliflower (gobi)
- Celery
- Cluster beans (guvar)
- Cucumber
- Drumsticks (surgavo)
- Eggplant (brinjal)
- Green beans
- Green papaya
- Greens, collard, kale, mustard, turnip
- Okra
- Onions (kanda)
- Peppers and chilies, green, yellow, red
- Radishes (muli)
- Ridge gourds (torai or turia)
- Spinach (palak)
- Tomatoes

Fruits
- Apples
- Apricots
- Bananas (many varieties)
- Figs
- Grapes
- Guava
- Jambu (also known as jamun)
- Lychee
- Loquat
- Mangoes (many varieties)
- Oranges
- Papayas
- Passionfruit
- Raisin, black or golden (kismish)
- Sweet limes

Milk products
- Condensed milk
- Dahi (homemade yogurt or curd)
- Lassi (buttermilk)
- Plain yogurt

Meats and meat substitutes
- Chicken
- Eggs
- Fish
- Shellfish
- Goat
- Lamb
- Lentils and other legumes
- Paneer (homemade cheese)

Fats and oils
- Butter
- Canola and peanut oil
- Ghee (clarified butter)
- Nuts: almonds (badam), cashews (kaju), peanuts (singdana)

(continued)

Box 8.1 *(continued)*

Herbs and spices

- *Amchur*
- Aniseed *(ajowain)*
- Asafoetida *(hing)*
- Bay leaf *(tej patta)*
- Black pepper *(kali mirchi)*
- Cardamom *(eliachi)*
- Chilies *(mirchi)*
- Chili paste *(sambal oelek)*
- Cinnamon *(dalchini)*
- Clove *(lavung)*
- Coconut *(nariyal)*
- Coriander, fresh (cilantro)
- Coriander seeds *(dhaniya)*
- Cumin *(jeera)*
- Dill *(suva bhaji)*
- Fennel *(saunf)*
- Fenugreek *(methi)*

- Garam masala (Indian spice blend)
- Garlic *(lasoon)*
- Ginger *(adarak)*
- Jaggery/palm sugar *(gur)*
- Mango powder *(amchoor)*
- Mint *(hara pudeena)*
- Mustard *(sarasoon)*
- Nutmeg *(jaiphal)*
- Onion seeds *(kalonji)*
- Parsley *(ajmood ka patta)*
- Pomegranate seeds *(anardana)*
- Poppy seeds *(khus khus)*
- Saffron *(kesar)*
- Sesame seeds *(til)*
- Tamarind *(imli)*
- Turmeric *(haldi)*

Table 8.1 · Traditional Indian and Pakistani Dishes, Breads, Beverages, and Desserts

Name	Description
Dishes	
Aviyal	South Indian dish of vegetables in gravy, with coconut and buttermilk
Channa	Chickpeas cooked in a tomato gravy with onions and spices
Chicken *tikka*	Pieces of boneless, skinless, broiled chicken marinated with spices
Chutney	Sweet or salty dip or relish
Curry	Dry vegetable or gravy dishes eaten with the main starch of the meal
Dal	Lentil dishes; many types of lentils are used individually or in combination, either dry or in gravy
Dhansak	Vegetable-lentil dish
Dhokla	Steamed dish made from lentils
Idli	South Indian steamed dish made from a fermented rice and lentil batter
Kebab	Generic term for broiled, skewered pieces of meat or vegetables, popular in Pakistan
Kadhi	Sauce made from diluted yogurt mixed with chickpea flour
Kheema	Spicy minced meat dish
Khichadi	Mixture of split mung and rice
Kofta	Round, deep-fried fritters made of cheese or vegetables and gram flour, soaked in gravy
Korma	Spicy curry dish consisting of different vegetables, sometimes a meat, and a gravy of yogurt and nuts
Matki usal	Sprouted mung bean dish with seasonings such as onions, garlic, and coriander
Poha	Beaten rice dish, which can also be prepared with vegetables
Raita	Light yogurt dish that often includes a vegetable, such as cucumber
Sambar	Spicy *toor* dal (yellow lentil) gravy from southern India, often made with vegetables and eaten with rice, *idli*, or *dosa*

(continued)

Table 8.1   *(continued)*

Name	Description
Tandoori chicken, fish, or lamb	Marinated meat in yogurt with a spice marinade, baked in a tandoor clay oven
Uppuma	Cereal dish made from cream of wheat seasoned with spices
Vada	Battered and fried vegetables served as an appetizer
Breads	
Batura	Mildly leavened bread made with added fat
Chapati	Flat bread, often made fresh just before the meal
Dosa	Southern Indian pan-fried crepe made from a soaked and fermented rice-mung dal batter
Naan	North Indian or Pakistani fermented bread made from flour and yogurt and baked and broiled in a clay oven
Papad/papadum	Indian flat bread similar in shape to a tortilla; can be deep-fried or roasted
Paratha	Shallow, fried wheat bread, which may be stuffed with vegetables, eggs, or meat
Pesrattu	Pan-fried lentil crepe, which may have added garnishes, such as onions
Puris	Deep-fried bread
Thepla	Flat bread made with wheat flour, gram flour, and spices
Beverages	
Chai masala	Spiced tea with added milk and sugar
Jheera pani	Watery drink made from cumin seeds
Kheer	Milk-based dessert drink with many additions, such as cereal, lentils, nuts, and fruits
Lassi	Buttermilk or yogurt drink, often diluted, to which salt or sugar is added for flavoring
Masala milk	Spiced milk
Rasam	Spicy, watery soup believed to help indigestion
Sharbat	Cool refreshing drink made from fruit juice
Desserts	
Halwa	Generic term for a common dessert made from wheat, nuts, sugar, and often vegetables; also can be made with carrots or beets
Ice creams, fruit-flavored	
Kulfi	Ice cream made from thickened milk with cardamom, saffron, slivered almonds, and often mango pulp
Laddu	Round, sometimes fried, sweet ball of lentil flour, semolina, or puffed rice
Mithai	Wide range of sweet snacks or desserts
Sooji	Semolina or cream of wheat

Northern Indian Meal Patterns

In northern India, breakfast and the midday meal may be a few servings of unleavened bread with a richly spiced meat, poultry, or fish curry or *dal;* a vegetable dish with yogurt; and spiced pickles. The evening meal is similar, although it typically includes an additional course of rice, a lentil dish, and a fresh salad or a cooked vegetable *(subji)*. Desserts are rich in whole milk, nuts, and ghee (clarified butter). Spiced, sweetened tea is a beverage of choice at any time of day. Popular cold summer beverages are freshly made sweetened lemonade *(nimbu-pani),* mango drinks, and other homemade fruit drinks. Cooking fats are hydrogenated vegetable oil and mustard oil (7).

Eastern Indian Meal Patterns

Bengal and Orissa are states in the eastern part of India. Bengalis tend to eat meals in courses, whereas this is not typical in Orissa. Rice is a staple food of this region. Fish curry, deep-fried and stewed vegetable dishes, and *dal* are typical. The food is not as heavily spiced as in other parts of India, although many dishes are seasoned with a mixture of mustard, coriander, and fenugreek seeds, and the Northern cuisines often incorporate hot, bitter, sour, and sweet flavors (7).

Southern Indian Meal Patterns

In southern India, meals are typically served on a freshly cut and washed banana leaf. Lunch and dinner typically include three courses with rice as the staple. The first two courses include lentil gravies as well as a stew of tomatoes, onions, and vegetables (eg, *sambar* or *aviyal*). The third course is *thair sadam,* a dish of rice and homemade yogurt or fresh curds. The condiments served with meals include pickles, chutneys, and fried wafers *(pappadums)*. Desserts are served on special occasions. Breakfasts include similar foods, but with less variation.

There are some subregional variations within southern India cuisine. For example, residents of Kerala use shredded coconut, coconut oil, fried plantain chips, and fish in a variety of dishes; the cuisine of Andhra Pradesh is especially spicy; and Karnataka cooking emphasizes dishes made with grains and lentils. Sesame, peanut, and hydrogenated vegetable oils are used as cooking fats (1).

Western Indian Meal Patterns

The states of Maharashtra, Goa, and Gujarat are on the coast of the Arabian Sea, and fish dishes are common in this region. In the coastal areas, individuals eat fresh fish. Salted, dried, and preserved fish are more common inland. A typical lunch or dinner begins with a course of boiled rice with *dal*, a teaspoon of ghee, and lemon; a curry of legumes, meat, poultry, or fish; a salad with yogurt; one or two vegetable dishes; and *puris* (fried bread). The next course is a rice or grain and vegetable mixture, such as *pulav*. Sesame seeds and peanuts are used in cooking. The meal ends with rice and buttermilk. Desserts are also served along with meals. Similar foods are eaten for breakfast, although the variety of dishes is usually more limited. The people of Gujarat are usually vegetarians and their cuisine includes many grain and lentil or vegetable and lentil dishes (1).

People from the Kutch district of Gujarat typically eat warm milk with sugar, *khakhada* (wheat wafer), and *makkhan* (clarified butter) for breakfast. Their lunch always includes a green chutney made of coriander leaves. Lunch and dinner both include *khichadi* (a mixture of split mung beans and rice), *kaddhi* (diluted yogurt mixed with chickpea flour), *baira no rotlo* (an iron-rich grain), *bijora nu athanu* (pickle), and *gur* (jaggery/palm sugar). Snacks include tea with milk, sugar, and masala (tea spices); *ukado* (diluted milk with special spices); *limbu pani* (lemon, sugar, and water); or coconut water.

Pakistani Meal Patterns

Wheat, rice, and corn are staples of the Pakistani diet. Wheat is the main ingredient in homemade breads, such as *chapatti, naan,* and *paratha. Dal* is a legume dish eaten with homemade breads. Chickpea flour is an ingredient in a variety of foods and also used in batter for frying fish, chicken, or vegetables. Muslim Pakistanis do not eat pork, but other types of meat—especially goat, chicken, and lamb—are popular. Kebabs (grilled meats), *kormas* (stews or casseroles), and deep-fried meat *koftas* are the most common meat dishes. Fish is popular in the coastal areas. Dairy items commonly include *dahi* (yogurt or curd), *lassi* (a diluted yogurt beverage), milk, and *paneer* (homemade cheese). Nuts, such as pistachios, cashews, and peanuts, are usually eaten in the winter months; they are also used in desserts and other dishes. Many herbs and seasonings, such as garlic, onions, ginger, and turmeric, are commonly used in food preparation.

Holiday Foods

Many South Asian holidays and religious observances involve fasting. Feasts, too, are important in Indian and Pakistani celebrations. Feasting and fasting activities are complex and vary greatly from person to person and group to group. (See Chapter 15 for more information on Islamic practices.) Feasts typically involve foods that are high in fat and sugar, and it may be socially unacceptable to decline foods.

Table 8.2 · Traditional Desserts and Sweets Consumed During Indian Holidays

Name	Description
Northern India and Pakistan	
Barfi	Similar to a bar cookie made with ghee, milk, and nuts
Gulab jamun	Doughnut-like balls soaked in a rose-flavored sugar syrup
Halwa	Sweet made with milk, sugar, ghee, and sometimes nuts
Jalebi	Fried in circle shapes, made with chickpea flour and dipped in sugar syrup
Peda	Sweet made with milk, ghee, and sugar
Rice kheer	Milk-based liquid dessert with many additions, such as cereals, lentils, nuts, and fruits
Southern India	
Ladu	Ball-shaped sweet made with chickpea flour and sugar
Payasam	Sweet dish made with milk, sugar, rice, or dal
Sweet *pongal*	Sweet cooked rice
Eastern India	
Mistidoi	Milk-based dessert
Rasogulla	Milk-based dessert in sugar syrup
Ras Malai	Milk-based dessert
Sandesh	Milk-based dessert
Western India	
Besan ladu	Made from besan flour and sugar
Dudhpak	Sweetened milk with dry fruit
Mango *ras*	Mango juice
Sutarfeni and *sev*	Sweet semolina
Shrikand	Milk-based dessert

Most Pakistanis are Muslims, and in the Islamic culture it is customary to give sweets to commemorate special events, such as including weddings, festivals, religious celebrations, or the birth of a child (1,7). Sweets are also popular at Indian holidays, such as the Hindi celebrations of Diwali and Holi. See Table 8.2 for traditional holiday desserts.

Traditional Health Beliefs

Religion influences the health beliefs and food choices of most Asian Indians and Pakistanis. Hindus may or may not be vegetarians, but most do not eat beef or pork. Muslims avoid all pork and pork products, but they are not vegetarians (see Chapter 15).

Orthodox Jains are vegetarians, who also avoid eating root vegetables (such as beet, carrots, garlic, ginger, *mogri, muda,* onions, and potatoes) because insects might be killed when the tubers are harvested (8). Jains also do not eat blood-colored foods. Traditional Jain beliefs clearly advocate moderation even when eating healthful foods. Obesity is discouraged, and the laws of food consumption dictate that the solid food should fill half the stomach, liquid one-fourth, and the remainder left for the process of digestion (1).

Current Food Practices

As Indians and Pakistanis in the United States become acculturated, their dietary patterns tend to shift from an emphasis on low-fat and high-fiber foods (such as vegetables and legumes) to a diet high in saturated fat and animal protein and low in fiber. Consumption of fast food and convenience foods also increases (9,10). In addition to increasing diabetes risk, these changes in diet may increase clients' risk for obesity, hypertension, cardiovascular disease, and certain types of cancer.

Counseling Considerations

Diabetes self-care is a challenge for any person with diabetes, but it can present distinctive challenges for Asian Indian and Pakistani clients (11). For example, they may not understand the connection between body weight and diabetes risk or accept the advice of health care providers regarding weight management. In an interview-based study of 106 Kashmiri men with diabetes in Leeds, United Kingdom, Naeem reported that most participants were overweight but did not believe that they were (12). It is important for registered dietitians (RDs) to consider cultural standards when counseling clients about body weight, BMI, and diabetes management.

Asian Indians and Pakistanis may have fatalistic attitudes about diabetes and its management. They may believe that the condition is caused by divine power and accept it as inevitable, making them less motivated for self-care (12,13). RDs working with this population should assess each client's understanding of the causes of diabetes and then educate clients on how their well-being will improve with self-care. It may be helpful to emphasize that self-care makes them better able to care for their families. In addition, if the client consents, the RD may wish to involve family members so they understand self-care concepts and can support the client's efforts.

Physical Activity

Compared with whites, Asian Indians and Pakistainis with low rates of physical activity have been found to have a greater risk for complications of diabetes (14). Although US research on this topic is limited, an analysis of data from the National Health Information Survey suggests that Asian Indians and Pakistanis with diabetes who reside in the United States were less physically active than non-Hispanic whites (15). RDs should assess the client's physical activity level and explain the rationale for regular physical activity and its role in diabetes management.

Feasting and Fasting

As noted in the section on holidays, feasts and fasts are a traditional part of South Asian religion and culture. RDs should ask clients about their fasting and feasting practices and determine what, when, and how much they plan to eat on occasions when they abstain from or celebrate with food. Use this information to advise clients about strategies to manage their blood glucose levels and diabetes medications.

Complementary and Alternative Medicine

India has a rich tradition of using foods for medicinal purposes. These practices stem from the traditional belief that the body consists of five humors, which, when kept in balance through a regulated lifestyle (including diet), can prevent illness. The use of herbs and vegetables as medicines is popular with Asian Indians and Pakistanis with diabetes (16).

In a study of patients with diabetes at an endocrine clinic in Allahabad, India, two-thirds of the study population (n = 493) used complementary and alternative medicine (CAM) and 30% used it their primary treatment for diabetes, without any other diabetes medication (16). The most common rationale cited for the use of CAM was "immediate relief." Participants usually obtained knowledge and information about CAM from family and friends.

In the United States, Asian Indians and Pakistanis typically use Western health care, and the use of CAM or home remedies is not necessarily detrimental to health. However, the use of certain herbal remedies or medicinal foods alongside prescribed medications could adversely affect blood glucose levels. For example, bitter gourd (*karela* in Hindi), is commonly used in India for its hypoglycemic effect (16). Individuals taking an oral diabetes agent or insulin could have hypoglycemia if they also consume bitter gourd. Grapefruit and okra are examples of other foods in South Asian cuisine that may have a hypoglycemic effect. RDs should therefore assess clients' food records and ask about use of supplements, herbs, and other types of CAM. Refer to Appendix C for questions to assess dietary supplement use.

Counseling Tips

When working with South Asian clients, the RD should assess each client's religious affiliation, degree of adherence to medical regimens, length of residency in the United States, degree of acculturation, and vegetarian or nonvegetarian food preferences. Important counseling objectives may include carbohydrate counting, portion sizes, modification of recipes to be higher in fiber and lower in fats (particularly saturated fats). Refer to Appendix B for medical nutrition therapy recommendations and related counseling messages/strategies.

In some counseling situations, it may be helpful to teach clients that people of Indian and Pakistani descent in the United States have higher rates of diabetes, obesity, and heart disease compared with their counterparts in their own country, and explain that eating habits may be one reason for the difference. This information can be a starting point in efforts to help clients blend traditional and Western cuisines to create a meal plan that is lower in total fat, saturated fat, animal protein, and dietary cholesterol (7).

Conclusion

The Asian Indian and Pakistani population in the United States is increasing, along with the prevalence of type 2 diabetes in this population. Information on the cultural practices, diabetes self-care knowledge, attitudes of Asian Indians and Pakistanis in the United States is limited. Research is essential to find out more about this population in the United States, including the barriers to self care.

Resources

American Association of Physicians of Indian Origin. http://aapiusa.org. Accessed April 2, 2009.
Gadia M: *New Indian Home Cooking.* New York, NY: Penguin Putnam, 2000. Includes information about diabetes, weight loss, and cholesterol management, as well as low-fat recipes with nutritional analyses and food exchanges.

References

1. *Indian and Pakistani Food Practices, Customs, and Holidays.* 2nd ed. Ethnic and Regional Food Practices series. Chicago, IL: American Dietetic Association; 2000.
2. Census of India 2001. *The First Report on Religion Data.* New Delhi, India: Registrar General & Census Commissioner; 2004.
3. Barnes JS, Bennett CE. The Asian population: 2000. Census 2000 Brief. February 2002. http://www.census.gov/prod/2002pubs/c2kbr01-16.pdf. Accessed April 2, 2009.
4. Abate N, Chandalia M. Ethnicity, type of diabetes, and migrant Asian Indians. *Indian J Med Res.* 2007;125:251–258.
5. Putting a number on India's diabetics. *India Abroad.* September 23, 2005.
6. Naser KA, Gruber A, Thomson GA. The emerging pandemic of obesity and diabetes: are we doing enough to prevent a disaster? *Int J Clin Pract.* 2006;60:1093–1097.
7. American Association of Physicians of Indian Origin. Indian Foods: AAPI's Guide to Health, Nutrition, and Diabetes. 2002. http://www.aapiusa.org/pdfs/Nutrition%20EBook.pdf. Accessed April 1, 2009.
8. Kittler PG, Sucher K. *Asian Indians: Food and Culture in America.* New York, NY: Van Nostrand Renhold; 1989.
9. Varghese S, Moore-Orr R. Dietary acculturation and health-related issues of Indian immigrant families in Newfoundland. *Can J Diet Pract Res.* 2002;63:72–79.
10. Raj S, Ganaganna P, Bowering J. Dietary habits of Asian Indians in relation to length of residence in the United States. *J Am Diet Assoc.* 1999;99:1106.
11. Hill J. Management of diabetes in South Asian communities in the UK. *Nurs Stand.* 2006; 20:57–64.
12. Naeem A. The role of culture and religion in the management of diabetes: a study of Kashmiri men in Leeds. *J R Soc Health.* 2003;123:110–116.

13. Stone M, Pound E, Pancholi A, Farroqi A, Khunti K. Empowering patients with diabetes: a qualitative primary care study focusing on south Asians in Leicester, UK. *Fam Pract.* 2005; 22:647–652.

14. Patel S, Popvich N. Prevalence of type 2 diabetes mellitus among the Asian Indian population. *U.S. Pharmacist.* 2003;28:11.

15. Mohanty S, Woolnhandler S, Himmelsteing D, Bor D. Diabetes and cardiovascular disease among Asian Indians in the United States. *J Gen Intern Med.* 2005;20:474–478.

16. Kumar D, Bajaj S, Mehrortra R. Knowledge, attitude and practice of complementary and alternative medicines for diabetes. *Public Health.* 2006;120:705–711.

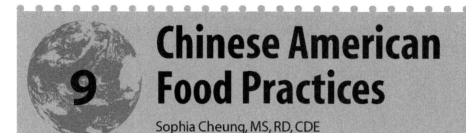

Chinese American Food Practices

Sophia Cheung, MS, RD, CDE

Introduction

In 2005, there were 3.4 million Chinese Americans (1.2% of the US population). Chinese Americans are the largest Asian American ethnic group, comprising 22.4% of the Asian American population (1).

The 1849 gold rush in California, the start of transcontinental railroad construction in 1854, the Immigration Act of 1990, and the transfer of Hong Kong from British to Chinese rule in 1997 each started waves of Chinese immigration to the United States (1). Many Chinese immigrants have worked as miners, railroad workers, cooks, launderers, and small business owners. Today, about 63% of Chinese Americans are first-generation immigrants from China, Taiwan, Hong Kong, and Macao (1). Younger generations of Chinese Americans participate in US mainstream job market; this population is also growing rapidly.

The largest Chinese American communities are in the western and northeastern states, particularly in California, New York, and Hawaii (1). Historically, many immigrants lived in Chinatowns and kept close contact with other Chinese Americans and people in Asia. First-generation Chinese Americans usually retain many traditional cultural values. Younger generations are more acculturated, have dispersed within the general US population, and tend to adopt a more Westernized lifestyle (2).

Chinese Americans are thus a very diverse minority group. They may be broken down into the following groups (3):

- Non-English-speaking peasants who emigrated from rural villages in the Toisan and Guangdong provinces in the southern part of mainland China. They are the strongest believers in Chinese folk culture, and their beliefs continue to influence the health practices of their immediate families.
- Bilingual students and professionals from Hong Kong, Macao, Taiwan, and mainland China who came to study and work in the United States.
- Ethnic Chinese who first immigrated to Vietnam, Laos, Cambodia, and other Asian countries and then came to the United States as refugees in the 1970s and 1980s.
- Second- and third-generation Chinese Americans who are acculturated and have adopted American dietary habits but follow certain Chinese dietary practices.
- Spouses or family members of Chinese Americans with US citizenship who immigrated to the United States to reunite with family.

Lifestyle, socioeconomic status, educational level, and attitudes and practices regarding diet, health, and health care vary widely among these groups. Health care providers should also note that Chinese Americans speak several distinct dialects, such as Mandarin, Cantonese, and Toisanese (the three most common dialects).

Diabetes Prevalence

The prevalence of type 2 diabetes in Asian Americans is estimated to be between 10% and 20% (4). After adjusting for age, body mass index (BMI), and gender, the prevalence of diabetes among the Asian Americans is 60% greater than prevalence in non-Hispanic whites (5). Diabetes prevalence in Asian Americans is similar to rates in more affluent Asian countries, such as Hong Kong, Taiwan and Macao, but much greater than prevalence in rural areas of China (6).

Between 1994 and 2001, the prevalence of diabetes in Asian Americans between the ages of 35 and 44 years increased by 88% (4). This data suggest that diabetes is a substantial health concern among Chinese Americans, and particularly among those who are in younger age groups. According to data from New York City's first Health and Nutrition Examination Survey (NYC HANES), Asian New Yorkers (43% of whom are Chinese Americans) have the highest rate (16%) of diabetes of all racial and ethnic groups in the city. Nearly half of all Asian New Yorkers have either diabetes or pre-diabetes. The rate is expected to double by 2050 (4).

Prevalence of type 1 diabetes in the Chinese is estimated to be 5% or less of total diabetes prevalence. Epidemiological studies suggest that Chinese people may be at lower risk for developing type 1 diabetes compared with whites (7).

Risk Factors for Type 2 Diabetes

Overweight

Being overweight and of Asian origin increases one's risk of developing type 2 diabetes. Notably, in Asians the risk for type 2 diabetes increases at a lower BMI (BMI ≥ 23) compared with other ethnic groups (BMI ≥ 25) (8–10). Therefore, optimal body weight standards for Asians may be lower than standards for other populations. Because a strong correlation exists between increased visceral adiposity and type 2 diabetes in Asian Americans (11), measuring waist circumference is often recommended to more accurately identify diabetes risk in Asian Americans who exhibit exhibit central obesity and have a BMI within the normal range. The waist circumference cutoff for identifying Asian Americans at risk of diabetes is 80 cm for both men and women (12).

Genetic Factors

Genetic factors play an important role in the development of diabetes in Chinese populations. In a study of familial early-onset of type 2 diabetes in young Chinese patients in Hong Kong, Ng and associates reported that genetic factors and obesity together contributed up to 70% of diabetes risk factors (13).

Traditional Foods and Dishes

To the Chinese, food's purpose goes beyond just nourishing the body. Food ingredients are carefully chosen and prepared to symbolize or wish for longevity, happiness, and luck. Food is a common gift when celebrating Chinese rituals, and it can be used as a signifier of one's social class. Most importantly, food is considered essential in treating and preventing illnesses. Doctors who practice traditional Chinese medicine often prescribe recipes of herbs, combined with food, to make soups or tea intended to relieve symptoms associated with diabetes, aid in health recovery, and prevent microvascular diabetes complications.

In the traditional Chinese diet, complex carbohydrates such as grains, legumes, vegetables, and other starches comprise up to 70% of energy intake. About 15% of calories come from protein (mostly from plant protein) and 15% from fat (14).

In southern China, rice is the staple food. Typically, a Chinese person consumes 2 to 3 cups or bowls of rice per meal. Long-grain rice is commonly used and prepared using one part rice to two parts water. Traditionally, rice is cooked in clay pots, and many restaurants still serve entrées over rice cooked in clay pots. However, electronic rice cookers are more commonly used because they are more convenient. Rice is cooked in different forms. The sticky, crusty portion *(guo ba)* that sticks to the bottom of the pot is often the favorite part of the meal. Porridge (congee), rice boiled in large quantities of water for a long period of time, is the common rice preparation in Guangdong or Canton province.

In northern China, the climate favors wheat production. Noodles, dumplings, and steamed buns are staples in this region.

Pork is the staple meat in the Chinese diet. Fresh poultry, eggs, fish, and seafood are consumed when and where available. Almost every animal part (including liver, kidneys, lungs, stomach, intestines, blood, marrow, brain, feet, and tail) is consumed as food or used as ingredients in traditional Chinese medicine.

The traditional Chinese diet includes plentiful quantities of fruits and vegetables. Vegetables are rarely eaten raw. They are usually stir-fried, steamed, or added to soups minutes before serving. The Chinese cook many edible plant parts, such as buds, fungi, flower petals, and sprouts. Lack of access to refrigeration and transportation led to the development of methods for preserving vegetables and fruits, including salting, pickling and drying. Preserved foods tend to be high in sodium, and sodium intake should be assessed when counseling the Chinese Americans.

Soy and soy products, legumes, and grains comprise 80% of the protein in the traditional Chinese diet. Soybeans are used dried, as sprouts, as tofu (soybean curd), or as soymilk, and they are fermented into seasonings and sauces.

Dairy products are not common in the traditional Chinese diet. The prevalence of lactose intolerance in the Chinese population is high (76% to 92%), as a consequence of a long history of little milk consumption. In addition, cattle are scarce, and most are used for work rather than for food. Limited intake of dairy products raises concerns about the sufficiency of calcium intake. It was believed that calcium deficiency might be less of a concern in older Chinese populations who enjoy eating tofu and fish, chicken, or pork bones in soup simmered for long periods, or in postpartum women who consume a concoction of pig feet cooked in sweet-and-sour broth of sugar and vinegar (3). However, the amount of calcium and vitamin D in these foods is small, and most modern Chinese Americans are moving away from these traditional practices. Furthermore, some Chinese women avoid direct sun exposure to keep a fair complexion. Limited intake of dairy products and minimal sun exposure increase the risk of calcium and vitamin D deficiency. Supplementation should be considered to ensure adequate levels calcium and vitamin D.

Although vegetable, peanut, sesame, and corn oils are increasingly popular for health reasons, lard is still commonly used in certain traditional pastries, instant noodle mixes, and special occasion foods such as *zong zi* (glutinous rice usually stuffed with beans, egg yolk and fatty pork wrapped in bamboo leaves). Chinese American restaurants frequently use chicken fat to braise vegetables and for added flavor.

Most Chinese drink hot tea. Types include green and black tea. Elderly Chinese prefer hot or lukewarm beverages to any cold beverages, such as soda, fruit juices or ice tea. In addition to traditional hot tea, younger generations drink coffee or cold milk tea, which is usually made with whole milk or condensed milk, added syrup, and tapiocas (*boba* milk tea). These drinks are as high in calories as frappes and cold beverages served at American coffee houses. See Box 9.1 and Table 9.1 for additional information on traditional foods. Refer to Appendix A for nutrient analyses.

Box 9.1 • Foods Used in Traditional Chinese Cuisine

Starches
- Cellophane noodles/vermicelli
- Glutinous (sticky) rice
- Rice
- Rice noodles

Starchy vegetables
- Corn
- Ginkgo seeds (apricot-like structures seeds having a shell that consists of a soft and fleshy section and a hard section)
- Lotus roots
- Pumpkin
- Sweet potatoes
- Tapioca
- Taro
- Water chestnuts

Soy foods, beans, and peas
- Broad beans
- Mung beans
- Red beans
- Soybeans
- Soymilk
- Tofu

Nonstarchy vegetables
- Bamboo shoots
- Bitter melon (bitter gourd)
- Black and white wood-ear (wood fungus, often used as vegetables in stir-fries and in soups; good source of soluble fiber)
- Brown mushrooms (eg, shitake mushrooms)
- Chinese spinach
- Chinese broccoli (Mandarin: *jie lan;* Cantonese: *gai lan*)
- Chinese cabbage (Mandarin: *bai cai;* Cantonese: *bak choy*)
- Chives
- Eggplant
- Garlic
- Napa cabbage
- Scallions
- String beans
- Watercress
- Winter melon

Fruits
- Banana
- Carambola/starfruit (glossy yellow pods marked with five longitudinal ribs that form a star shape when the fruit is sliced; the skin is edible, and the flesh is translucent, crisp, and juicy, with a tart to sweet taste)
- Dragon fruit *(pitaya)*
- Durian
- Grapes
- Guava
- Lychee/litchi/litchee (small, round fruits that contain brilliant orange red skin and delicious opaque, white flesh; commonly canned in syrup.)
- Longan (small and round with smooth, brown skin and clear pulp, this fruit comes in clusters when fresh, but is more commonly found canned in syrup)
- Mango (delicate, sweet-flavored tropical fruit, the mango is oval to round in shape; the skin color varies from green to yellow, and the interior is golden-yellow)
- Oranges
- Papaya
- Passion fruit (round or oval fruits with green-orange pulp and sour-sweet flavor)
- Pineapple
- Pomelo/shaddock/Chinese grapefruit (citrus fruit that is green yellow, or pink in color; can grow to several inches in diameter)
- Tangerines

(continued)

Box 9.1 *(continued)*

Meats

- Beef
- Chicken
- Chinese sausage
- Eggs
- Fish and seafood
- Oxtail
- Ox tongue

- Pork
- Pig blood pudding or cake (blood cooked until it is thick enough to congeal when cooled; the cooled blood is then cut into rectangular pieces and served with soups or noodles soup)
- Pork intestine
- Tripe, beef

Seasonings and spices

- Bouillon cubes
- Chinese chili pepper
- Coriander
- Fermented tofu
- Five-spice powder
- Ginger
- Monosodium glutamate (MSG)

- Mustard seeds
- Oyster sauce
- Sesame seeds, black and white
- Soy sauce
- Star anise
- Szechuan peppercorn

Table 9.1 · Traditional Chinese Dishes, Beverages, and Desserts

Name	Description
Dishes from China	
Beef or pork ribs with bitter melon	
Buddhist delight	Stir-fried vegetables, mushrooms, black fungus, and dried tofu
Dumplings	
Hot pot	Meats, seafood, vegetables, wontons, dumplings, and other ingredients cooked at the table in a pot of simmering stock and then dipped in sauce
Mantou	Steamed buns
Ma po tofu	Szechuan bean curd with minced pork
Peking duck (Beijing roast duck)	Roast duck served with lotus leaves, pancakes, and sweet sauce
Scallion pancakes	
Steamed fish with ginger, scallions, and soy sauce	
Taiwanese Dishes	
Beef noodle soup	
Blood pudding with sticky rice	
Marinated pig ears	
Minced pork with marinated egg over rice	
Oyster and scallion pancake	
Salted soymilk with fried dough	
Stinky tofu	Fermented tofu served as a snack or side dish
Tea egg	Egg boiled in tea and soy sauce
"Three cups" chicken	Chicken marinated in a sauce of a cup each of rice wine, sesame oil, and soy sauce
Hong Kong and Macao Dishes	
Baked seafood, pork chop, or chicken	
Barbecue pork	

(continued)

Table 9.1   *(continued)*

Name	Description
Beef *chow-fen*	Stir-fried rice flat noodles with soy sauce, beef slices & scallions
Eggplant and salted fish over rice baked in a clay pot	
Fish cake and noodle soup	
Ha mun–style vermicelli	Stir-fried vermicelli with pork slices and vegetables
Lo mein	Stir-fried dry egg noodles with shredded pork or beef
Pineapple bun, cream bun, and egg custard	Hong Kong–style pastries, often an afternoon tea snack
Rice congee	Rice porridge
Roast duck	
Soy sauce chicken	
Stir-fried shrimp with scrambled eggs	
Tomato and beef over rice	
Wife cake	Crispy crust, Hong Kong–style pastry with almond paste
Wonton noodle soup	Broth soup with stuffed wonton dumplings
Dim Sum	
Dim sum	Small steamed basket or plates of meat/seafood/vegetables/desserts and fruits
Char siu bao	Barbecue pork bun
Fung zhao	Chicken feet
Har gao	Shrimp dumpling
Shu mai	Pork dumplings
Beverages	
Dessert and sweet soups	
Flavored tea	May be made with added fruits, mixed with whole milk and syrup
Horlicks	Malted milk drink; in Hong Kong and Macao, this is often considered a nutritious drink
Milk teas	Common in Taiwan, Hong Kong, and Macao
Milo	Chocolate and malt; in Hong Kong and Macao, this is often considered a nutritious drink
Soups, herbal soups	
Tea and herbal tea	
Desserts	
Almond gelatin	
Egg custard	
Egg puff	Flour mixture with egg, baked in between hot plates that contain molds in the shape of an egg
Lotus seeds and lily bulb soup	Slightly sweetened Chinese herbal soup
Mango pudding	
Red bean soup	Sweet soup, often mixed with other beans and tapioca
Shaved ice	Usually topped with condensed milk or syrup; other toppings include red bean, egg yolk, fruits and ice-cream; originated in Taiwan
Sweet glutinous rice ball with sesame filling in sweet soup	
Tofu pudding	
White wood ear with papaya soup	May be topped with coconut milk, which is believed to smoothen one's complexion

Traditional Meal Patterns and Holiday Foods

Mainland China

In China, people traditionally eat breakfast, lunch, and dinner, and usually a snack after dinner. Breakfast typically includes rice, congee, noodles in soup, or steamed buns. Preserved vegetables and minced meat are often served as side dishes. Lunch consists of stir-fried vegetables and meat served with noodles or rice. Dinner, which is usually the main meal of the day, includes a clear broth soup, rice or noodles, and two or three stir-fried meat-and-vegetable dishes. A soup of clear broth boiled with herbs, vegetables, and a protein is served before the meal starts. Regional cuisines reflect differences in climate, food availability, religion, and custom. In northern area, including Beijing, dishes are characterized by the use of garlic, leeks, and scallions. In eastern coastal area around Shanghai, food is commonly braised with large amounts of soy sauce and sugar. Pickled and salted vegetables and meat are often used as seasonings. Thus, Shanghai cuisine tends to be high in sodium. The western region, including Sichuan and Hunan, is known for the use of chili peppers and hot pepper sauces, and foods tend to be spicy and oily. The Guangdong (Canton) province, located in the southern part of China, serves Cantonese dishes, many of which are steamed or stir-fried. Dim sum, literally translated as "a touch of heart," is well known for including a variety of Chinese dishes in small steamed baskets.

Hong Kong and Macao

As colonies of Britain and Portugal, Hong Kong and Macao encountered Western dietary influences in the 19th century. Dietary patterns in these populations are a fusion of both Western and Eastern diets. Dairy products are more commonly consumed than in mainland China. People typically eat breakfast, lunch, an afternoon tea snack, dinner, and a late evening snack called *shiu ye*. Breakfast could include pastries, milk tea, oatmeal, and bread; steamed flat rice noodles; stir-fried egg noodles; congee; or even macaroni in soup served with minced meat and preserved vegetables. Lifestyles are busy, and people commonly dine out or buy take-out for lunch and dinner. Typical choices are Cantonese, Indonesian, American, and Portuguese cuisines. Because of the region's proximity to coastal areas, seafood is the predominant source of protein. Western-influenced high tea, also referred to as a "midafternoon snack," usually happens around 3 or 4 PM and includes a pastry with milk tea or coffee. Popular pastries are pineapple buns and egg tarts. Other choices include French pastries, cake, pie, and sandwiches. Many restaurants and fast-food chains are open until dawn (some for 24 hours) to accommodate the nightlife of the population. Desserts are usually sweet soups made from tapioca, red beans, Chinese herbs, and sugar. During weekends, dim sum is a popular brunch for the whole family.

Taiwan

Taiwan combines a variety of southern Chinese and Japanese cuisines. Similar to Hong Kong, Taiwan has a lively nightlife, including night food markets where young people socialize. Restaurants and street food vendors serving a variety of cuisines group together in one area and serve a variety of finger foods (eg, fried or steamed meat-filled buns, oyster-filled omelets), drinks, sweets, as well as sit-down dishes. Taiwanese individuals tend to eat two or three small meals a day with snacks in between.

Holiday Foods

Annual Chinese holidays include the following:

- Chinese New Year
- *Qing Ming*—celebrated annually April 4 to 6, this holiday involves a cemetery ritual that nourishes and remembers ancestral spirits
- Dragon Boat Festival—this festival, which occurs from late May to mid-June, honors the death of a patriotic poet, Wut Yuen, who drowned on the fifth day of the fifth lunar month in 277 BC. At that time, Chinese citizens threw bamboo leaves filled with cooked rice into the water so the fish would eat the rice instead of their hero. From this event, it became customary to eat *Zhong zhi* and rice dumplings.

Table 9.2 • Traditional Foods Consumed During Chinese Holidays

Holiday	Foods
Chinese New Year	• Bird's nest soup
	• Chinese black mushrooms
	• Chinese broccoli
	• Chinese long string beans
	• Dried bean curd
	• Dried oysters
	• Glutinous rice cake (usually cut into small square pieces and pan-fried with eggs)
	• Lily buds
	• Long-grain rice or noodles
	• Lotus seeds
	• "Monk's" vegetarian dish (assorted stir-fried nonstarchy vegetables)
	• Peanuts, candies, red dates, dried longan, tangerines, and walnuts
	• Poultry served whole with feet and head
	• Shark's fin soup
	• White cloud ears (wood ears; edible fungus)
	• Whole fish with head and tail
Qing Ming	• Crispy-skinned roast pork
	• Custard tarts
	• Golden sponge cake
	• Oranges and apples
	• Steamed pork buns
	• Steamed rice
	• Whole boiled chicken
Dragon Boat Festival	• *Zhong zhi/Joong* (glutinous rice with meat, green beans, egg yolk and lard filling wrapped in bamboo leaves)
Midautumn Festival	• Mooncakes (dense pastries usually filled with a paste made with lotus seeds)
	• Pomelo
	• Snails
	• Taro

- Midautumn Festival. During this September festival, the Chinese offer thanksgiving and celebrate a bountiful harvest.

Christmas and Easter holidays are also celebrated in Hong Kong and Macao. See Table 9.2 for traditional holiday foods. For more information on this topic, see reference 15.

The Chinese also consume or avoid certain foods at special occasions. For example, pregnant women avoid lamb, shellfish, bananas, and watermelon. During the first postpartum month (ie, the Sitting Month), new mothers are believed to be "cool" (*leung* in Cantonese), and they use dietary methods to restore the internal balance of *yin* (cool) and *yang* (hot). Ginger, wine, and black vinegar are the key ingredients used to invigorate the new mothers' strength. These ingredients are believed to generate heat and aromas that warm the body. Dishes that are served during the Sitting Month include the following:

- Chicken wine soup: This soup contains black mushrooms, lily buds, wood ears, chicken, large pieces of ginger, red dates, rice wine or gin, and rock sugar.
- Black vinegar pig's feet: This stew contains pig's feet, black vinegar, water, large pieces of ginger, brown sugar bars, and hard-boiled egg.

Box 9.2 • *Yin* (Cool) and *Yang* (Hot) Foods	
Yin	
• Bananas	• Seaweed
• Cold drinks	• Soybeans, soymilk
• Fish	• Vegetables
• Juices	• Watermelons
• Rice water	
Yang	
• Beef	• Liver
• Chicken	• Nuts
• Coffee	• Vinegar
• Fried foods	• Wine
• Ginger	

- Red eggs: Hard-boiled eggs dyed red. Eggs are a symbol of fertility, birth, and life, whereas red symbolizes happiness and good luck.
- Pickled ginger roots: The ginger roots are either dyed red or pink and pickled in brine. This food represents a family's strong, deep roots that their grandchildren perpetuate.

Traditional Health Beliefs

Classic Chinese medicine involves the concepts of *yin* and *yang*, two opposing forces that interact with one another to maintain balance and harmony. *Yin* represents the feminine, phoenix, moon, water, passivity, coolness, mystery, even numbers, north, and west. *Yang* is the masculine, dragon, sun, fire energy, heat, directness, odd numbers, south, and east. To maintain good health, one must balance *yin* and *yang* forces within the body. Illness is a result of the imbalance. Frequently, the terms "cold and wet" refer to *yin* forces and "hot and dry" refer to *yang* energy.

Depending on the type of energy they yield when metabolized, foods and herbs are classified as *yin* or *yang*. See Box 9.2.

Current Food Practices

In China, which has a history of famine, the consumption of fatty foods is considered to be luxurious and nutritious (the Chinese translate "nutritious" as *bu*, which actually means "replenishing and nourishing the body"). As the population becomes more affluent, the Chinese prefer fatty and well-marbled cuts of meat. Excessive added fat in cooking may contribute to overconsumption of saturated fat and cholesterol. Many soups that are considered to be nutritious are simmered for hours with pork, whole chickens, and meat bones. Registered dietitians (RDs) may want to counsel Chinese clients to skim the fat off the soup. Lard and chicken fat are commonly used in Chinese American restaurants. Fried chicken wings, chicken fingers, egg rolls, and fortune cookies are dishes invented for the American palate. Foods are topped with oil to provide a glossy appearance.

The following factors influence the food practices and meal patterns of Chinese living in the United States (16–18):

- Degree of acculturation
- Socioeconomic status
- Length of stay in the United States
- Place of origin

- Food availability
- Access to food purchasing and/or preparation
- Health beliefs
- Participation in government food programs

Acculturation patterns as well as the languages spoken at home determine, to a great extent, whether individuals consume Americanized foods. Multiple studies provide insight into current food practices of Chinese Americans living in the United States. Grivetti et al (19) examined the diets of first-, second-, and third-generation Chinese Americans in northern California and found that seafood and duck consumption sharply decreased as time in the United States increased. Frequency of rice consumption also decreased, whereas hamburgers, hotdogs, and hot and cold breakfast cereals gained popularity. Yang and Fox (16) reported that most Chinese Americans tend to adopt American-style breakfast and lunch foods but continue to eat a traditional Chinese dinner. In a cross-sectional study of 399 subjects in Pennsylvania, Lv and colleagues (20) found that acculturation was positively associated with intake of fruits, fats/sweets, and soft drinks. Individuals with better English proficiency consumed grains, fruits, meats and meat alternatives, and fats and sweets more frequently than those with limited English.

Counseling Considerations

Demonstrating Courtesy and Respect

When working with a non-English-speaking client, start each session with a simple, linguistically appropriate greeting, such as *ni hao* (Mandarin) or *nei hou* (Cantonese). This suggests that you are willing to address cultural differences. Many Chinese Americans, particularly those who do not speak English, prefer to choose a provider of the same culture because they believe that the provider will understand their background and lifestyle as an immigrant.

Interpreting Clients' Nonverbal Communication

Ethnic Chinese clients may interpret eye contact differently than Western health care providers. Whereas the Western therapist may believe that a Chinese client avoids eye contact because he or she has low self-esteem or is not telling the truth, the Chinese client considers a lack of eye contact to signify politeness and respect.

Chinese Americans with either limited English proficiency or low health literacy and a high respect for their health care provider may not be able to verbalize their lack of comprehension about the treatment modality. Clients may respond "yes" or "no" even though they do not clearly understand the content of the counseling session. Asking open questions is critical. For example, instead of asking the yes-or-no question, "Do you understand what foods to choose now?" try the question, "Could you tell me two diet changes you will make when you get home?"

Inquiring About Clients' Understanding of Diabetes

Many Chinese Americans believe that heredity and eating too many sweets cause diabetes. Elderly Chinese may feel that a diagnosis of diabetes burdens the family and one should keep diabetes management to oneself. When health care providers discuss insulin use, these individuals may refuse because they believe they can control their diabetes solely with diet.

Chinese American clients may believe that Western medicines are "too strong" and cause too many adverse effects. Some individuals refuse to take diabetes medicines because they fear kidney or liver damage. Clients sometimes begin an insulin regimen without sufficient education on how, when, and why to take it. This can lead to unnecessary hypoglycemic events and contribute to the perception that Western medicines are too strong. There can be a stigma attached to the use of needles. Questions such as, "What do you think caused your diabetes?"or "Do you talk to anyone about your diabetes issues?" can help identify a client's misconceptions about diabetes and barriers to quality diabetes care.

Discussing Clients' Use of Complementary and Alternative Medicine

In China, approximately 70% of the people use Chinese herbal medicine (CHM) for diabetes (21). Many use a combination of CHM and Western treatments because they believe that Western medicine controls blood glucose levels while CHM addresses the cause of diabetes and prevents microvascular complications. Traditional Chinese medical doctors often prescribe a recipe containing approximately 10 types of herbs, which are boiled in water for up to 3 to 8 hours. A classic Cantonese recipe boils herbs in 4 cups of water for 1 hour, reducing the mixture to yield 3 cups. See Tables 9.3 and 9.4 for common CHM treatments (21).

Pills and capsules that contain CHM herbs are available as alternatives to herbal soups, which usually have a bitter or unpleasant aftertaste. Many products marketed as traditional Chinese medicine have sulfonylurea as the main ingredient.

Refer to Appendix C for questions to assess dietary supplement use. When counseling patients using CHM, health care providers may also ask:

- Have you seen other practitioners for the treatment of diabetes and its related conditions?
- What treatments or remedies are you taking? How long have you been taking them?
- What differences have you noticed since you started taking these remedies?

Considering Family Demands and Dynamics

Family dynamics are an important counseling consideration. Elderly Chinese Americans often live with younger generations of their family and try to integrate their lives with the family routine without causing disruption. Family traditions and customs usually take precedence over one's own health. To partake in a family social gathering, elderly Chinese may abandon their diabetes meal plan in favor of food choices selected by other family members.

Table 9.3 • Single-Herb Remedies Used by Chinese Americans for Diabetes Treatment

Chinese Name[a]	English Name
Bai zhu	Ovate atractylodes
Bai shao	White peony root
Ban xia	Pinellia
Bian dou	Hyacinth bean
Can e	Silkworm moth
Cang zhu	Atractylodes root
Chai hu	Bupleurum root
Chi shao	Red peony root
Chi xiao dou	Adsuki bean
Chuan xiong	Ligusticum root
Da huang	Rhubarb
Dang gui	Angelica
Dang shen	Codonopsis root
Dan pi	Mountain bark
Dan shen	Salvia root
Di gu pi	Lycium root bark
Du zhong	Eucommia bark
E zhu	Zedoary
Fu ling	Poria
Gan cao	Licorice root
Ge gen	Pueraria root

(continued)

Table 9.3 *(continued)*

Chinese Name[a]	English Name
Gou ji	Cibotium root
Huai niu xi	Achyrathes root
Huang bai	Phellodendron bark
Huang jing	Polygonatum root
Huang lian	Coptis root
Huang qi	Astragalus root
Huang qin	Scutellaria root
Jiang can	Silkworm
Jin ying zi	Cherokee rose fruit
Li he	Lychee pit
Mai dong	Ophiopogon tuber
Niu bang zi	Arctium seed
Ren shen	Ginseng
Sang pi	Mulberry root bark
Sang piao xiao	Mantis egg-case powder
Sang shen zi	Mulberry
Sang ye	Mulberry leaf
San qi	Notoginseng root
Shan dou gen	Root of straight sophora
Shan yao	Dioscorea root
Shan zha	Crataegus fruit
Shan zhu yu	Asiatic cornelian cherry fruit
Sha ren	Amomum fruit
She chuang zi	Cnidium seed
Sheng di huang	Dried rehmannia root
Sheng shai shen	*Panax* ginseng
Shi gao	Gypsum
Shi hu	Dendrobium
Shu diu huang	Cooked rehmannia root
Tai zi shen	Pseudostellaria root
Tao ren	Peach kernel
Tian dong	Arisaema tuber
Tian hua fen	Trichosanthes root
Wu wei zi	Schisandra berry
Xian ling pi	Epimedium herb
Xi yang shen	American ginseng
Xuan shen	Scrophularia root
Yi mi	Coix seed
Yi mu cao	Leonurus
Yu zhu	Solomon's seal root
Ze sie	Alisma tuber
Zhi mu	Anemarrhena root
Zhu ling	Polyporus

[a]Mandarin pin yin only.
Source: Data are from reference 21.

Table 9.4 · Herbal Recipes Used by Chinese Americans for Diabetes Treatment

Name (Description)	Ingredients
Baihu tang (white tiger decoction)	*Shi gao* (gypsum), *zhi mu* (wind-weed rhizome), *gan cao* (prepared licorice root), *gen mi* (polished, round-grained, nonglutinous rice)
Buyang huanwu tang (decoction invigorating *yang* for recuperation)	*Huang qi* (astragalus root), *dang gui* (Chinese angelica root), *chi shao* (red peony root), *chuan xiong* (Chuanxiong rhizome), *tao ren* (peach kernel), *hong hua* (safflower), *di long* (earthworm)
Liuwei dihuang wan (bolus of rehmannia six)	*Shu di huang* (prepared rhizome of rehmannia), *shan zhu yu* (dogwood fruit), *shan yao* (dried Chinese yam), *ze xie* (oriental water plantain), *fu ling* (poria), *mu dan pi* (mountain bark)
Shen qi wan (bolus invigorating the kidney *qi*)	*Di huang* (dried rehmannia), *shan yao* (dried Chinese yam), *shan zhu yu* (dogwood fruit), *ze xie* (oriental water plantain), *fu ling* (poria), *mu dan pi* (mountain bark), *gui zhi* (cinnamon twig), *fu zi* (prepared aconite root)
Yu quan wan (jade spring bolus)	*Ge gen* (pueraria root), *tian hua fen* (trichosanthes oot), *mai dong* (ophiopogon tuber), *sheng di huang* (dried rehmannia root), *Geng mi* (polished, round-grained, nonglutinous rice), *gan cao* (prepared licorice root), *wu wei zi* (Schisandra berry)

Source: Data are from reference 21.

Some clients may neglect taking their insulin if they believe the regimen upsets the family routine. Similarly, Chinese American women may prioritize their families' dietary preferences over their own needs. A female client may prepare a meal that appeals to the family first and make a separate "healthy" meal for herself.

Engaging Others in Counseling Sessions

Health care providers should inquire about clients' support systems. If possible, encourage clients to invite friends and relatives to be part of the goal-setting process. Once family members understand the importance of treatment, they are more likely to help clients achieve successful outcomes. Health care providers may want to engage the use of community health workers, if available.

Using the "Replenish" and "Balance" Concepts in Diabetes Counseling

Like many other ethnic groups, Chinese Americans may worry about the perceived side effects of insulin injections, including the possibility of harming body organs. A very common concern is how insulin affects the liver. When educating clients about insulin injections, health care providers may want to describe insulin as a "natural" medicine that has minimal adverse effects when used properly. Explain to clients who cannot produce insulin themselves that they need insulin injections to replace (replenish) what the body is missing.

The "balance" concept may be used to teach clients about carbohydrate counting. During the first few sessions, focus on how to achieve consistent amounts of carbohydrate at meal times and how to balance and adjust starch portions with fruits. These topics are more useful to clients than calorie restrictions.

Nutrition Counseling

Appendix B offers selected medical nutrition therapy recommendations for individuals with diabetes and general counseling suggestions that support those recommendations. The following are culturally specific nutrition counseling strategies for Chinese American clients:

- Chinese culture teaches that food has curing and nourishing properties and certain foods can be used to treat specific diseases of certain organs. For example, eating pig's pancreas supposedly helps increase endogenous production of insulin. RDs may want to take advantage of this concept and try teaching food groups in the context of their functions in the body.

- Chinese American immigrants are usually unfamiliar with the nutrition data on food labels. Educate clients about how to read and interpret the carbohydrate, fiber, protein, and fat information on food labels.

- Although Nutrition Facts panels are an important tool for choosing healthful food options in US supermarkets, clients should be cautioned that food labels on imported foods are not as reliable. Therefore, ingredients lists on imported products should be checked to ensure the selection of healthful choices.

- For clients accustomed to a traditional Chinese diet, provide a meal plan that includes moderate amounts of rice; egg, rice, or mung bean noodles; root vegetables; and fruits.

- If the client wishes to eat more fruit at a meal, emphasize the importance of eating smaller portions of starches. For snacks, encourage clients to choose fruit instead of packaged foods like crackers.

- Encourage the consumption of traditional foods that are high in fiber and other nutrients, such as brown rice, dried beans, soy, chickpeas and peas, mushrooms and fungus, and nonstarchy vegetables such as Chinese broccoli and bitter melon. Suggest that clients eat oatmeal or brown rice congee instead of congee made with white rice.

- If clients dislike the taste of brown rice, suggest they try mixing white and brown rice or use another type of whole grain.

- Clients may refer to sugar-free foods as "free" or "diet" foods. Emphasize that these foods are not necessarily calorie- nor carbohydrate-free.

- Encourage clients to choose low-fat vegetable soups instead of pork bone–based soups. Also, teach clients to refrigerate or freeze soups made with meat or bones, and then skim off the top layer of fat.

- Provide a list of sources of saturated fat, including traditional foods like Chinese sausage, organ meats, and fatty pork.

- Explain that many Chinese bakery products are high in saturated and *trans* fats and encourage clients to limit consumption of these treats.

- Emphasize that shrimp and lobster do not have more cholesterol than chicken or many other meats, so clients do not need to completely eliminate shellfish from their diet. However, organ meats should be eaten only occasionally and in small portions.

Challenges and Barriers to Dietary Compliance

Chinese American clients may face the following challenges and barriers to dietary compliance:

- Difficulty saying no when food is offered: Eating is a big part of Chinese culture and is essential in all events and celebrations. Offering foods to others is a very common gesture to show appreciation and love toward others, and accepting the foods is a gesture to show appreciation for the efforts. It is considered impolite if one rejects eating the foods offered.

- Inability to control portion sizes.

- Limited availability of healthful food choices in the local area.

- Budgetary/economic constraints: For example, clients may rely on Food Stamps and/or Meals on Wheels.

- Reliance on others to prepare meals: For example, older adults may not choose what they eat when younger family members cook food for the household.

- Poor dental health: Dental problems are common and clients may not recognize them to be an issue until discussed with a counselor.

- Poor health status; lack or limited health insurance.

- Lack of English proficiency.

- Low literacy—in either English or Chinese.

Counseling Tips

The following tips can improve nutrition counseling of Chinese Americans:

- Dietary assessment should be specific. Many clients say they eat a bowl of rice, green vegetables, and meat. For a more detailed picture of what the client eats, ask how the food was prepared, including the ingredients used.

- Encourage clients to keep a food record for a few days to learn their dietary and blood glucose patterns.
- Ask patients to bring food labels, purchased-food containers, and supermarket fliers for ethnic foods to counseling sessions.
- To teach portion control, use food replicas and pictures. It is also helpful to determine the volume of utensils and dishes the client commonly uses, such as a standard rice bowl, lunch box, or teacup.
- When working with clients with limited English and/or health literacy, use visual tools instead of written examples and handouts. Clients with limited literacy want simple, practical, and relevant information on what foods to eat and how to prepare them. They typically prefer hands-on activities that are enjoyable and allow them to share ideas and experiences.
- Assess the importance of religion in the client's understanding of health issues.
- Recommend economically available and acceptable foods. Provide a shopping list and ideas for meal preparation that include acceptable substitutions.
- Explain how food intake and activity levels affect blood glucose levels, and how to make adjustment with medications.
- Review and explain the importance of properly timing medications and insulin.
- Become familiar with cultural myths about health and be prepared to demonstrate the differences between myth and facts.
- Set specific, concrete, and attainable goals at the end of each session. Focus on changes that are feasible, sensible, and practical for the client and client's family.

References

1. US Census Bureau. American Community Survey 1 year estimates. 2007. http://factfinder.census.gov/servlet/DatasetMainPageServlet?_program=ACS. Accessed March 10, 2008.
2. Chang I. *The Chinese in America: A Narrative History*. New York, NY: Penguin Books; 2003.
3. *Chinese Americans Food Practices, Customs, and Holidays*. Ethnic and Regional Food Practices Series. Chicago, IL: American Dietetic Association; 1999.
4. New York City Department of Health and Mental Hygiene. More than 100,000 New Yorkers Face Complications Due to Seriously Out-of-Control Diabetes (press release). January 30, 2007. http://home2.nyc.gov/html/doh/html/pr2007/pr002-07.shtml. Accessed March 10, 2008.
5. McNeely MJ, Boyko EJ. Type 2 diabetes in Asian Americans: results of a national health survey. *Diabetes Care*. 2004;27:66–69.
6. International Diabetes Federation. Diabetes Atlas. http://www.eatlas.idf.org/atlasff5d.html?id=0. Accessed May 20, 2009.
7. Park Y. Why is type 1 diabetes uncommon in Asia? *Ann N Y Acad Sci*. 2006;1079:31–40.
8. Pan WH, Flegal KM, Chang HY, Yeh WT, Yeh CJ, Lee WC. Body mass index and obesity-related metabolic disorders in Taiwanese and US whites and blacks: implications for definition of overweight and obesity for Asians. *Am J Clin Nutr*. 2004;79:31–39.
9. McNeely MJ, Boyko EJ, Shofer JB, Newell-Morris L, Leonetti DL, Fujimoto WY. Standard definitions of overweight and central adiposity for determining diabetes risk in Japanese Americans. *Am J Clin Nutr*. 2001;74:101–107.
10. World Health Organization Expert Consultation. Appropriate body mass index for Asian populations and its implications for policy and intervention strategies. *Lancet*. 2004;363:157–163.
11. Wen CP, David Cheng TY, Tsai SP, Chan HT, Hsu HL, Hsu CC, Eriksen MP. Are Asians at greater mortality risks for being overweight than Caucasians? Redefining obesity for Asians. *Public Health Nutr*. 2008;12:1–10.
12. Wildman RP, Gu D, Reynolds K, Duan X, He J. Appropriate body mass index and waist circumference cutoffs for categorization of overweight and central adiposity among Chinese adults. *Am J Clin Nutr*. 2004;80:1129–1136.
13. Ng MC, Lee SC, Ko GT, Li JK, So WY, Hashim Y, Barnett AH, Mackay IR, Critchley JA, Cockram CS, Chan JC. Familial early-onset type 2 diabetes in Chinese patients: obesity and genetics have more significant roles than autoimmunity. *Diabetes Care*. 2001;24:663–671.
14. Campbell TC. Energy balance: interpretation of data from rural China. *Toxicol Sci*. 1999; 52:87–94.
15. Gong R. *Goodluck Life: The Essential Guide to Chinese American Celebrations and Culture*. New York, NY: Harper Collins; 2005.

16. Yang GI, Fox HM. Food habit changes of Chinese persons living in Lincoln, Nebraska. *J Am Diet Assoc.* 1979;75:420–424.
17. Kim KK, Yu EX, Liu WT, Kim J, Kohrs MB. Nutritional status of Chinese-, Korean-, and Japanese-American elderly. *J Am Diet Assoc.* 1993;93:1416–1422.
18. Satia JA, Patterson RE, Kristal AR, Hislop TG, Yasui Y, Taylor VM. Development of scales to measure dietary acculturation among Chinese-Americans and Chinese-Canadians. *J Am Diet Assoc.* 2001;101:548–553.
19. Grivetti LE, Patterson MB. Nontraditional ethnic food choice among first generation Chinese in California. *J Nutr Educ.* 1978;10:109–112.
20. Lv N, Cason KL. Dietary pattern change and acculturation of Chinese Americans in Pennsylvania. *J Am Diet Assoc.* 2004;104:771–778.
21. Zhao HL. Traditional Chinese medicine in the treatment of diabetes. *Nestle Nutrition Workshop and Clinical Performance Program.* 2006;11:15–29.

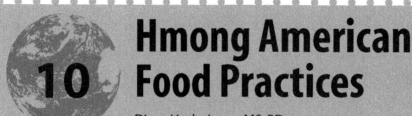

Hmong American Food Practices

Diane Veale Jones, MS, RD

Introduction

Most Hmong Americans are immigrants, or the children of immigrants, from the mountainous areas of northern Laos, Vietnam, and Thailand. Their ancestors migrated southward from China about 300 years ago and settled in remote areas that were not extensively populated. Traditionally, they farmed, hunted, and fished to sustain themselves. Because the form of agriculture they practiced tended to deplete the soil, they moved their villages to new sites every 4 to 6 years.

During the Vietnam War, the US Central Intelligence Agency recruited and trained the Hmong to fight for the United States in the "secret war" in Laos. Many Hmong died in this conflict. Their 15-year involvement in US military operations led to their persecution by the Communist Pathet Lao and the Vietnamese after the United States pulled out of Southeast Asia and the Royal Lao government collapsed. Many Hmong were killed, but a sizeable number escaped to refugee camps in Thailand. In 1976 the US Refugee Program allowed Hmong to come to the United States.

According to the 2000 US Census, 169,428 Hmong lived in the United States (1). In 2001, the estimated number of Hmong Americans was 300,000 (2). The largest Hmong communities outside of Southeast Asia are in California, Minnesota, and Wisconsin. Hmong people also live in Massachusetts, North Carolina, and Michigan, as well as small numbers in other states (2). Hmong tend to locate in metropolitan areas. However, in Minnesota, for example, they maintain their agricultural roots by growing gardens and selling produce at farmer's markets (3,4).

Diabetes Prevalence

Approximately 8% of Americans have diabetes (5). Research on the prevalence of diabetes among Hmong Americans is scarce (6). One study found that diabetes prevalence in Hmong Americans was higher than in the general population (7). A cross-sectional survey conducted by Her and Mundt found that 41% of Hmong Americans in Wisconsin were "potentially at risk for developing" diabetes (7). The prevalence of diabetes in the Hmong before they moved to the United States is unknown. However, Hmong participants in a study by Devlin and coworkers indicated that diabetes was uncommon in their homeland (8).

Risk Factors for Type 2 Diabetes

Overweight

Adults who are overweight (body mass index [BMI] ≥ 25) and those who are of Asian and Pacific Islander origin are considered to be at increased risk of developing type 2 diabetes (9). Information on the weight status of the adult Hmong American population is limited.

Her and Mundt studied 144 adult Hmong Americans and found 62% of women and 35% of men had a BMI greater than 27 (7). Another study of 50 Wisconsin Hmong Americans found that the mean BMI for men and women was 26.8 (10). According to data from the University of California Los Angeles School of Public Health, prevalence of overweight in Asian and Pacific Islanders in the United States increases with the number of years since immigration (11).

Evidence is increasing that Hmong American children and adolescents are overweight. High blood pressure and obesity were observed in Hmong children in the early 1990s (12,13). In California the prevalence of overweight Asian and Pacific Islander children increased from 7% in 1994 to 15% in 2003 (14). Among second-generation Asian American adolescents, the obesity rate is more than double the rate for first-generation adolescents (11,15). In a study that focused on food and weight patterns of US-born Hmong American and non-Hispanic white adolescents, 28.6% of Hmong American males had a BMI equal to or greater than the 95th percentile for age and sex, compared with 12.7% of non-Hispanic white males (15). In the same study, there was no difference in obesity rates between Hmong American and non-Hispanic white female adolescents (15).

Compared with whites, the risk of insulin resistance in the Hmong may be associated with a lower BMI (16). Therefore, it may be prudent to routinely check Hmong clients, especially overweight youths, for glucose tolerance (16).

Many Hmong Americans recognize that being overweight is not healthy and understand the value of physical activity and healthful eating (17). There are efforts to promote healthful eating and exercise among Hmong Americans. For example, the Minnesota Hmong Health Resource Group's 2008 initiative included three important messages (18):

- The body likes healthy foods . . . Go walking 30 minutes.
- Eat a variety of foods . . . Run until you sweat.
- A healthy body makes you happy . . . Go biking.

Ancestry

Genetics is linked to diabetes for Mexican Americans and Japanese Americans. It is also likely that Hmong ancestry increases the risk for diabetes (6).

Psychological and Social Factors

Obesity is associated with food insecurity in refugee populations (6). Individuals who experienced malnutrition and starvation may overeat due to past and current stress (6,19). Many Hmong suffer from depression due to separation from their homeland (20,21), and mental health issues can complicate treatment of diabetes (6,22).

The degree of acculturation, education levels, and age affect the incidence of diabetes in the Hmong American population. Some researchers posit that diabetes is associated with "New World syndrome"—ie, the American lifestyle with a diet that is high in fat and simple sugars, and with a lack of physical activity (6,15,17,23,24).

In addition, "a lot of Hmong parents show love by feeding their kids," according to Yer Moua Xiong, a medical resident in Minnesota, who further noted, "another problem is that for new immigrants with a lot of kids nutrition is not the primary goal, just getting food on the table, as cheaply as possible is the concern" (18).

Low socioeconomic status is also associated with lack of access to medical care and healthful foods (6,10). Language barriers and differences between Western medicine and traditional Hmong health/illness practices affect diabetes treatment (6,25–28). Traditional Hmong health beliefs and practices are discussed later in this chapter.

Traditional Foods and Dishes

The traditional Hmong diet is high in complex carbohydrates and low in refined sugar. White rice is the staple of the Hmong diet and may comprise as much as half of a typical day's energy intake (23). It is served at every meal (2 cups per meal is typical), and no meal is considered complete without it. Hmong families usually purchase rice in 100-lb sacks. Noodles made from rice, wheat, or mung beans are also popular.

The Hmong are familiar with a wide variety of fruits and vegetables. Some of the fruits they consumed in their homeland, such as the jackfruit, are not generally available in the United States, and the high cost of other traditional choices (eg, mango, papaya, coconut, guava, and pineapple) limits their consumption.

Families often grow vegetables in community gardens or on other small plots of land available to them. Unusual varieties of eggplant, squash, pumpkin, and edible gourds are among the vegetables cultivated. The young, tender vines and leaves of these plants are simmered in water to make a broth to sip at mealtime.

The Hmong value freshness in food. They did not can or freeze food in their homeland, and refrigeration was unavailable. Pickling and drying were the only methods of food preservation the Hmong used. In the United States, the Hmong continue to prefer fresh food; families typically purchase canned, frozen, or convenience foods only when fresh items are not available. Families who have a garden usually freeze their Hmong vegetables for later use.

Among types of meat, the Hmong prefer pork. It is not unusual for a family to purchase a live pig, butcher it, freeze it, and then eat the meat over an extended time period. They also like chicken and eat it regularly. Families may butcher their own fresh chickens or get them from chicken farms. Large quantities of fresh beef, venison, and fish may also be frozen for future use. Turkey is not popular, but some families may eat turkeys if they receive them as gifts at Thanksgiving and Christmas. The Hmong eat beef less often than pork or chicken, but they do eat it. They enjoy eggs and freshwater fish and frequently consume tofu (29).

Boiling, grilling, steaming, deep-frying, and stir-frying are the basic methods of food preparation. Meat may be broiled or roasted in the oven or grilled over charcoal. Older homemakers do not use measuring cups or spoons for food preparation, and they may be unfamiliar with such common household measurements as teaspoons, cups, and ounces. The Hmong do not traditionally eat casseroles, but stews and soups are common.

In stir-fries, the Hmong usually use pork lard as the fat, although some home cooks have learned to use vegetable oil. The Hmong may eat salad dressing and mayonnaise. A typical Hmong salad dressing includes lemon juice, fish sauce, ground peanuts, boiled eggs, and vegetable oil.

The most commonly consumed beverage at mealtime is the broth in which vegetables have been cooked; the Hmong sip it from a small bowl or cup. They drink cold water to quench thirst and do not customarily consume alcoholic beverages before or as part of a meal. Alcohol is consumed by men on social occasions, but women usually do not drink it. See Table 10.1 and Box 10.1 (30) for more information on traditional Hmong foods. Refer to Appendix A for nutrient analyses.

Traditional Meal Patterns and Holiday Foods

Hmong families eat two or three meals a day; if money for food is limited, they are more likely to eat only two meals (29). Snacking is not common among adults, but children snack. Hmong eat most meals at home. A typical meal is rice, vegetables (usually greens), and chicken, pork, or beef. The food is put into bowls and placed in the center of the table for family members to serve themselves. Spoons and forks are common eating utensils.

For everyday meals, all family members eat together. However, they may eat at different times due to school or work schedules.

The Hmong celebrate one major holiday each year, the New Year, which generally takes place in December or January. The community usually holds a large New Year's celebration lasting several days and including traditional dancing, music, and games. Displays of Hmong artistry—such as *pa ndau,* a complicated reverse appliqué needlework, and handmade silver jewelry—are also part of the festivities. Preparation for the holiday begins months earlier because everyone, especially teenagers, must have new clothing and jewelry. In 2004 Hmong Americans celebrated their 29th Hmong New Year in Minnesota. The 2-day

Table 10.1 · Foods Used in Traditional Hmong Cuisine

Food	Comments
Starchy vegetables	
Cassava	
Plantains	
Pumpkin	
Nonstarchy vegetables	
Bamboo shoots	Fresh bamboo shoots are not available in the United States. They are usually purchased canned in water and used in stir-fries or other mixed dishes.
Bitter melon	A cucumber-like vegetable with a bumpy green surface and bitter flavor.
Cucuzzi squash/spaghetti squash/suzzamelon	This large, edible gourd is round to oval with a pale yellow skin. The flesh forms translucent strands similar to spaghetti when cooked.
Lutta squash or gourd	This vegetable has a green, ridged body and a firm, sweet interior.
Mung beans	Tiny dried beans that can be sprouted to grow mung bean sprouts.
Mustard greens	This dark-green, leafy vegetable with a somewhat bitter taste is a staple in the Hmong diet and may be eaten daily. Greens may be stir-fried, simmered in water, or pickled with salt.
Summer squash	
Thai round green eggplant	This type of eggplant does not look at all like the dark-purple variety that is common in the United States. Small, with a striated green skin, it is usually eaten raw with rice at the main meal of the day. Sometimes it is cubed and stir-fried with bite-size pieces of chicken or fish. It can also be used in fish soup and served with *nqaij liab*.
Yard-long beans	Looking much like 1.5-to-2-foot-long green beans, yard-long beans have the same crunchy texture as green beans.
Rice and noodles	
Cellophane or mung bean noodles	Thin, translucent noodles made from mung beans
Hmong rice patty	A traditional food also eaten as a snack with either molasses or caramel syrup. Hmong rice patty is made by heavily pounding on cooked sticky rice, which is then separated and shaped into small patties to be wrapped with banana leaf or aluminum foil. This is also a nostalgic food for elders.
Once-cooked rice	Rice that has been boiled with water until half done and then transferred to a rice steamer to steam until done. In the United States, most young families cook rice using an automatic rice cooker.
Rice flour	Typically used to make desserts.
Rice sticks	Opaque noodles made from rice flour.
Spring roll wrapper or rice paper	Thin sheets, larger than wonton wrappers, made from rice flour. Because they are rather stiff, they need to be soaked in warm water to soften before they can be used to wrap food mixtures.
Sticky rice (sweet or glutinous rice)	A short-grained rice that is much more glutinous (the grains adhere together) and more expensive than regular short-grain rice .
Fruits	
Apple pear (Asian pear)	This large, light-yellow, apple-shaped fruit has a crunchy texture.
Guava	An oval fruit that resembles a rough-surfaced lemon. The skin color ranges from yellow to green. The flesh, which can be white, yellow, pink, or red, has a grainy texture because of the presence of small seeds.
Jackfruit	An oblong fruit with a greenish-yellow to brown surface covered with hard points. The flesh is bright yellow.
Mango	
Papaya	The Hmong use green-fleshed papaya as an ingredient in some dishes, such as the popular papaya salad.

(continued)

Table 10.1   *(continued)*

Food	Comments
Spices and seasonings	
Cilantro/Chinese parsley/coriander	This flat-leafed parsley has a pungent, musky flavor. The leaves are scattered over many foods for flavoring and can also be used as an ingredient in salads or spicy dipping sauce. Chinese parsley is sometimes used as a medicine for chicken pox.
Dill	
Fish sauce	A sauce made by fermenting small, salted fish in wooden casks for several months and draining the liquid.
Garlic	
Ginger, fresh	
Green onions	
Lemon and lime juice	
Lemongrass	A tall, wide-bladed grass that emits a lemony odor when torn and is used or seasoning.
Monosodium glutamate (MSG)	
Soy sauce	
Thai chili peppers	Small, hot red peppers that are dried and used for seasoning.
Meat	
Beef	
Chicken	
Freshwater fish	
Pork	
Tofu/bean curd	A smooth, custardlike curd made by pureeing soybeans, precipitating the soybean milk with calcium sulfate, vinegar, lemon juice, or another coagulating agent, and then transferring the curd to a mold to form square cakes. Hmong frequently consume tofu. The Hmong made their own tofu in their homeland, but most in the United States buy it from local stores.
Venison	

Box 10.1 • Traditional Hmong Dishes, Beverages, and Desserts

Dishes

- Baked striped bass with tomatoes and herbs[a]
- Noodle soup
- Pea vine salad
- Pork and mustard greens soup[a]
- Stir-fried chicken or pork
- Stuffed bitter melon[a]
- Tofu and chicken soup

Beverages

- Vegetable broth
- Water

Desserts

- Cassava root and plantain tapioca dessert[a]
- Pumpkin pudding
- Steamed sweet rice cakes

[a]Recipes can be found in reference 30.

Box 10.2 • Traditional Foods Consumed During the Hmong New Year

- *Nqaij liab:* mixture of ground pork, chili peppers, green onion, Chinese parsley, rice flour, and monosodium glutamate (MSG). A small amount is served on a bed of lettuce or a cabbage leaf. (the pork may be served raw)
- Noodles
- Papaya salad
- Smoked pork
- Sticky rice
- Sticky rice cakes wrapped in banana leaves
- Sweet drinks

---

gathering of more than 70,000 Hmong was "the celebration of freedom and liberty, along with the maintenance of thousand year-old traditions" (31). In California the 2006 Hmong New Year celebration contrasted traditional music and dancing with contemporary music and dance styles (32).

Traditionally, men and boys do most of the food preparation during the New Year's celebration, whereas women generally are responsible for daily food preparation. The men customarily eat first at holiday time, which is not usually the case in the home. Box 10.2 lists traditional New Year's foods. Vendors at the Hmong New Year celebration also offer a variety of American foods, including ice cream, tacos, donuts, and fried chicken (33).

Traditional Health Beliefs

Traditional Hmong beliefs regarding health and illness are inseparable from spiritual beliefs. The Hmong believe three souls reside in the body, but one or more can move in and out of it, depending on the balance and harmony among the souls. Upon death, the souls take three routes: one is with the ancestors, one stays in the body, and one goes to the spirit world. Although the Hmong recognize natural and physical causes of sickness, they attribute most illnesses to problems in the spirit world. Disharmony with the spirit world results in the loss of one or more of the individual's three souls (34–38). This loss results in a range of afflictions, such as pain, depression, headaches, vomiting, rashes, and infertility (34,35). The traditional system of dealing with sickness involves several types of healers (21,34–36):

- Shamans (*tus txiv ua neeb* or *neng*): A shaman is a man, woman, or child who is "chosen" *(yuav ua neeb)* as a spiritual healer, usually following a serious illness. He or she serves as a mediator between a Hmong person and the spirit world, performing healing ceremonies and negotiating with spirits by using spirit money or exchanging an animal soul for a human one.
- Soul callers *(tus hu plig)*: A soul caller is a man or woman who calls the lost soul and returns it to the body in a soul-calling ceremony that involves chanting, the burning of incense, and offerings of food. One learns the practices from other soul callers.
- Magic healers (*tus ua khawv koob* or *dug u ker kong*): These healers are not "chosen" ones. They use magic incantations to treat nonspiritual illnesses.
- Herbalists (*kws tshuaj* or *kau chua*): Most herbalists are women. They treat nonspiritual illnesses and have knowledge of medicinal plants.

Many Western physicians view shamanism as positive therapy to counteract anxiety and other psychic and psychosomatic disorders (20). The herbal medicines can have nutritional effects as well as medicinal properties. Corlett and colleagues found that Hmong Americans in California grew 25 medicinal herbs in urban gardens. These herbs contributed minerals such as calcium, zinc, and iron to the diet (39).

The Hmong define a serious illness as a condition that renders the individual incapable of eating, drinking, or getting out of bed (35). An individual who can still function, even at a low level, is considered to be only mildly ill. Thus, Hmong may not seek medical attention until they are very ill by Western standards.

In interviews with Hmong individuals in the central valley of California, Ikeda and colleagues discovered that some were concerned that Western medicines are "too strong" for the Hmong because they "are little people and Americans are big people" (29). According to Culhane-Pera and Her, some Hmong clients feel weaker and sicker when they take Western medicines (19).

In a 2002 health survey of Hmong Americans in Orange County, California, 74% indicated that they went to a shaman when ill (40). Although many Hmong are Christian, they consult both physicians and traditional healers (10,26,36,41). Second- and third-generation Hmong Americans are typically comfortable with Western medicine (42).

Current Food Practices

With acculturation, some Hmong Americans have changed their traditional diet. Today, the Hmong eat more fat, sugar, salt, and meat than they traditionally ate (19,24). Consumption of refined carbohydrates such as soft drinks, pies, cookies, and cakes has also increased (10,29). Bread is eaten to a limited degree. Older Hmong homemakers may not be aware that there are different kinds of flour (whole-wheat and white) with different nutritional properties.

Cereals were introduced to the Hmong, primarily the children, via the Special Supplemental Nutrition Program for Women, Infants, and Children (WIC) program. Parents will often purchase a cereal requested by their children or one advertised heavily on television.

In the United States, the Hmong typically eat oranges, apples, peaches, bananas, cantaloupe, grapes, pears, grapefruit, and watermelon. They drink orange juice and apple juice; grape juice and pineapple juice are favorites. Some Hmong may be unfamiliar with reading food labels and not know the difference between 100% fruit juice and fruit-flavored drinks.

In their homeland, the Hmong usually did not consume tea or coffee. In the United States, the Hmong occasionally enjoy coffee with condensed milk and sugar or plain tea. Adults generally do not drink milk, but some children do. Children also consume hamburgers, hot dogs, corn dogs, pizza, spaghetti, tacos, sandwiches, and ice cream.

School nutrition programs such as the National School Lunch Program are among the major forces introducing new foods to Hmong Americans. Most Hmong children receive a free school lunch, and some receive free breakfast as well. In this way, they are served many foods that are new to them, and with repeated exposure they often learn to like them.

Some parents have reported anxiety about marketing and school-day influences on their children's eating habits (14). Many Hmong associate changes in their traditional diet with being "out of balance" (19). Focus group research suggested that some Hmong think their health was better when they ate a traditional diet and did physical labor (8). Participants mentioned that city living directly affected their activity level, "In Laos, we could work and sweat; we had places to be active and we could eat anything" (8).

Counseling Considerations

Demonstrating Courtesy and Respect

Studies suggest health providers can earn the trust of Hmong clients by carefully listening to their clients' experiences with diabetes and the ways they manage it (7,8). Many Hmong clients use spirituality and traditional medicines to treat diabetes, and health professionals need to respect that these approaches may help to restore balance to the client's lives (8).

Hmong people consider the following behaviors rude (42–45):

- Direct eye contact
- Laughing

- Speaking loudly
- Waving hands
- Pointing
- Winking
- Declining offers of food or drink
- Assuming familial relationships
- Touching without permission
- Making comments about children

The Hmong do not traditionally shake hands when greeting others, and women may be uncomfortable doing so, especially with a man. Men and women avoid close proximity to one another (44,45). Elders are respected, and children are expected to defer to them and their parents and to be well behaved.

There may be generational differences in expectations of courtesy and respect. Today, many second- and third-generation Hmong Americans follow American customs. Most of them also respect their Hmong heritage and practice Hmong traditions. In response to the question, "What makes you Hmong?" one individual replied, "I think what makes me Hmong is practicing Hmong culture unconsciously when I interact with people; when I say Hmong, I mean the food, clothes, rituals, clan relationships and many more things" (46).

Interpreting Clients' Nonverbal Communication

Traditionally, Hmong people are humble and do not demonstrate emotions in front of others. When counseling clients, look for nonverbal actions that may indicate a lack of understanding, such as glazed eyes, looking off to the side, shifting uncomfortably, or giggling (47).

Inquiring About Clients' Understanding of Diabetes

Several studies report that many Hmong Americans misunderstand diabetes (19,48,49). Perez and Cha used focus groups to learn about Hmong American knowledge of diabetes. They found an "overwhelming lack of knowledge about diabetes mellitus among study participants" (48). There is no word for diabetes in the Hmong language. However, two of the participants told the interviewer that diabetes was *ntshav qab zib* ("blood sweet" or "sweet blood") and they did not understand what caused the condition (48). Interviews with 11 Hmong shamans in California who had diabetes and/or hypertension revealed that they did not understand the condition or its relationship to diet (49). On the other hand, a study by Culhane-Pera and Her found that Hmong participants with diabetes knew that they need to practice portion control, especially when eating rice, and restrict consumption of sugar, alcohol, sodium, fat, soft drinks, and fruit (19).

As a sign of respect to the health care provider, Hmong clients may be reluctant to ask questions or to say "no" to a question. Most likely, a client will respond to a question with a nod, a "yes," or a "maybe" even if he or she disagrees or does not understand (43,45,50).

The following factors may make it difficult to determine a client's understanding of diabetes (6,15,19,25,38,51):

- Language barriers
- Client's unfamiliarity with the concept of a chronic disease
- Lack of appropriate interpreters
- Lack of culturally appropriate health care
- Client's mistrust of the Western medical system

Like other new immigrants and refugees to the United States, the Hmong may have difficulty communicating because they do not speak, read, or understand English. Older Hmong may have limited education and English-language skills and must rely on interpreters or their children to talk with English speakers. Because there was no written Hmong language until the 1950s, many older Hmong do not read or write Hmong or English. Traditions were handed down through oral stories.

Diabetes and other chronic diseases may be difficult for the Hmong to comprehend. Many Hmong do not understand human anatomy or physiology, and the Hmong vocabulary does not include words for many medical concepts (25). Furthermore, they may not understand reasons for invasive procedures, such a finger pricks, or the purpose of medications (34).

Using analogies to something familiar in Hmong culture improves client's understanding of diabetes. For example, Peterson and colleagues used the process of making tofu to explain how insulin functions in the body, drawing comparisons between the need for lemon juice in the tofu-making process and the role of insulin in controlling glucose in the body (23). The authors acknowledge that individualized counseling is required to determine whether clients understand the analogy.

Federal law requires that health professionals make an interpreter available to Hmong clients (52). However, some interpreters are unfamiliar with the Hmong language or medical terminology, and some families rely on children to translate (6), even if the topics discussed are not appropriate for their age (53).

One interviewer of Hmong clients noted that "the Hmong traditionally understand there to be potential cures for all illnesses." Therefore, telling a Hmong person that diabetes (or another disease is chronic, "is at best like saying that you are giving up on the patient and at worst is like putting a curse on them" (28).

The lack of health-related concepts in the Hmong language can limit a Hmong client's understanding of diabetes (37). Health care providers who are unfamiliar with Hmong beliefs and practices can hinder communication with Hmong clients.

Some researchers report that Hmong distrust the Western medical system because the US government failed to keep promises following the Vietnam War (8). Hmong Americans may also believe that health care professionals withhold treatment from them or use them for medical experimentation (25,28).

Culhane-Pera and colleagues developed a Hmong Cultural Model to address their patients' view that their life in the United States was unbalanced compared with life in Laos (19). With awareness of traditional Hmong culture, the model "connects personal bodily experiences of diabetes with a traditional model of balance, and a shared social suffering of refugees living in a country where they do not fit" (19). Another effort to treat Hmong clients with diabetes found that they benefited mentally from group visits to the community health facility, but this contact did not lead to better control of diabetes (22).

Discussing Clients' Use of Complementary and Alternative Medicine

Ask the client whether he or she uses any traditional Hmong health practices. Many Hmong Americans may use both Hmong remedies and Western medicines. Herbs are used to treat a broad range of symptoms and are usually the first remedy a family tries. If herbal preparations do not work and symptoms persist or worsen, the Hmong consult a shaman.

Many Hmong realize that health care providers view their traditional health beliefs as incompatible with Western medicine. This may make clients reluctant to seek assistance from US health care providers. To secure greater success with Hmong clients, health care providers should not automatically discourage the use of traditional methods of diagnosis and healing. Instead, look for ways to present Western medical procedures as a complement to traditional methods. This approach may be more successful than advocating the abandonment of Hmong health practices in favor of Western medicine.

Although it is well documented that Hmong use herbs for treatment of health problems, specific herbs are not usually identified. Specific home remedies for diabetes treatment have not been adequately described in medical research, but some information about the treatment of children is available. For example, Hmong parents have been warned that a traditional medicine, *pay loo ah,* contains lead and can poison their children (54). See Table 10.2 for additional information about Hmong forms of alternative and complementary medicine (36,38). Refer to Appendix C for questions to assess dietary supplement use.

Table 10.2 · Remedies Used by the Hmong for Self-treatment

Hmong Name	Description	Uses	Administrator
Hu plig	Soul-calling ceremony	Cure for illness	Head of household
Kav	Rubbing with a spoon	Pain relief	Adult
Khi huluas tes	Wrist string tying	Treatment for illness; also used in celebrations (eg, marriages, births)	Elder family member
Nchos ceeb	"Fright release" (parent massages a child to reduce his or her fear)	Reduction of fear in infants and children	Adults
Npaus	Pinching	Headache relief	Adults
Txhuav	Cupping	Pain relief	Adult

Source: Data are from references 36 and 38.

Considering Family Demands and Dynamics

Family, both nuclear and extended, is extremely important to the Hmong. A traditional household consists of a husband and wife and their children and grandchildren. It may also include elderly relatives of the husband or wife. Children are taught to revere their fathers. Male family members usually address issues related to health or other family matters (55). It is customary to greet family members according to age and gender, acknowledging the oldest male first. Although wives are involved in the decision-making process, they are traditionally expected to defer to their husbands in final decisions. However, some Hmong women question traditional views of femininity and gender identity (56), and Hmong American youth may challenge traditional parental relationships and family obligations. A focus group of Hmong youth revealed that many felt their parents were "inflexible, overprotective, controlling, and isolated from community resources" (57).

Engaging Others in Counseling Session

According to Perez and Cha, diabetes should "not be treated as a personal disease" (48). The Hmong belong to patrilineal kinship groupings (clans) and these groups are of utmost importance in Hmong culture, even in the United States. The Hmong pay deep respect to clan membership, and a system of mutual obligation and respect links clan members (23). A clan leader, chosen by consensus, is often the eldest male head of household and represents each clan. The Hmong community looks to clan leaders for guidance. Families may consult clan leaders when making a major decision, such as whether a family member should have surgery or to submit to some other Western medical procedure.

It is important for health professionals to recognize the typical influence of the male head of household on all aspects of family life. It may be appropriate to include the head of the household in counseling sessions when diet or lifestyle changes are discussed because he may have the final word as to whether the changes are implemented. If possible, individuals who shop for and prepare the meals should also be included in the counseling session.

Nutrition Counseling

Most Hmong understand that eating too much causes weight gain, but some may not understand that high-fat foods contribute to overweight. Older Hmong Americans may be unfamiliar with the concept that food contains calories or nutrients.

Appendix B offers selected medical nutrition therapy recommendations for individuals with diabetes and general counseling suggestions that support those recommendations. The following are culturally specific nutrition counseling strategies for Hmong American clients:

- The goal of nutrition counseling for Hmong clients should be to limit but not eliminate consumption of unhealthful traditional foods (48). For example, given the centrality of white rice in the Hmong diet and culture, it may be unrealistic to ask clients to switch to brown rice. Instead, emphasize portion control and encourage clients to try other foods, such as whole-grain bread and cereal products, that provide the nutrients found in brown rice (29).

- Offer clients actual food items to taste, because they likely cannot afford to purchase a variety of whole-grain breads and cereals to determine their preferences. Also, show them the food packaging—Hmong often buy items based on visual recognition of the product.
- Encourage clients to have sticky rice only occasionally, and eat long-grain rice more often. Also, advise them to have smaller portions of rice if they are eating noodles in the same meal.
- Use actual foods or Asian food models and measuring tools (eg, Asian-style bowls) to teach portion control, particularly when working with older Hmong, who do not traditionally use recipes and are likely unfamiliar with food measurements.
- Encourage consumption of healthful traditional foods, especially fresh fruits and vegetables and vegetable broth.
- Explain that it is not necessary to have meat at every meal.
- Demonstrate how to trim fat from meat, remove skin from chicken, and skim fat from soups and stews.
- Encourage clients to replace lard with heart-healthy oils; stir-fry foods in small amounts of oil; and steam foods.
- Suggest that clients limit their intake of organ meats and eggs.
- Promote daily activities such as gardening and walking.
- Encourage clients to drink plain water or vegetable broth instead of soft drinks.

Challenges and Barriers to Dietary Compliance

When working with Hmong clients, the following may be obstacles to dietary compliance (19,51):

- The client is unwilling or unable to eat foods different from what the family eats.
- The client's food budget is limited.
- Medical care is expensive or limited in availability.
- The client is not proficient in English.
- Appropriate interpreters are unavailable.
- The client feels isolated.
- The client is confused about diabetes and its treatment.

Counseling Tips

As you work with Hmong clients, the following tips may help facilitate counseling: (51,55,58,59):

- Allow sufficient time for listening to clients' concerns.
- Provide simple, basic information about diabetes.
- Be positive, honest, and hopeful about the client's ability to manage diabetes, while avoiding insincere flattery.
- Be respectful of religious and traditional health practices.
- Avoid stereotypes and generalizations about the Hmong culture; individualize care.
- Consider group counseling.
- Use hands-on learning techniques.
- Personalize your points with stories from your own life, if you feel comfortable doing so.
- Encourage clients to share the ways they manage diabetes.
- Ask clients to bring food labels from products they have purchased to counseling sessions.

Conclusion

The prevalence of type 2 diabetes among Hmong Americans is linked to ancestry, weight gain, and social factors. Acculturation favors the Western diet over the traditional diet of rice, fresh vegetables, and small amounts of meat. Although Hmong Americans know that being overweight is unhealthy; understanding of diabetes is often limited.

Hands-on activities, use of analogies and stories, and group sessions are techniques that improve Hmong American clients' knowledge of type 2 diabetes. Furthermore, effective dietary counseling requires cultural sensitivity to Hmong family structure and an understanding of the traditional health beliefs and practices of the Hmong.

Resources

Hmong and Diabetes. http://www.diabetesyouth.com/hmong.htm. Accessed February 24, 2009.

Hmong Health Website. http://www.hmonghealth.org. Accessed February 24, 2009.

Hmong Home Page. http://www.hmongnet.org. Accessed February 24, 2009.

Hmong Studies Internet Resource Center. http://www.hmongstudies.org. Accessed February 24, 2009.

Selected Patient Information in Asian Languages (SPIRAL). Patient Information by Topic: Hmong Hmoob. http://www.library.tufts.edu/hhsl/spiral/hmong.shtml. Accessed February 24, 2009.

Symonds PV. *Calling the Soul: Gender and the Cycle of Life in a Hmong Village.* Seattle: University of Washington Press; 2004. (This book covers birth and death rituals of the Hmong in their homeland.)

Working with Hmong Audiences: A Collection of Resources for Nutrition Education. University of Minnesota Extension Service and Wisconsin Nutrition Education Program, University of Wisconsin. http://www.uwex.edu/ces/wnep/hmong. Accessed February 24, 2009.

References

1. US Census Bureau. Hmong Fact Sheet, 2000. http://factfinder.census.gov/home/saff/main.html?_lang=en. Accessed March 9, 2002.

2. Pobzeb V. Hmong Population and Education in the United States and the World. Lao Human Rights Council Web site. 2001. http://www.laohumanrights.org/2001data.html. Accessed March 30, 2004.

3. Carlson G. Asians in Minnesota, 2000. *Population Notes.* Minnesota State Demographic Center; 2002. http://www.demography.state.mn.us/DownloadFiles/pdf/AsiansMN2000.pdf. Accessed March 2, 2009.

4. Vang CY. *The People of Minnesota: Hmong in Minnesota.* St. Paul, MN: Minnesota Historical Society Press; 2008.

5. American Diabetes Association. Total prevalence of diabetes and pre-diabetes. http://www.diabetes.org/diabetes-statistics/prevalence.jsp. Accessed March 27, 2008.

6. Southeast Asian Subcommittee of the Asian American/Pacific Islander Work Group, National Diabetes Education Program. Silent trauma: diabetes, health status, and the refugee Southeast Asians in the United States: issues and recommendations for approaches to reduce the burden of diabetes in this vulnerable population; June 2006. http://ndep.nih.gov/resources/SilentTrauma.htm. Accessed March 27, 2008.

7. Her C, Mundt M. Risk prevalence for type 2 diabetes mellitus in adult Hmong in Wisconsin: a pilot study. *West J Med.* 2005;104:70–77.

8. Devlin H, Roberts M, Okaya A, Xiong YM. Our lives were healthier before: focus groups with African American, American Indian, Hispanic/Latino, and Hmong people with diabetes. *Health Promot Pract.* 2006;7:50.

9. American Diabetes Association. Standards of medical care in diabetes—2006. *Diabetes Care.* 2006;29(Suppl 1):S4–S42.

10. Chang PG. Anthropometrics, dietary habits, and feelings about health among Wisconsin Hmong-Americans. *UWL Journal of Undergraduate Research.* 2005;8:1–6. http://www.uwlax.edu/URC/JUR-online/PDF/2005/chang.pdf. Accessed March 2, 2009.

11. Kagawa-Singer M. A case for an AAPI 5-a-day and physical activity campaign. California Asian American Nutrition and Physical Activity Campaign. 2006. http://www.ph.ucla.edu/cehd/Documents/Kagawa_Singer___2006_CORICA.pdf. Accessed July 7, 2008.

12. Himes JH, Story M, Czaplinski K, Dahlberg-Luby E. Implications of early obesity in low-income Hmong children. *Am J Dis Child*. 1992;1:67–69.

13. Munger RG, Gomez-Marin O, Prineas J, Sinaiko AR. Elevated blood pressure among Southeast Asian refugee children in Minnesota. *Am J Epidemiol*. 1991;12:1257–1265.

14. Obesity increasing among Asian Americans. *Medical News Today*. October 23, 2004. http://www.medicalnewstoday.com/printerfriendlynews.php?newsid=15362. Accessed July 8, 2008.

15. Stang J, Kong A, Story M, Eisenberg ME, Neumark-Sztainer D. Food and weight-related patterns and behaviors of Hmong adolescents. *J Am Diet Assoc*. 2007;107:936–941.

16. McCarty DJ. Glucose intolerance in Wisconsin's Hmong population. *WMJ*. 2005;104:13–14.

17. Harrison GG, Kim LP, Kagawa-Singer M. Perceptions of diet and physical activity among California Hmong adults and youth. *Prev Chronic Dis*. 2007;4:A93.

18. Doeun A. Hmong healthy eating and exercising initiative. *Hmong Times*. February 13, 2008:12.

19. Culhane-Pera KA, Her C, Her B. "We are out of balance here": a Hmong cultural model of diabetes. *J Immigr Minor Health*. 2007;9:179–190.

20. Bliatout BT. Guidelines for mental health professionals to help Hmong clients seek traditional healing treatment. In: Hendrick GL, Downing BT, Deinard AS, eds. *The Hmong in Transition*. New York, NY: Center for Migration Studies of New York; 1986:349–363.

21. Muecke MA. Caring for Southeast Asian refugee patients in the USA. *Am J Public Health*. 1983; 174:431.

22. Culhane-Pera KA, Peterson KA, Crain AL, Center BA, Lee M, Her B, Xiong T. Group visits for Hmong adults with type 2 diabetes mellitus: a pre-post analysis. *J Health Care Poor Underserved*. 2005;16.2:315–327.

23. Peterson KA, Vang ML, Xiong YM. Type 2 diabetes in the Hmong community. In: Culhane-Pera KA, Vawter DE, Xiong P, Babbit B, Solberg MM, eds. *Healing by Heart: Clinical and Ethical Case Stories in Hmong Families and Western Providers*. Nashville, TN: Vanderbilt University Press; 2003.

24. Lee MM, Huang S. Immigrant women's health: nutritional assessment and dietary intervention. *West J Med*. 2001;175:133.

25. Johnson SK. Hmong health beliefs and experiences in the Western health care system. *J Transcult Nurs*. 2002;13:126–132.

26. Warner ME, Mochel M. The Hmong and health care in Merced, California. *Hmong Stud J*. 1998;2:1–29. http://www.hmongstudies.com/HSJ-v2n2_Warner.pdf. Accessed March 2, 2009.

27. Gensheimer L. Learning from the experience of Hmong mental health providers. *Hmong Stud J*. 2006;7:1–31. http://www.hmongstudies.org/Gensheimer.pdf. Accessed March 2, 2009.

28. Henry RR. *Sweet Blood, Dry Liver: Diabetes and Hmong Embodiment in a Foreign Land* [dissertation]. Chapel Hill, NC: University of North Carolina; 1996.

29. Ikeda JP, Ceja D, Glass R, Harwood JO, Lucke K, Sutherlin J. Food habits of the Hmong in central California. *J Nutr Educ*. 1991;23:168–174.

30. Lee S, Scripter S. *Cooking from the Heart: Hmong Cooking in America*. St. Paul, MN: University of Minnesota Press, 2009.

31. Bringing in the new: Hmong New Year celebrations. *Asian Week*. December 2-8, 2004;26:9.

32. Millbourn T. Hmong culture is stepping out New Year festival honors traditions, and bends a few. *The Sacramento Bee*. November 26, 2006:B1.

33. Yang K. An assessment of the Hmong American New Year and its implications for Hmong-American culture. *Hmong Stud J*. 2007;8:1–8. http://hmongstudies.org/KYangHSJ8.pdf. Accessed March 2, 2009.

34. Her C, Culhane-Pera KA. Culturally responsive care for Hmong patients: collaboration is key component. *Postgrad Med*. 2004:116:39–46.

35. Thao X. Hmong perception of illness and traditional ways of healing. In: Hendrick GL, Downing BT, Deinard AS, eds. *The Hmong in Transition*. New York, NY: Center for Migration Studies of New York; 1986:365–378.

36. Plotnikoff GA, Numrich C, Wu C, Yang D, Xiong P. Hmong shamanism: animist spiritual healing in Minnesota. *Minn Med*. 2002;85:29–34.

37. Vang XX. *Awareness of Hmong Religious Practices and Rituals in Regards to Counseling Hmong Students* [thesis]. Stout, WI: University of Wisconsin-Stout; 2007.

38. Nuttall P, Flores FC. Hmong healing practices used for common childhood illnesses. *Pediatr Nurs*. 1997;23:247–251.

39. Corlett JL, Clegg MS, Keen CL, Grivetti LE. Mineral content of culinary and medicinal plants cultivated by Hmong refugees living in Sacramento, California. *Int J Food Sci Nutr*. 2002; 53:117–128.

40. Vang G, Ichinose T, Murrieta S. Hmong Health Care Practices in Orange County: Results from a Hmong Health Survey. County of Orange Health Care Agency, Public Health Services Web site. Summer 2002. http://www.ochealthinfo.com/docs/AgcyPubs/phs/hmong_survey_02.pdf. Accessed March 27, 2008.

41. Gilman SC, Justice J, Saepham K, Charles G. Cross-cultural medicine a decade later: use of traditional and modern health services by Laotian refugees. *West J Med*. 1992;157:310–315.

42. Veale Jones D. Hmong Americans. In: *Ethnic Foodways in Minnesota*. 2nd ed (unpublished manuscript).

43. Hmong for Health Care Workers. Kern Resource Center. http://www.health-careers.org/resources/Hmong%20Handbook%20Revised%203-06.pdf. Accessed July 9, 2008.

44. Vujongyia K. Hmong Information Sheet. University of Minnesota, Extension Web site. http://www.extension.umn.edu.

45. Lee TP, Pfeifer ME. Cultural Etiquette for Interacting with Traditional Hmong. Building Bridges: Teaching about the Hmong in our Communities. Hmong Cultural and Resource Center; 2006. http://www.hmongstudies.org/BuildingBridgesGeneralPresentation2006Version.pdf. Accessed June 30, 2008.

46. Vang N. What makes you Hmong? *Hmong Times*. May 16, 2007:1–2.

47. Cultural Competency: Working with the Hmong. 1977 Lao Family Community of Minnesota. http://lapfamily.org/culture/culture info5.htm. Accessed March 9, 2004.

48. Perez MA, Cha K. Diabetes knowledge, beliefs, and treatments in the Hmong population: an exploratory study. *Hmong Stud J*. 2007;8:1.

49. Helsel D, Mochel M, Bauer R. Chronic illness and Hmong shamans. *J Transcult Nurs*. 2005;16:150–154.

50. Betancourt D. Cultural Diversity: Eating in America: Hmong. Ohio State University Extension Fact Sheet. 2006. http://ohioline.osu.edu/hyg-fact/5000/5254.html. Accessed July 17, 2008.

51. *Voices from the Community: Focus Groups with African American, American Indian, Hispanic, and Hmong People with Diabetes*. St. Paul, MN: Minnesota Department of Health, Minnesota Diabetes Control Program; 1998.

52. Cultural and Medical Traditions: Hmong Culture and Medical Traditions. Children's Hospital and Clinics. 2003. http://expedo02.children.org. Accessed March 30, 2004.

53. Immigration in Minnesota: Discovering Common Ground. The Minneapolis Foundation; 2004. http://www.minneapolisfoundation.org/immigration/home.htm. Accessed June 30, 2005.

54. These home remedies contain lead and are very dangerous. Alameda County Community Development Agency, Lead Poisoning Prevention Program. 2007. http://www.aclppp.org.homerem.htm. Accessed July 17, 2008.

55. Pinzon-Perez H. Health issues for the Hmong population in the U.S.: implications for health educators. *Int Electronic J Health Educ*. 2006:9:122–133.

56. Julian R. Hmong transitional identity: the gendering of contested discourses. *Hmong Stud J*. 2004–2005;1–23.

57. Xiong ZB, Detzner DF. Southeast Asian adolescents' perceptions of immigrant parenting practices. *Hmong Stud J*. 2004–2005;5:1–20.

58. Vujongyia K. Supporting Positive Dietary Changes in Diverse Audiences. Presentation at the Minnesota Dietetic Association's annual meeting, St. Cloud, MN; May 2, 2003.

59. Hmong Culture. Hennepin County, Minnesota. 2008. http://www.co.hennepin.mn.us/portal/site/HCInternet/menuitem.3f94db53874f9b6f68ce1e10b1466498/?vgnextoid=888b60a6bb9fc010VgnVCM1000000f094689RCRD&vgnextfmt=default. Accessed July 14, 2008.

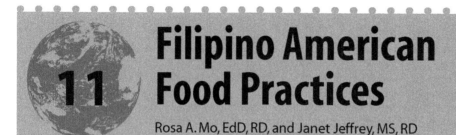

Filipino American Food Practices

Rosa A. Mo, EdD, RD, and Janet Jeffrey, MS, RD

Introduction

The Philippines consists of 7,107 islands situated southeast of mainland Asia and separated from it by the South China Sea. Other bordering seas include the Philippine Sea and the Pacific Ocean on the east, the Celebes Sea on the south, the Sulu Sea on the southwest, and the South China Sea on the west. The three main islands are Luzon, Visayas, and Mindanao. Manila, the capital of the Philippines, is located on the island of Luzon.

The number of Filipinos in the United States has increased substantially since 1965, when laws were changed to permit more immigrants from the Philippines. Two-thirds of Filipino immigrants qualified to come to the United States as professional or technical workers. In the 2000 US Census (1), 2 million respondents identified themselves as either Filipino alone or Filipino in combination with one or more Asian groups or other races. Among these respondents, more than 75% indicated they were Filipino only (1). The Filipino population was the second largest Asian population in the United States, following the Chinese group. The Filipino population is greatest in the western United States, particularly in Hawaii and California (1).

Filipino Americans are a very heterogeneous group, who originate from many cultural subgroups within the Philippines. Although they may speak many different dialects, Filipino Americans typically speak English and their educational attainment is high. They have not formed large, homogenous neighborhoods comparable to the Chinatowns in many US cities.

Diabetes Prevalence

Data about the prevalence of diabetes in this ethnic group are limited. However, a cross-sectional study of a convenience sample of Filipino Americans, age 20 to 74, in Houston, Texas, estimated the prevalence rate of type 2 diabetes to be 16.1% (2). This rate was much higher than the 1998 US diabetes prevalence rate of 6.5% (2). Similarly, a study of Filipino Americans in Daly City, California, estimated the prevalence of diabetes in Filipino Americans to be 34.7%, vs 24.1% prevalence in whites (3). The same study also found Filipino Americans were at greater risk for developing type 2 diabetes (3). In a study in San Diego County, California (4), the prevalence of type 2 diabetes in Filipinas was 36%, vs 9% in white women, and the prevalence of metabolic syndrome in Filipinas was 34%, vs 13% in white women. Whereas 33% of the white subjects with diabetes were obese, 10% of the Filipinas with diabetes were obese (4). The high prevalence of diabetes in nonobese Filipinas suggests the need to further study diabetes in various non–Northern European ethnic populations (4).

Visceral adipose tissue (VAT)—ie, fat located around internal organs—is associated with insulin resistance and glucose intolerance. Araneta et al (5) used glucose levels, anthropometric measurements, and computed tomography to compare VAT and the risk for type 2 diabetes in 55- to 80-year-old Filipina, African American, and white women without known cardiovascular disease. VAT was greatest among Filipina women, but they had the lowest age-adjusted body mass index (BMI). BMI and waist circumference were weaker predictors of VAT in Filipina and African American women than in whites. The occurrence of age-adjusted type 2 diabetes was higher in Filipinas (32.1%) than in white women (5.8%) or African American women (12.1%). After adjusting for age, VAT, exercise, education, and alcohol intake, Filipinas had the highest risk for type 2 diabetes compared with African Americans and whites (5).

Risk Factors for Type 2 Diabetes

Age

Increasing age is the strongest risk factor for diabetes in Filipino Americans, and diabetes prevalence in Filipinos increases between the ages of 30 and 39 years. The sharpest increase in prevalence in Filipinos is in the 65- to 74-year age range (2).

Family History of Diabetes

Among Filipino Americans, familial clustering of diabetes is more common than in the second US National Health and Nutrition Examination Survey (NHANES) population (2). Cuasay and associates conducted a cross-sectional survey of 831 Filipino Americans between the ages of 20 and 74 in the Houston, Texas, metropolitan statistical area from September 1998 to March 2000 (2). In this survey of Filipino American participants, 37.5% reported that one parent had diabetes, 6% reported diabetes in both parents, and 20% reported diabetes in one or more siblings. In contrast, the 1982–1983 Diabetes Mellitus Survey in the Philippines, which surveyed 12,297 Filipinos aged 20 to 65 found that 30% of native Filipinos had one or both parents with diabetes and 14% had siblings with diabetes (2).

Overweight and Obesity

In the second NHANES population, the prevalence of obesity was high in individuals with diabetes. However, obesity alone does not explain the high prevalence of diabetes in Filipino Americans. The mean BMI of individuals with diabetes in the second NHANES study was 28.1 vs a mean BMI of 26.1 for Filipino Americans with diabetes in the Houston, Texas, survey by Cuasay et al (2). In the Houston survey, the mean BMI for Filipino Americans without diabetes was 24.4 (2).

Acculturation

An increased risk of diabetes has been demonstrated in epidemiologic studies of immigrant groups who adopted a Western lifestyle and diet. The length of stay in the United States, however, was not associated with prevalence of diabetes in the study of Filipinas living in San Diego County (4). These results are consistent with the observations of Mexican, Puerto Rican, and Cuban immigrants (6). The Philippines, Mexico, Puerto Rico, and Cuba were colonies of Spain for more than 300 years. In addition, the Philippines and Puerto Rico became US colonies in 1898. These shared cultural factors and exposure to Western lifestyle prior to US immigration may explain why the length of stay in the United States does not affect the risk of diabetes for these groups (4).

Traditional Foods and Dishes

The traditional foods and cuisine of the Philippines evolved through the process of indigenization—ie, the process in which a food or dish arrives in a country through trade or colonization and over time becomes native to the country. Filipino food is a melding of Malay, Chinese, Spanish, and American influences. For example, *pancit* originated as a Chinese noodle dish and is now a signature Filipino dish. Another dish entrenched in the native cuisine is *adobo*. In Spain, *adobo* is a pickling sauce of olive oil, vinegar, garlic, thyme, laurel, oregano, paprika, and salt. After native Filipino cooks adapted it, *adobo* became a mixture of vinegar, garlic, bay leaf, peppercorns, and soy sauce.

Many Filipino dishes use vinegar to tenderize meat, lengthen the dish's shelf life without need for refrigeration, and contribute the slightly sour flavor that is common in Filipino foods. The Filipino method of sautéing *(pag-gigisa)* is the foundation of many dishes and can turn mundane vegetables or leftovers into delicious dishes. This cooking process consists of the following steps: heat oil, brown garlic, sauté onion until translucent, and add tomatoes; then add vegetables, leftovers, or other ingredients and sauté until fully cooked.

The use of dipping sauces *(sawsawan)* is a hallmark of Filipino cuisine. Filipinos manipulate the flavor of dishes to suit their individual preferences by using various ingredients such as vinegar, garlic, *calamansi* (similar to lemon juice), soy sauce, *patis* (fish sauce), and *bagoong* (fermented sauce) (7).

Box 11.1 lists foods commonly used in traditional Filipino cuisine, and Table 11.1 lists traditional Filipino dishes, beverages, and desserts (8,9). Refer to Appendix A for nutrient analyses. Because Filipino cuisine varies greatly by region, these food lists are not comprehensive.

Box 11.1 • Foods Used in Traditional Filipino Cuisine

Starches

- Egg bread *(pan monay)*
- Glutinous, sticky or sweet rice *(malagkit)*
- Rice
- Rice vermicelli or rice sticks *(bihon)*
- Roll *(pan de sal)*
- Soybean or silky noodle *(sotanghon)*
- Steamed rice cakes *(puto)*

Starchy vegetables

- Beans *(abitsuwelas,* garbanzos, mung beans)
- Corn
- Green peas *(gisantes)*
- Plantain
- Potatoes
- Purple yams *(ube)*
- Taro *(gabi)*
- Yam or sweet potato *(camote)*
- Yuca (cassava)

Nonstarchy vegetables

- Bamboo shoots
- Banana blossoms
- Beets
- Bitter gourd, Asian gourd, or bitter melon
- Bottle gourd *(upo)*
- Cabbage *(pechay)*
- Carrots
- Cauliflower
- Chayote
- Chinese chard cabbage (bok choy or *pechay)*
- Cucumber
- Eggplant
- Green and red peppers
- Green beans
- Hearts of palm or young coconut tree bud
- Horseradish tree *(malunggay)*
- Jicama *(sinkamas)*
- Leek
- Mung bean sprouts
- Mushroom
- Okra
- Onions
- Pepper leaves *(dahong sili)*
- Snow peas *(sitsaro)*
- Sponge gourd *(patola)*
- Spinach
- Squash blossoms
- String beans *(sitaw)*
- Swamp cabbage *(kangkong)*
- Tamarind
- Tomatoes
- Wax gourd *(kondol)*

(continued)

Box 11.1 *(continued)*

Milk and milk products
- Edam cheese *(queso de bola)*
- Evaporated milk
- Farmer's cheese *(quesong puti)*

Fruits
- Avocado
- Banana
- Grapes
- Guava
- Jackfruit *(langka)*
- Lime *(calamansi)*
- Mango
- Orange *(naranghita)*
- Pears
- Pineapple
- Pomelo
- Raisins
- Sapodilla *(chico):* a round fruit, 2–4 inches in width with brown skin. The flesh is described as resembling a pear and its color ranges from yellow to dark brown.
- Soursop *(guyabano)*
- Star apple *(kaimito)*
- Star fruit
- Strawberry
- Sugar apple fruit *(atis)*
- Watermelon

Meats and meat substitutes
- *Balut* (cooked fertilized egg)
- Beef
- Chicken
- Fish:
  - Anchovy *(dilis)*
  - Carp *(gurami)*
  - Catfish (*hito* or *kanduli*)
  - Codfish *(bacalao)*
  - Flounder *(dapa)*
  - Grouper *(lapulapu)*
  - Mackerel (*hasa-hasa* or *tanguingge*)
  - Milkfish *(bangus)*
  - Milkfish, dried *(daing na bangus)*
  - Mudfish *(dalag)*
  - Pompano (*pompano* or *cavalla*)
  - Red snapper *(maya-maya)*
  - Sardines
  - Shark fish
  - Tilapia
- Organ meats (heart, kidney, lungs, brains, liver, tongue, tripe, blood pudding)
- Pork:
  - Bilbao sausage *(chorizo de Bilbao):* a spicy sausage from Bilbao, Spain
  - Cured pork *(tocino)*
  - Ham
  - Pork crackling *(chicharones)*
  - Pork sausage *(longaniza)*
- Salted egg
- Shellfish and other seafood:
  - Prawns *(sugpo)*
  - Shrimp *(camaron)*
  - Clams *(halaan)*
  - Crab *(alimango)*
  - Eel
  - Oysters
  - Squid *(pusit)*

Nuts
- Cashews
- Peanuts

Herbs, spices, and other flavorings
- Anise seeds
- Annato seeds *(achuete)*
- Bay leaf
- Black beans, fermented *(tausi)*
- Cinnamon
- Ginger
- Fish paste, fermented *(bagoong)*
- Fish sauce *(patis)*
- Hot pepper
- Peppercorn

(continued)

Box 11.1   (continued)

- Cloves
- Coriander
- Curry powder
- Garlic

Fats

- Butter
- Canola oil
- Coconut cream: coconut milk first extracted from freshly shredded coconut then diluted with water
- Coconut oil (latik): precipitate of boiled coconut milk

- Saffron
- Soy sauce
- Turmeric

- Lard
- Margarine
- Olive oil
- Peanut oil
- Vegetable oil

Table 11.1 · Traditional Filipino Soups, Dishes, Beverages, and Desserts

Name	Description
Soups	
Albondigas	Meatball soup with noodles
Misua soup	Fine white noodle soup with chicken
Munggo gisado masabaw	Mung bean soup with cubed or sliced pork and shrimps
Pansit molo	Filipino-style wonton soup
Picadillo soup	Soup with ground pork or chicken and vegetables such as chayote or upo (bottle gourd)
Tinolang halaan or tulya	Shellfish soup with ginger and generous amounts of fresh vegetables such as upo (bottle gourd), chayote, pepper leaves (dahong sili), green cabbage (pechay), and horseradish tree (malunggay) leaves
Meat dishes	
Adobo	Pork and chicken simmered in vinegar, soy sauce, and garlic
Asado	Filipino-style beef pot roast
Bacalao	Salted, dried codfish
Bistec	Sliced beef marinated in lemon (calamansi) juice and soy sauce, pan-fried and served with pan-fried sliced onions
Caldereta	Cubed goat meat sautéed with potatoes, peas, bell peppers, and seasonings
Callos de garbanzos	Ham hocks, tripe, or oxtail and chorizo de Bilbao with chickpeas
Embotido	Roll of ground meat wrapped in leaf lard
Empanada	Meat turnover
Escabeche	Sweet-sour fried fish
Mechado	Similar to asado, but with narrow strips of fat inserted into the beef and cooked in a clay pot in tomato sauce
Menudo	Ground beef with diced liver or tripe, peas, carrots, and chickpeas
Morcon	Rolled flank steak stuffed with ham, sausage, hard-cooked eggs, and olives
Pochero	Beef, chicken, or pork stewed with chorizo de Bilbao, ham hocks, vegetables, and plantains
Tapa	Thinly sliced pork or any other meat cured, salted, and dried, then pan-fried
Vegetable dishes	
Bulanglang	Mixture of several vegetables simmered with fish and seasoned with bagoong
Lumpia	Eggroll stuffed with fresh vegetables
Pinakbet	Stew of bitter gourd, okra, eggplant, and tomatoes

(continued)

Table 11.1 *(continued)*

Name	Description
Breakfast and merienda *dishes*	
Bibingka	Baked coconut and rice dessert made with rice flour, brown sugar, butter, and condensed milk; may be garnished with salted egg
Champorado	Rice porridge flavored with chocolate
Cuchinta	Steamed snack made with powdered rice, sugar, and lye water, which lends a brown color to the finished soft product
Esaimada	Sweet roll with cheese
Espasol	Sweet rice flour cake with coconut milk and sugar
Halo-halo	Literally translated as "mix-mix"; layers of various beans, tropical fruits topped with shaved or crushed ice and *leche flan;* eaten with condensed milk or milk and sugar
Itlog na maalat	Salted duck egg
Lugao	Sweet concoction of rice and other ingredients, with coconut milk
Palitaw	Glutinous rice dough balls flattened to a tongue-like shape, boiled and rolled on a mixture of sugar-toasted sesame seeds and shredded coconut
Polvoron	Shortbread
Puto	Fluffy glutinous rice cake
Sitsaron	Deep-fried pork or chicken skins
Tsokolate	Chocolate
Beverages	
Pandan tea	Tea made from the aromatic screw pine leaves
Salabat	Gingered tea
Desserts	
Buko	Fresh immature coconut with gelatinous meat
Guinataan	Starchy vegetable cooked in coconut milk
Gulaman	Gelatin from seaweeds sold in dehydrated bars
Leche flan	Custard topped with caramelized sugar
Maja blanca	Sweet, gelatin-like dessert made from rice flour and milk
Suman sa ibus	Boiled glutinous rice wrapped in banana leaves and eaten dipped in white sugar
Taho	Soft soybean that is served with syrup and tapioca pearls

Source: Data are from references 8 and 9.

Traditional Meal Patterns and Holiday Foods

The Filipino traditional meal pattern consists of a large breakfast, lunch, and dinner, as well as a midafternoon snack called a *merienda.* Breakfast is typically a starchy food and a protein dish. Starchy foods include rice, bread, or native *kakanin. Kakanin* is derived from the word *kanin* (rice) and refers to foods made from different kinds of rice (eg, regular, sticky, or sweet) that are baked, boiled, or steamed. Types of *kakanin* include *puto, kuchinta,* and *suman,* which are sweet dishes prepared with rice flour or sticky rice and coconut milk. Rice at breakfast is always leftover from the night before and may be fried with garlic. Another breakfast dish, *champorado,* is rice cooked in cocoa and coconut milk. Breakfast bread, called *pan de sal,* may be substituted for rice. Another popular breakfast bread is a yeast roll called *ensaimada,* which is baked and then sprinkled with shredded cheese and sugar. The protein dish may be fried eggs, vienna sausage, a pork sausage called *longganiza,* or dried fish *(daing).* Breakfast beverages include hot chocolate, hot ginger tea *(salabat),* or hot coffee.

Table 11.2 · Traditional Foods Consumed During Holidays

Name	Description
Arroz caldo	Thick rice soup with tripe or chicken
Bibingka	Glutinous rice flour cake steamed with coconut milk
Ensaimada	Brioche-like cakes buttered, sugared and cheese-sprinkled
Jamon en dulce	Honey cured ham
Kari-kari	Beef shank or oxtail sautéed in shrimp paste *(bagoong)* with vegetables, with sauce thickened with ground peanuts or peanut butter and color enriched with annatto *(achuete)*
Lechon	Roasted pig
Pandan tea	Tea made from the aromatic screw pine leaves
Relleno	Stuffed and boneless chicken or fish
Salabat	Gingered tea
Tsokolate	Hot, thick chocolate beverage
Ukoy	Shredded vegetables dipped in batter and deep fried then served with shrimp for garnish

Source: Data are from references 8 and 9.

Lunch and dinner are hot meals and similar to each other in the amount and kinds of dishes served. The typical meal consists of soup, a hot entrée, vegetables, and a noodle dish or rice, which is always a staple. Fresh fruit or dessert ends the meal. Homes with a strong Spanish tradition serve the courses consecutively. In contrast, homes with a heavy Filipino influence serve the courses family-style.

The traditional *merienda* is part of the casual style of living and the hospitality of Filipinos. It is common for friends to drop in for a friendly conversation after a siesta (afternoon nap) to share leftover *kakanin* from breakfast, freshly prepared banana fritters, *empanadas* (a meat-filled pastry), *lumpia* (similar to an egg roll), or *guinataan,* which is a combination of various boiled starchy vegetables and fruits (8).

Major holidays celebrated by the Filipinos are typically related to the Catholic faith and include Christmas, Easter, the feast days of patron saints *(fiestas),* and the New Year. The Christmas celebration in the Philippines begins on December 16 with attendance at the first of nine predawn Masses called *Misa de Aguinaldo.* The celebration continues until the Feast of the Epiphany on January 6. Refer to Table 11.2 for foods served during the Christmas holiday (8,9).

Filipino Americans are well known for their hospitality. They will go to great lengths in food preparation, including serving *lechon* (roasted pig) on holidays and special occasions (8). In the Philippines, Christmas coincides with the rice harvest, and therefore Christmas celebrations typically include many native rice cakes and foods with sticky rice. Some examples of these foods include *puto bungbong* and *bibingka,* as well as *ensaimadas* to dip in *tsokolate.* Apples, oranges, chestnuts, and walnuts, commonly eaten in Europe during Christmas time, are also included in Philippine holiday celebrations (7).

Traditional Health Beliefs

Influenced by an excellent public health system while under American colonization, Filipinos today generally respect modern medicine. However, they also have traditional beliefs and health practices that can affect their care and compliance. They may seek culturally specific alternative therapies for certain maladies (10).

Traditional health beliefs and behaviors vary among the different ethnic groups within Filipino culture, but there are some commonalities, which are described here. *Bahala na* is the concept that life is controlled by the will of God or a supernatural power. Whatever happens is predetermined, and therefore *bahala na* encourages a sense of security that God will take care of everything. *Bahala na* justifies the Filipino's sense of resignation to whatever comes, a faith that it is their bad luck or destiny to have the disease. It can also be an escape from decision-making and social responsibility (10).

Filipinos view their health and wellness from the perspective of balance *(timbang)*. They believe that adherence to proper social and cultural behaviors can prevent health problems, whereas illness is associated with social conflicts, assaults to cultural practices, and negative dealings with the supernatural (10). According to traditional Filipino health beliefs, humans, nonhumans, or divine retribution can cause illness. For example, a health imbalance may be caused by a witch or a sorcerer, ghost, dead ancestor, evil spirit, or all-powerful supernatural being (10). The concept of balance centers on *hotness* and *coldness* as related to bodily humors, food, and air balances. Quick changes from hot to cold can disrupt balance. For humoral balance, Filipinos maintain a warm condition. For example, if the body is hot after performing strenuous activities, Filipinos will not wash their hands or body in cold water until the body cools down. Sudden shifts in balance may cause temporary paralysis, muscle spasms, or bulging of blood vessels. Similarly, Filipinos avoid exposure to cold air from a blowing fan or draft because this can upset the body's equilibrium and potentially trigger colds, fever, rheumatism *(rayuma)*, or respiratory tract infections (10). In addition, Filipinos aim to maintain food balance. For example, they may stay away from cold drinks early in the morning because they believe that cold drinks cause abdominal pain *(masisik-mura)*. Overeating late at night is a form of food imbalance; Filipinos believe it can cause sudden abdominal cramps *(bangungut)* that lead to death (10).

Filipinos highly value personal hygiene. It is common for Filipinos to take multiple baths each day to maintain the proper balance of hot and cold in the body. They believe baths of warm or cool water infused with herbs restore balance. Washing and not just wiping after voiding maintains balance. Filipinos seek to maintain regular bodily functions, sleep patterns, eating routines, and bathing practices to avoid illnesses and sustain balance. They believe what goes around comes around. Thus, if they have been habitually careless in their appearance *(burara)*, they will pay for it in terms of illness (10).

Current Food Practices

As in many cultures, food is essential to Filipino social life. Spanish, Mexican, Malaysian, Chinese, American, and Indian cooking have influenced Filipino food practices (11).

Three basic principles in Filipino cooking are as follows:

- Never cook any food by itself.
- When frying, use garlic in olive oil or lard.
- Foods should have a sour, cool, and salty taste.

Regular mealtimes are observed and include three meals a day (breakfast, lunch and dinner) along with one snack *(merienda)* in the midafternoon (see Traditional Meal Patterns section earlier in this chapter). Some Filipinos may eat a second breakfast *(segundo almuerzo)* at approximately 10:30 AM.

Individuals coming from a rural background will make lunch their main meal, whereas those with an urban background will emphasize the evening meal. The amount of meat or fish eaten in meals will depend on what the family can afford to buy. A typical meal consists of the following:

- Soup
- Viand *(ulam)*
- Fried or boiled rice *(kanin)*
- Pork, seafood, or chicken
- Native fruits
- Dipping sauces

The most common cooking methods are sautéing, stewing, boiling, braising and frying. Fried food will often be left on the *kawali* (wok) longer to allow the food to absorb more fat. Baked dishes are rarely served. During hot days, cold drinks *(sa malamig)* made from watermelon, cantaloupe, mango and other tropical fruits are often consumed.

Counseling Considerations

Cardiovascular disease is the leading cause of death in Filipino Americans, and Filipino diets are high in total fat, saturated fats, and cholesterol. Therefore, special attention should be given to clients' lipid levels as well as their blood glucose values (A1C, fasting blood glucose, and postprandial glucose) (12).

General counseling considerations include the following (13):

- Keep a nonjudgmental attitude and open mind.
- Determine the client's primary language and preferred communication and learning styles. If necessary, use a trained interpreter in counseling sessions.
- Provide information that is pertinent to the client.
- Assess the client's current diet and food preferences before giving dietary advice and making nutrition recommendations.

Demonstrating Courtesy and Respect

When greeting Filipino Americans, make eye contact, smile, and shake hands. Avoid any other type of touching, and place your hands by your sides, not in your pockets. Always request permission before addressing an individual by his or her first name. Filipino Americans consider it inappropriate and disrespectful to call an elderly client by his or her first name. This is particularly true if the health care provider is young. A positive attitude and expression are culturally expected. Therefore, Filipino Americans tend to avoid confrontation and prefer communication that is polite and formal (14).

Interpreting Clients' Nonverbal Communication

In Filipino culture, nonverbal communication is very important. The counselor should focus on the following (15):

- Pace of conversation: Allow for short moments of silence during the counseling session so the client can process information.
- Physical distance: Give the client enough personal space—a distance of 1 to 2 feet is customary.
- Eye contact: Sit at eye level with the client, so the client does not have to look up at you, and make brief and frequent eye contact. Older clients may look down or away as a sign of respect to an authority figure. Prolonged eye contact between a Filipino male client and a female clinician may be considered flirtatious.
- Emotional responsiveness: Notice facial expressions. Elders may sometimes smile or chuckle at what seem like inappropriate moments because they are nervous.
- Body movement: Frequent hand gestures may be used. Elders may cover their mouths with one hand when speaking or smiling if they feel shy or embarrassed. Nodding one's head has many meanings, such as "I hear you" or "Yes I'll cooperate."
- Touch: Elderly Filipina women may touch an arm or give a hug to express appreciation.

Inquiring About Clients' Understanding of Diabetes

Ask your clients, "Why do you think you developed diabetes?" The client's response may indicate that he or she understands the pathophysiological process. However, he or she may believe that diabetes is a supernatural punishment or caused by external, unbalanced conditions such as moving from a warm to a cool climate (14).

Discussing Clients' Use of Complementary and Alternative Medicine

Traditional healers in the Philippines include the following:

- Midwives
- Curers, who diagnose disease through the pulse
- Shamans, who use folk remedies to cure diseases
- *Arbularyos* (herbalists), who use thyme, marjoram, and chamomile to treat diabetes
- Faith healers, who cure disease through prayer by transmitting sacred healing energy

Table 11.3 · Selected Medicinal Plants Used in the Philippines

Names	Uses
Akapulko *(Cassia alata)*—bayabas-bayabasan (ringworm bush)	Treatment for ringworm and fungal infections
Ampalaya *(Momordica charantia)*—bitter gourd or bitter melon	Blood glucose control
Bawang *(Allium sativum)*—garlic	Cholesterol and blood pressure control
Bayabas *(Psidium guajava)*—guava	Antiseptic; also used as a mouthwash to treat dental cavities and gum infection
Lagundi *(Vitex negundo)*—five-leaved chaste tree	Cough suppressant and treatment for asthma
Niyog-niyogan *(Quisqualis indica L.)*—Chinese honeysuckle	Treatment for intestinal Ascaris and Trichina worms
Sambong *(Blumea balsamifera)*—Blumea camphora	Diuretic for the excretion of stones
Tsaang gubat *(Ehretia microphylla Lam.)*—Wild tea	Treatment for intestinal motility; also used as a mouthwash (contains fluoride)
Ulasimang bato *(Peperomia pellucida)*—pansit-pansitan (shiny bush or clearweed)	Treatment for arthritis and gout
Yerba buena *(Clinopodium douglasii)*—Peppermint	Treatment for aches and pains

Source: Data are from reference 16.

Through the *timbang* principle, an unbalanced person may be predisposed to illnesses. To correct this imbalance, many traditional healers use the following three practices:

- Heating: Filipino Americans traditionally believe that a warm body prevents illness. To achieve warmth, a person must expose himself or herself to the sun or another heat source, and eat the correct proportion of hot and cold foods. For example, cooling foods include orange juice and tropical fruits, vegetables, milk and dairy products, eggs, fish, and lean meats. Avocados, chili peppers, spices, alcoholic beverages, nuts, legumes, and fatty meats are examples of hot foods.

- Protection: Barriers are used to shield the body from natural and supernatural forces. For example, body fat prevents the body from external cooling. Filipino Americans traditionally believe that wind spreads disease, which is then absorbed by pores in the skin. They use coconut oil as an ointment for the skin to help close pores to disease.

- Flushing: Types of flushing, such as perspiration, flatulence, vomiting, and menstrual blood, are supposed to remove impurities from the body. A mixture of vinegar, water, salt, and chili peppers is used as a flushing treatment to stimulate sweating.

See Table 11.3 for examples of medicinal plants traditionally used in the Philippines (16). Refer to Appendix C for questions to assess dietary supplement use.

Considering Family Demands and Dynamics

Many Filipino American families are composed of members from multiple generations, with grandparents acting as surrogate parents for young families. When counseling clients, pay attention to how the individual's diabetes self-management fits within the context of the family network. Children are expected to show respect for older family members, such as *lola* (grandmother) and *lolo* (grandfather). Interdependence and care of the elderly are part of Filipino culture. Extended families are very common; they include all maternal and paternal family members, family elders, and unmarried siblings. Friends, coworkers, and neighbors may also be considered part of the extended family. The term *compadrazgo* is used to describe the relationship between a child, his or her parents, and the *compadre* (godfather) *or comadre* (godmother). This relationship is established when individuals act as sponsors to a marriage and as godparents at baptism.

Engaging Others in Counseling Sessions

For Filipinos, food symbolizes sharing and reciprocity and is used as a way to reestablish relationships. It is customary to serve foods to guests. Not eating the host's food is perceived as a rejection of social ties. When food is refused, the host may feel offended and ashamed.

These customs can be obstacles for diabetes self-management—clients may disregard dietary measures when facing a difficult social situation. Consider asking the client to invite family members or close friends to counseling sessions to keep everyone informed and create a supportive network (13).

Nutrition Counseling

Refer to Appendix B for medical nutrition therapy (MNT) recommendations for diabetes management as well as general nutrition counseling strategies. In addition, consider the following points when providing nutrition counseling to Filipino American clients (13,17):

- With the consent of the client, dietary counseling should include family members who are in charge of purchasing food and preparing meals.
- Counseling should focus on positive messages, including ways to improve well-being, prevent complications, and regain one's sense of balance.
- Clients must be part of the problem-solving discussion. Be aware that clients may feel ashamed when the counselor points out the areas in need of modification.
- Milk and dairy products are not staples in the traditional Filipino diet. Help clients get sufficient calcium by advising them to eat plenty of green leafy vegetables, nuts, legumes and soy products.

Challenges and Barriers to Dietary Compliance

Individuals with low health literacy or educational levels may require simple, pictorial-based instructions about what to eat, whereas other clients can comprehend more complex nutrition concepts and medical explanations about diabetes. Some may accept illness as part of their fate and will tolerate symptoms until they become severe. A client may consult neighbors, family members, friends, or traditional healers before obtaining medical services. This could delay the achievement of optimal glycemic control and contribute to diabetes-related complications (14).

Some Filipinos believe that fat protects them from becoming too cold and losing energy. This perception may be a barrier to even a modest weight loss, because being overweight is preferred to being too thin (15).

Counseling Tips

A trained interpreter should be used when the health care provider and client do not speak the same language. Clients may be more receptive and attentive to diabetes education when the discussion occurs in their native language. It is important, however, to ask the client whether an interpreter is needed. Some may be offended by the presence of a interpreter if they believe they have mastered the English language (13).

Conclusion

Given their high levels of education and English fluency, Filipino American clients can typically understand the advice of their diabetes counselors. However, diabetes management may be challenged by traditional beliefs in fate, supernatural forces, and the curing powers of faith, prayer, and sacred healing energy. One approach is to appeal to the Filipino culture of strong family ties. A diabetes counselor may be most effective by discussing diet modifications with family members as well as the client, while taking into consideration the individual's degree of acculturation, his or her traditional health beliefs, and personal food habits (13).

Resources

Epicurious.com: http://www.epicurious.com. Accessed May 27, 2009. (Database of more than 4,000 food terms and resource for ethnic and cultural foods.)

Quirante RE, Serrano-Claudio V, eds. *Filipino American Cookbook for Calorie Controlled Diets.* Audubon, IA: Jumbo Jack's Cookbooks; 1993.

References

1. US Census Bureau. Summary File 1. 2000 Census of Population and Housing. Technical Documentation. July 2007. http://www.census.gov/prod/cen2000/doc/sf1.pdf. Accessed March 3, 2009.
2. Cuasay LC, Lee ES, Orlander PP, Steffen-Batey L, Hanis CL. Prevalence and determinants of type 2 diabetes among Filipino-Americans in the Houston, Texas metropolitan statistical area. *Diabetes Care.* 2001;24:2054–2058.
3. Ryan C, Shaw R, Pilia M, Zapolanski AJ, Murphy M, Valle H, Myler R. Coronary heart disease in Filipino and Filipino-American patients: prevalence of risk factors and outcomes of treatment. *J Invasive Cardiol.* 2000;12:134–139.
4. Araneta MR, Wingard DL, Barrett-Connor E. Type 2 diabetes and metabolic syndrome in Filipina-American women: a high-risk nonobese population. *Diabetes Care.* 2002;25:494–499.
5. Araneta MR, Barrett-Connor E. Ethnic differences in visceral adipose tissue and type 2 diabetes: Filipino, African-American, and white women. *Obes Res.* 2005;13:1458–1465.
6. Harris MI. Epidemiological correlates of NIDDM in Hispanics, whites, and blacks in the U.S. population. *Diabetes Care.* 2006;14:639–648.
7. Fernandez DG. Culture ingested: notes on the indigenization of Philippine food. *Gastronomica.* 2003;3:61–71.
8. David-Perez E, ed.. *Recipes of the Philippines.* Philippines: National Book Store; 1973.
9. Quirante RE, Serrano-Claudio V, eds. *Filipino American Cookbook for Calorie Controlled Diets.* Audubon, Iowa: Jumbo Jack's Cookbooks; 1993.
10. Spector R. Health traditions. In: *Cultural Diversity in Health and Disease.* 6th ed. Upper Saddle River, NJ: Prentice Hall; 2004.
11. Anderson JN, Cross-cultural medicine: health and illness in Pilipino. *West J Med.* 1983; 139:811–819.
12. Southeast Asians and Pacific Islanders. In: Kittler P, Sucher K, eds. *Food and Culture.* 5th ed. Belmont, CA: Thomson Wadsworth; 2004:361–389.
13. Brown T. Meal planning strategies: ethnic populations. *Diabetes Spectrum.* 2003;16:190–192.
14. Rodell P. Marriage, family, and gender. In: *Culture and Customs of the Philippines.* Westport, CT: Greenwood Press; 2001:119–138.
15. McBride M. Health and Healthcare of Filipino American Elders. Stanford University School of Medicine. http://www.stanford.edu/group/ethnoger/filipino.html. Accessed August 1, 2007.
16. Ten (10) Herbal Medicines in the Philippines Approved by the Department of Health (DOH). Philippine Herbal Medicine Web site. May 14, 2007. http://herbal-medicine.philsite.net/doh_herbs.htm. Accessed September 10, 2007.
17. Nutrition recommendations and interventions for diabetes: a position statement of the American Diabetes Association. http://care.diabetesjournals.org/cgi/reprint/30/suppl_1/S48. Accessed September 3, 2007.

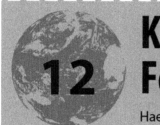

Korean American Food Practices

Haewook Han, PhD, RD, CSR, Jennifer Kwon, MS, RD, and Linda C. Ro, MS, RD

Introduction

Korea is an East Asian peninsula at approximately the latitude of northern California and covered with low mountains. For 3 years after the end of World War II, the Soviet Union occupied the northern half of the country while the United States controlled the southern half. After those years of outside control, Korea remained divided, with the Democratic People's Republic of Korea in the north and the Republic of Korea in the south. South Korea's population is almost 50 million, with 12 million people living in the capital Seoul. Approximately 82% of the population lives in urban areas.

Koreans began immigrating to the United States in the late 19th century, and US immigration became even more popular in 1970s. Many Koreans came to the United States to study; others were hoping to follow the "American Dream," especially after the Vietnam War. According to the 2000 US Census, more than 12.1 million individuals of full or partial Korean heritage live in the United States (1).

Korean immigrants often achieved high levels of education while in Korea, and then came to the United States between the ages of 20 and 40 years. However, many first-generation Korean Americans were not able to work in their chosen fields in the United States because of both US licensing laws and their limited English skills. An alternative was to own small retail businesses, such as dry cleaners and convenience food stores. These businesses are often unable to afford health insurance premiums, so Korean Americans are among the ethnic groups with the lowest rates of insurance coverage. The lack of insurance and limited English skills both contribute to low levels of health care utilization (2).

Korean immigrants tend to settle in already established Korean American communities. There are large populations of Korean Americans in California, New York, and New Jersey (3). Those living in large cities tend to socialize within the Korean American community, where Korean newspapers and Korean-language television programs are available. These media are popular with Korean Americans but may limit their use of English and can isolate them from English-speaking American culture (2). Most Korean Americans shop in Korean food stores. If they live in smaller cities where Korean stores are not available, they may drive long distances to visit these shops.

Diabetes Prevalence

Being of Asian heritage can be a risk factor for diabetes. The International Diabetes Federation lists the prevalence of diabetes in Korea in 2003 as 5% to 8% and forecasts a prevalence of 8% to 11% in South Korea by 2025 (4). Specific prevalence statistics for the United States are not available; Korean Americans are typically included within the Asian grouping in national health data.

Risk Factors for Type 2 Diabetes

Overweight and Obesity

Researchers have found that the longer an immigrant lives in the United States, the greater the risk of being overweight or obese. Cho and Juon list several factors that may contribute to these findings (2): individuals may increase their intake of high-fat, calorie-dense foods common in the United States (such as fast food); they may lead a more sedentary lifestyle and drive more; their income may decline; and they may work more than 40 hours per week.

McNeely and Boyko found that Asian Americans have an increased risk for diabetes at a lower body mass index (BMI) than non-Hispanic whites (5). In other words, Asian Americans develop diabetes at lower body fat levels than their white, non-Hispanic counterparts.

Lifestyle Factors

Heavy smoking and alcohol consumption are issues for some Koreans. In addition to diabetes, common chronic illnesses include hypertension and liver disease (2).

Traditional Foods and Dishes

Korea's geography has influenced its cuisine—fish and other seafood are abundant; the heavy rains of the hot summer coincide with the growth of the rice crop; and the topography makes small rice paddies more practical than large farms. Beef was not widely available in Korea until global transportation of foods became possible, but chicken and pork were a part of traditional Korean cuisine.

Japan occupied Korea for almost 40 years early in the 20th century, and the Japanese have had some influence on Korean eating habits. For example, Koreans eat raw fish (sashimi and sushi) and tempura (deep-fried fish, shellfish, or vegetables).

There are regional cuisines of the north and especially the south. However, during the Korean War, millions of North Korean refugees fled into South Korea, bringing their dietary habits with them. Therefore, there is now less regional variation. Southern Korean cuisine traditionally favors hot, salty foods because food preservation is more difficult in the warmer southern climate.

Traditional cooked foods are prepared on a stove. Foods are often boiled, sautéed, or fried in a variety of vegetable oils. Rice, soups, stews, and boiled vegetables are mainstays. Koreans rarely use ovens, and baked goods are not part of traditional Korean cuisine. To "bake" items such as sweet rice cakes, Koreans use a large, covered cast iron pan placed on a stove.

Refrigeration was not widely available until the 1970s. Until that time, Koreans had to salt and dry perishable foods to preserve them. This method of preservation gave foods a unique taste of salt and fermentation that Koreans enjoy. To make kimchi, the Korean national dish, vegetables such as Korean cabbage and radishes are combined with salt and red pepper; over time, the vegetables ferment and become crisp from the salt. Traditionally, the fermentation of kimchi took place in huge clay jars placed in the ground to be stored over the winter. In recent decades, however, more and more Koreans have moved to apartment buildings that do not allow residents to store kimchi in the ground. A few Korean electronics companies therefore sell a "kimchi refrigerator" that can be used instead. Commercially made kimchi is also widely available in Korea and major United States cities.

Many Korean foods are very spicy due to hot peppers, hot bean or pepper pastes, ginger, chopped scallions, and garlic. The traditional Korean diet contains many vegetables and few meats and sweets. Packaged snack foods were nonexistent until recent years. The diet is typically high in sodium because of the consumption of soy sauce; bean and hot pepper pastes; and dried fish.

The traditional Korean diet is rich in carbohydrates, including the following foods:

- Rice: Koreans eat large quantities of white glutinous or "sticky" rice, sometimes with brown rice, red beans, or barley added. Rice is typically eaten at two or three meals a day, in portions that are larger than usual American side-dish portions.

- Cakes of rice boiled in soup.
- Cakes of rice with red beans or soybeans.
- *Mandoo*: Similar to wontons, these dumplings are steamed, fried, or added to soup.
- Noodles: Many varieties are used in soups or mixed dishes.
- Beans: Soy, mung, and red beans are used in a variety of ways.
- Starchy vegetables such as sweet potatoes, potatoes, and corn on the cob.
- Several dessert items made from rice.
- Many kinds fresh fruit, often consumed as dessert.

See Table 12.1 and Table 12.2 for more information about traditional foods and dishes. Refer to Appendix A for nutrient analyses.

Table 12.1 · Foods Used in Traditional Korean Cuisine

Food	Description
Breads, cereals, and grains	
Noodles	Made from mixtures of buckwheat, wheat, soy bean, mung bean, sweet potato, or potato flour, Korean noodles can look like thick spaghetti. They may be served in soup; boiled and served with sesame oil, vegetables, and hot red pepper sauce without the liquid; or served in *chop chae,* a mixed dish with vegetables, beef, or pork. Popular noodles include udon (thick chewy noodles), somen (thin flour noodles), and soba (thin buckwheat noodles).
Rice cakes *(duk)*	White rice flour that is steamed and formed into sticks and cut into 1-inch-thick slices. *Duk* (pronounced "Ttuck") are added to broth to make the soup *duk gook,* a traditional New Year's dish.
Wheat and buckwheat	Common grains in the Korean diet.
White rice *(bap)* and sweet rice	Short-grain, glutinous white rice is the staple food for Koreans. White rice is typically prepared in electric rice cookers that store rice for a long time without altering the taste. Koreans frequently add beans or barley to the rice. This adds to the protein found in the rice and increases the fiber and vitamin content. Sweet rice is a different grain than white rice. Both grains are used in numerous types of sweets and desserts.
Beans	
Red beans	Ground red beans are made into soups or porridge or may be used to top sweet rice cakes.
Soybeans	A major part of the Korean diet. Soybeans are boiled and then ground, or made into bean paste, tofu, or soy sauce.
Starchy vegetables	
Corn on the cob	Eaten steamed without butter.
Potatoes	Potatoes are baked, boiled, steamed, or made into flour. The flour is used to make noodles.
Pumpkin	Pumpkin is boiled and made into soup; sliced, dried, and fried; or mixed with sweet rice for a dessert bar.
Sweet potatoes	Sweet potatoes are boiled and eaten by hand with the skin peeled back—similar to eating a banana.
Fruits	
Apples, pears, mandarin oranges, oranges, strawberries, bananas, grapes, peaches, plums, nectarines, pomegranates, many varieties of melons, and persimmons	Fruits are peeled, sliced, and served on a tray as dessert. Pears may also be added to kimchi—especially the summer water kimchi (*see* Nonstarchy vegetable section of this table). Koreans drink several varieties of fruit juices. Persimmons are eaten fresh or dried or brewed with ginger, cinnamon, and brown sugar into a tea.

(continued)

Table 12.1 *(continued)*

Food	Description
Sweeteners	
Honey	
Sugar	Sugar is added in small amounts to some meat marinades (eg, *bulkogi*). The amount of sugar consumed would be small unless a very large portion was eaten.
Sweet rice syrup	This syrup can be either a liquid or a thick product similar to toffee.
Nonstarchy vegetables	
Garlic and scallions	Chopped garlic and scallions/green onions are used as seasoning in many dishes.
Herbs and greens	Koreans harvest the early tender shoots of many wild herbs. They are boiled and dried to be used throughout the year. When boiled, they look almost like cooked spinach. First-generation Korean Americans have gardens, if possible, or may harvest leafy greens when they walk in parks or open areas. Salt, hot pepper, chopped garlic, sesame oil, soy sauce, and/or bean paste may be added to greens.
Kimchi	Staple vegetable in Korean diet. It now comes in several varieties, but the traditional kimchi is a mixture of Korean cabbage and radish, scallions, hot pepper, garlic, ginger and salt to crisp the vegetables. Many South Korean people make kimchi with various *jut-ga* (salted and fermented seafood including shrimp, anchovies, and other small ocean fish). In the United States, Korean Americans may substitute Vietnamese fish sauce or squid sauce if *jut-gal* is not available. Kimchi is fermented and has a strong, distinctive fragrance—which becomes stronger as it ages. Before refrigeration was available, kimchi was made each fall and put into clay pots then placed in the ground to preserve it for use all winter. It is now made in large glass jars and stored in a separate "kimchi refrigerator." Nuts and fruits are added to one variety of kimchi.
Lettuce	Koreans use large lettuce leaves as a wrapper for rice, bean paste, and meats. They hold the leaf cupped in their hand, wrap it, and then eat it.
Seaweed	Kelp is made into soup and is traditionally consumed three times each day by new mothers; many in the United States follow this custom. Other seaweeds are made into flat sheets called *gim* and used to wrap seasoned rice, chopped vegetables, sliced egg omelet, and perhaps chopped meat or tiny shrimp, rolled into a log and then sliced similar to Japanese *futomaki* rolls. Koreans call this dish *gim bap,* or seaweed rice.
Other nonstarchy vegetables	Any meal can include several side dishes of greens, sliced zucchini, bean sprouts, sliced carrots, sliced green peppers, sliced raw cabbage—all highly-seasoned or plain with bean paste added during the meal.
Meat and meat substitutes	
Eggs	Eggs are scrambled, cut into strips, and added to seaweed-rice rolls or *chop chae*. Eggs are also used in savory custard made with scallions and sometimes salted shrimp. They may also be slurred into several different soups.
Fish and seafood	Fish and seafood can be served plain, salted with soy sauce and a variety of spices, or coated with flour. Cooking methods include boiling, grilling, frying, and or "baking" in cast iron pans over a fire. Seafood stews with fish, squid, shellfish, vegetables, tofu, vegetables, and lots of hot pepper are very popular. Small fish serve are eaten whole, including the bones, and are therefore a calcium source.
Meats	Traditionally, Koreans used chicken, pork, or beef almost as a condiment by making a broth with a small amount of the meat. They also cut up small amounts of meat for *mandoo* or seaweed-rice rolls. As the economy has improved, portions of meat have increased in size. Meats are boiled, grilled, fried or "baked" in cast iron pans over a fire. Marinated sliced beef *(bulkogi)* and short ribs *(kalbi)* are grilled and served as special dinners.
Nuts	Chestnuts and peanuts are toasted or boiled and eaten as a snack. Chestnuts eaten as an addition to kimchi and other banquet foods.
Squid	Squid is often dried, salted, seasoned with pepper and eaten as a snack. Dried squid is grilled over an open flame and eaten as a snack or served as a side dish with beer. Thinly sliced dried squid can also be used as a salty and spicy side dish with steamed rice when it is cooked with hot pepper paste, soy sauce and sugar.

(continued)

Table 12.1   *(continued)*

Food	Description
Tofu and boiled soybeans	Pieces of tofu are added to many soups and stews along with vegetables and meat, fish or seafood. Tofu may also be fried.
Fats	
Butter and margarine	These are not traditional Korean foods because dairy cows were rarely found in Korea. However, their use has increased with the changing dietary habits in both Korea and the United States.
Sesame, soy and sunflower oils	Used in meat marinades, as seasoning for vegetables, and for frying. Since sesame oil has a low smoking point, they use other vegetable oils for frying. Sometimes sesame oil is added afterward for flavor.
Condiments and seasonings	
Bean paste	Bean paste comes in two forms—hot *(gochu jang)* and not-hot *(dwen jang)*. *Gochu jang* is made from ground soybeans, hot peppers, sweet rice, salt, and a small amount of sugar. *Dwen jang* is also made with salt and added to soups and stews as a flavoring. The two bean pastes may be mixed with garlic, sesame oil, chopped scallions, and sugar to be used as condiment for fresh lettuce wrapped around grilled meat. This mixture is *Ssam-jang.* (*Ssam* means "wrappers.")
Soy sauce	A common ingredient in Korean cooking. It is used for meat marinades, Korean pancakes, and many other dishes that need salt.

Table 12.2 · Traditional Korean Dishes, Beverages, Sweets, and Desserts

Food	Description
Dishes	
Chop chae	Udon, somen, or soba noodles mixed with vegetables, beef, or pork.
Korean pancakes	Mung bean flour and water are combined to form a batter and then mixed with chopped meats, fish, shrimp, squid, and/or slivered vegetables. They are then fried in oil and served as a side-dish. Soy sauce may be an accompanying seasoning.
Mandoo	Dumplings made with a refined wheat flour skin filled with finely chopped vegetables, tofu and sometimes beef, pork or chicken. They are boiled in broth to make *mandoo gook*. The carbohydrate content of the soup depends on the number of *mandoo* in the serving. *Mandoo* are also steamed or fried and served for dinner or at parties and celebrations.
Beverages	
Alcoholic beverages	Korean rice wine (*mak-gull-ly* or *dong dong ju*) is popular among elderly Koreans. The Korean word for liquor is *sool*. The most popular liquor among Korean men is *soju*, which is made from potatoes and similar to Russian vodka. Its alcohol content is over 21% proof, so it is often mixed with sliced lemon or cucumber to mask its strong alcohol smell.
Instant coffee	May be served with or without cream and sugar.
Teas	Types of tea include herbal, ginseng, green, and persimmon-ginger. Koreans use herbal teas for medicinal purposes.
Water	Water is the beverage usually consumed with meals.
Desserts and sweets	
Cakes	Cakes used to be less popular and were used only for special occasions. However, many Korean stores and bakeries have developed a new type of cake with a mixture of Korean and Western flavors that may Koreans, including those in the United States, prefer.
Rice cakes *(baram duk)*	Balls of sweet rice with sweetened ground red beans in the center. The rice may be colored pink or green.
Rice cakes *(si-ru duk)*	Sweet rice is cooked, pounded into large squares, topped with cooked, ground red bean or soybean flour, and then cut into smaller squares. *Si-ru duk* are served as treats for holidays, weddings, and other special occasions.
Other desserts	The traditional Korean dessert is fruit. There are more than 50 different types of desserts made from rice or rice flour. Usually, Korean Americans buy these rice-based desserts from Korean supermarkets.

Table 12.3 · Traditional Foods Consumed During Holidays

Holiday	Foods
Lunar New Year	*Duk gook* (rice cake soup), *chal duk* (sweet rice cakes), fruit, rice wine, fish, and meats.
Big Moon Celebration (January 15)	Rice with five different grains (*oh-gok-bap*) and seven different dried vegetables from the prior year are eaten for a long life. Nuts are eaten to prevent bad luck.
Chu-suk (Korean harvest festival; mid-October)	Families take newly harvested foods such as *song-pyun* rice cakes, fresh pears, apples, or grapes, rice wine, and other foods to complete the meal to the gravesites of family members to honor their ancestors.

Traditional Meal Patterns and Holiday Foods

The traditional Korean meal pattern is three meals a day. Each meal consists of rice, soup, and several side dishes, including cooked vegetables, meat, fish, and kimchi. Water is drunk with meals. Coffee may be served after a meal.

In traditional Korean households, women took care of the housework, including cooking. The evening meal was a time when all members of the family were usually together. Korean men worked long hours so the meal was typically quite late. This custom can have implications for scheduling diabetes medications.

Confucianism influences the traditional meal patterns and holiday foods of Korean Americans. The basic concepts of Confucianism include respect and obedience toward authority and elders at all times; separate roles for men and women; the importance of status and dignity; the privileging of hierarchy rather than equality; the value of families over individuals; the significance of loyalty; and saving money. Many Koreans in the United States still follow these tenets, which can affect their eating habits, especially on holidays and at family gatherings.

Traditional Korean holidays center on the Lunar New Year and *Chuk-Suk,* the harvest festival. Meals are larger at these times of year, and special foods are served. Lunar New Year is celebrated by visiting family and friends. People will eat several times a day as they move from house to house. The Western calendar's New Year is also celebrated in the same way, but on a lesser scale. *Chu-Suk* is celebrated after the harvest, typically in mid-October. Families take newly harvested foods to the gravesites of family members to honor their ancestors. Recent generations of Korean Americans may be less likely to celebrate *Chu-Suk* because it follows the lunar calendar and therefore does not land each year on a set date in the Western calendar. However, Korean Americans celebrate American Thanksgiving; their Thanksgiving meals are often a combination of traditional American holiday fare and special Korean foods.

During the past century, a great number of Koreans have become Christians. They celebrate Christmas and Easter along with traditional Korean holidays. For Christian Korean Americans, these holidays tend to focus on worship celebrations, but special meals are often included. Again, Korean Americans will celebrate with meals combining the holiday's American foods with traditional Korean fare. See Table 12.3 for foods served on holidays.

Traditional Health Beliefs

Traditional Korean medicine has a long and successful history. Many Western health care providers may be skeptical about non-Western practices; but the establishment of the National Center for Complementary and Alternative Medicine within National Institutes of Health suggests that Western practitioners are beginning to give more respect to Eastern medical wisdom.

Korean practices include acupuncture, reflexology, and use of herbal medicines. Do not refer to these interventions as "Chinese" in the presence of Korean clients. The Koreans developed their own expertise, and Chinese clients frequently come to Korea to be treated with both traditional and Western forms of medicine.

Current Food Practices

Within the lifetimes of older Koreans, South Korea has changed from a developing to developed nation. The transition has brought about several dietary changes, including the availability of refrigeration, increased portions of meat, access to ready-to-cook foods, the presence of US chain restaurants, and the custom of frequently eating out.

In Korea, an improved economy and the importation of beef have encouraged Koreans to eat more meat. American foods, such as bread, dairy foods, baked goods and fast foods, have also influenced dietary habits in Korea.

The degree to which Korean Americans follows a traditional Korean diet is influenced by their degree of acculturation and their age/generation. Older, first-generation immigrants tend to follow Korean food patterns more than middle-aged and younger Korean Americans. Younger generations enjoy Korean foods, but they may not think it is worth the effort to prepare them. When younger-generation Korean Americans marry non-Koreans, family meals may become a blend of traditional Korean dishes and American dishes.

Traditionally, Koreans ate three meals prepared in the home. Now, more families consume a quick breakfast of doughnuts, toast, or pastries, and coffee. Cereal with milk is consumed by children, but it is not popular among older adults due to the high prevalence of lactose intolerance. Yogurt may be consumed as a beverage.

Family gatherings and social functions usually involve eating out, instead of preparing foods at home. Most Korean American families prefer either Korean or Chinese restaurants. After Sunday services, Korean American churches frequently have potlucks with the women preparing traditional Korean foods. This tendency to eat away from home is a concern for clients who need to control energy intake.

In both Korea and the United States, it is now common for both men and women work to work outside the home. As a result, food preparation time has become limited and convenience and fast foods are consumed in both countries.

Most Korean Americans purchase prepared vegetables, meats, rice cakes, and *mandoo* (Korean dumplings) from Asian grocery stores. Korean foods are chopped into small pieces and eaten with chopsticks and spoons. Knives are not placed on the table, so buying ready-to-cook foods saves a great deal of time for the cook. Side dishes are usually placed in the center of the table and shared by the whole family. Therefore, portion estimates of foods eaten by an individual family member may be inaccurate.

In the United States, the availability of pre-made Korean foods including kimchi varies according to the Korean population in the area. Registered dietitians (RDs) should ask their clients if they buy pre-made Korean foods or make their own.

The diet of a Korean American child will depend in part on whether his or her mother works outside the home. If she does, the child may eat fast-food meals frequently. If she does not, the child's diet is more likely to be traditionally Korean.

Traditionally Koreans ate fruit for dessert. That tradition continues in Korean American families, but they have also learned to like chocolate, candy, ice cream, cookies, brownies, and pies. Older Korean American clients may not consume many American sweets, but that will vary from client to client.

Counseling Considerations

Demonstrating Courtesy and Respect

As a sign of respect to your clients, begin each conversation with formal greetings. Always address Korean American clients as Mr., Miss, or Mrs. followed by their surname, even if the client has adopted a European first name. This is especially important if you are younger than the client. Within the Korean culture, even good friends address each other as Mr. and Mrs. When shaking the client's hand, bow slightly as a sign of respect.

At the start of counseling, ask nonthreatening, polite questions about neutral topics. For example, ask what foods they enjoy, the times when they eat, and what foods they eat at those times. A counselor with a positive attitude toward Korean food is more likely to establish good rapport and the trust needed for an effective intervention.

Korean Americans have great respect for health care professionals, especially physicians. As with any medical nutrition therapy (MNT) intervention, suggest that clients try one or two changes at first and then progress to others. It is important that the client understand the rationale for changes and how the diabetes food plan can be part of the overall Korean diet. If they do not understand this, they may think you are asking them to adopt an American eating pattern.

Interpreting Clients' Nonverbal Communication

To understand Korean Americans' nonverbal communication, it is important to recognize *Kibun*—ie, one's mood, feelings, and state of mind. Maintaining *Kibun* promotes one's inner peace. Therefore, to effectively communicate when interacting with Korean Americans, health care providers have the responsibility to assess their clients' *Kibun*. This outward assessment is known *nunchi*. The state of *Kibun* is easily disturbed, such as when a young person shows disrespect toward an elder (6).

Koreans do not commonly communicate feelings through facial expressions. At a first meeting, Korean Americans may be reluctant to make eye contact, especially when the encounter is between people of different genders, ages, and/or social status. However, among familiar persons, Korean Americans may feel more comfortable making eye contact and speaking in the first person. Meaningful conversation, as opposed to small talk, is valued. Smiling and joking are acceptable in certain conditions and situations. If used inappropriately, however, such expressions are interpreted as a lack of intelligence and respect (6).

Korean Americans understand that health care professionals may need to touch them in the process of providing care. They will allow you to physically examine them if they believe you intend to improve their health (6).

Inquiring About Clients' Understanding of Diabetes

Research about Korean Americans' perceptions of diabetes is limited. Counselors should recognize that Korean Americans may believe that they will develop an illness if they do not adhere to Confucianism or Christian spiritual beliefs (7). Also, among Korean Americans, chronic illness is often perceived as one's fate, and hospitalization may be seen as sign of impending death.

Discussing Clients' Use of Complementary and Alternative Medicine

Korean Americans often use Asian pharmaceutical and herbal products. Now that Korean hospitals practice Western medicine and use equipment as up to date as that in the United States, Koreans see no contradiction in combining Western and traditional options.

Herbal teas are common treatments for many conditions, including diabetes. Commonly used teas include green, persimmon-ginger, and assorted herbal varieties. Ginseng may also be used in tea. Koreans consider this herb to be an energy and immune system booster, a treatment for high blood pressure, a preventive measure for cancer and dementia, and an aphrodisiac. In addition to tea, ginseng may be an ingredient in candies or it may be ground, mixed with honey, and eaten by the spoonful.

In Korea, pharmacists and herbalists are permitted by law to prescribe and dispense herbal and Western medications, including antibiotics and treatments for diabetes and high blood pressure. They typically prescribe several herbals for diabetes. Now, however, Koreans take insulin and Western oral agents even if they also take traditional herbals.

Given this history of positive experiences with herbals, Korean American clients tend to be more likely than their European American counterparts to use "natural" products in the treatment of many medical conditions. RDs should ask all clients whether they take vitamin and mineral or herbal supplements and if they drink any special teas. Many Korean American clients are likely to say yes—and the herbals they use may include types that are not traditionally Korean. Although many herbal products have positive pharmacological effects, their safety profiles have not been adequately evaluated. Whether RDs decide to accept or discourage the use of these products, they need to do so with respect, not disdain. See Appendix C for questions to assess dietary supplement use.

Considering Family Demands and Dynamics

Korean Americans have a strong family orientation and value the opinion of their relatives (7). Therefore, the RD may gain additional insight by asking the client to invite family members to counseling sessions.

Learning the family's schedule is important. When both spouses work outside the home, meal schedules can be hectic. This is even more likely if children live at home, because it is important to Korean Americans that their children be active at school.

In Korean American households, the wife usually is in charge of the kitchen. Therefore, you may wish to encourage married male clients to bring their wives to counseling sessions. It also can be helpful to have the husbands of married women with diabetes join sessions. If the husband does not cooperate with dietary changes, his preferences may trump any advice the RD gives.

If a Korean American client or his or her spouse is not convinced of the need for dietary changes, it may be helpful to include the eldest or most successful son in the counseling sessions (with the client's consent). Older Koreans often listen more to their sons than to their spouse, especially if the son has done well financially or academically.

Older clients may have special needs, whether or not they live with their adult children. In large cities, older, widowed Korean Americans may live in senior citizen apartment buildings. Some will not have easy access to a supermarket with Korean foods. Creative solutions can be used to find traditional foods, or the client can be taught to prepare simple foods for successful MNT.

Nutrition Counseling

Refer to Appendix B for MNT recommendations for diabetes as well as general counseling strategies. The following are culturally specific suggestions for nutrition counseling of Korean American clients:

- Evaluate whether clients are familiar with US tools for measuring portions, such as measuring cups and tablespoons. If they do not already use these tools in food preparation, explain their use.

- Suggest that clients bring to the rice bowls and plates they use at home to a counseling session so you can use them to teach portion sizes for rice and other dishes.

- The major source of carbohydrate in the Korean American diet is rice. However, the RD should assess and discuss the individual client's carbohydrate intake and preferences. The client may be willing to add brown rice to white rice or to try the mixed grains sold in most Korean markets. These changes will increase intake of fiber and some minerals.

- If a client's current meal pattern includes soup with noodles or rice cakes (especially sweet rice) in addition to rice as a main dish, the carbohydrate content of the meal may be especially high. Advise clients to decide whether they prefer decreasing their rice intake enough to compensate for the carbohydrates in the soup, or if they prefer to eat rice, meat, vegetables, and kimchi. Another option is to encourage clients to eat more *bibimbop*, which is a mixed dish of meat, vegetables and rice.

- When clients adopt American eating habits, their diet may be high in carbohydrates from fast food, pizza, and sweets. If clients are receptive, encourage them to revive the traditional Korean pattern of some rice, meat, and lots of vegetables, with fruit for dessert.

- Encourage clients to enjoy traditional foods such as fish, tofu, bok choy, kale, tangerines, persimmons, Korean pears, and melon.

- Koreans typically eat kimchi, a high-sodium food, several times a day. However, the salt in kimchi is not just a flavoring; it is used to crisp the vegetables. Therefore, reducing the amount of salt in the preparation would result in mushy, unpalatable kimchi. It is more practical to suggest that clients have smaller servings of regular kimchi along with larger servings of other vegetables seasoned with red pepper/garlic and/or eat *mul* (water) kimchi. Some clients may find lettuce/cabbage *gukjuli*, which is prepared with fresh vegetables and not marinated in salt, to be an acceptable substitute for kimchi.

- Assess the client's use of traditional Korean condiments, such as bean pastes, soy sauce, sesame oil, and/or sliced garlic cloves preserved in soy sauce. Hot bean paste has more than 110 mg sodium per teaspoon. (Reduced-sodium bean pastes are not available.) This condiment is used to season many kinds of Korean foods. A small amount is added to the food after serving, or a person might dip a bite of food into a small dish at the table. Many clients will use less than 1 teaspoon at a meal, and they may therefore be able to include bean paste in a reduced-sodium diet. Others, however, will use considerably more. Soy sauce is used much like bean paste/hot bean paste; however, more soy sauce is needed for the same amount of flavor because it is a liquid. Some brands of regular soy sauce exceed 1,000 mg sodium per tablespoon. In comparison, reduced-sodium soy sauce has about 575 mg sodium per tablespoon. Encourage clients to try reduced-sodium soy sauce and control the amount they use.
- People from southern South Korea often add dried salted fish *(jut-gal)* to their kimchi. Encourage clients to omit this ingredient.
- Koreans prefer highly seasoned foods. Using seasonings such as red pepper, garlic, chopped scallions, and limited amounts of bean paste or hot bean paste will help them decrease the use of salt and soy sauce. Encourage clients to try salt substitutes as well as lemon for any of traditional dishes other than kimchi itself. These substitutions can be a first step in getting used to a less salty flavor.
- Most Koreans like fresh fish. Counsel clients to eat more fish and reduce portions of the high-fat cuts of beef and pork used for popular dishes such as *bulkogi* (thinly sliced marinated beef), *kalbi* (marinated short ribs), and uncured bacon. (Traditionally, Koreans eat the fat.)
- Koreans are used to walking and are great hikers. Therefore, Korean Americans who grew up in Korea will be familiar with walking and may be receptive to suggestions that they walk more to increase their physical activity levels. In addition, yoga or tai chi may be appealing options for the elderly population.

Challenges and Barriers to Dietary Adherence

Korean Americans, particularly if they are older adults, may be reluctant to express disagreement with any recommendations made. It is important to ask respectfully whether a certain suggestion will work for the client. Recognize that it can be difficult for Korean American clients with diabetes to follow MNT recommendations because their traditional diet is high in carbohydrates, sodium, and fat. Try starting with an easily implemented change that fits within Korean food habits. This approach may make clients more receptive to future changes.

To establish good rapport, the counselor should demonstrate great respect for the client, show interest in and knowledge of the client's culture and ethnicity, and collaborate with him or her to implement changes one at a time. Cultural awareness will also give the RD insight into why certain practices occur and increase MNT success.

Resources

National Library of Medicine, National Institutes of Health. Asian American Health: Materials in Asian Languages—Korean. http://asianamericanhealth.nlm.nih.gov/Alkorean.html. Accessed March 6, 2009.

Seattle and King County Public Health. http://www.kingcounty.gov/healthServices/health/languages/korean.aspx. Accessed May 9, 2009.

Selected Patient Information Resources in Asian Languages (SPIRAL). http://spiral.tufts.edu. Accessed March 6, 2009.

References

1. US Census 2000. http://factfinder.census.gov/servlet. Accessed September 21, 2008.
2. Cho J, Juon HS. Assessing overweight and obesity risk among Korean Americans in California using World Health Organization body mass index criteria for Asians. *Prev Chronic Dis.* 2006; 3(3):A39.
3. Kim MT. Healthy Korean American Project. Johns Hopkins University School of Nursing. http://www.son.jhmi.edu/research/Korean-American/index.htm. Accessed September 21, 2008.

4. International Diabetes Federation. Diabetes Atlas, Executive Summary. 2nd ed. 2003. http://www.eatlas.idf.org/webdata/docs/Atlas%202003-Summary.pdf. Accessed March 6, 2009.

5. McNeely MJ, Boyko EJ. Type 2 diabetes prevalence in Asian Americans. *Diabetes Care.* 2004; 27:66–69.

6. Beller T, Pinker M, Shapka S, Van Dusen D. Korean-American health care beliefs and practices. 2004. http://www3.baylor.edu/~Charles_Kemp/korean.htm. Accessed September 21, 2008.

7. Rim Shin K, Shin C, Lanoie Blanchette P. Health and health care of Korean-American elders. http://www.stanford.edu/group/ethnoger/korean.html. Accessed September 21, 2008.

Acknowledgments: Thanks to Jamie Futterman, Outclient Dietitian and Diabetes Educator with Washington Adventist Hospital in Takoma Park, Maryland, for editorial assistance. Thanks also to Young Sik Lee from Canfield, Ohio, for providing information about Korean foods.

Cajun and Creole Food Practices

13

Colette Guidry Leistner, PhD, RD, and Lauren Hirschfeld, MS, RD

Introduction

The dietetics profession learned valuable lessons from Hurricanes Katrina and Rita, which hit the Gulf coast in August and September 2005. The number of displaced residents from New Orleans and southwest Louisiana is a reminder that registered dietitians (RDs) should be prepared to meet the needs of all clients at all times. The information contained within this chapter will help RDs in their work with individuals in and from Louisiana (1–6).

Southern Louisiana is the home of two complex and fascinating American cultures—the Cajun and the Creole. Those outside these communities may not fully understand how multifaceted and rich these cultures are. As a result, stereotypes regarding at least two aspects of culture—the people and the cuisines—persist. Although they have evolved side by side for more than 300 years and share such influences as economics, politics, geography, climate, and Roman Catholicism, the two cultures and their cuisines are not synonymous. The variations may be unnoticeable to others, but they are noteworthy to residents of southern Louisiana.

Cajuns descend from French settlers called the Acadians, who were expelled by the British from Acadie (present-day Nova Scotia). The Acadians eventually settled in southern Louisiana between 1756 and 1788. Predominately Roman Catholic, Cajuns have traditionally been a rural people with close family ties. The nuclear family and extended family continue to be dominant features of Cajun culture. While fluent in English, many Cajuns still speak or at least understand Louisiana French (7–9). Familiarity with the French language is especially true of older individuals.

Most Cajuns live in a 22-parish (county) area of southern Louisiana that does not include New Orleans. In 1971 the Louisiana legislature designated this region *Acadiana* in recognition of its enduring French-Acadian culture, traditions, and language. Today, common livelihoods among the Cajuns include farming, ranching, fishing, trapping, and occupations in the oil industry, as well as white-collar positions (7).

To define Creole to everybody's satisfaction is virtually impossible. The term describes a culture, people, cuisine, and language. The Creole culture in the United States is historically associated with New Orleans. To some, the term Creole brings to mind the descendants of Louisiana's early European settlers and suggests wealth and aristocracy. To others, it refers to the descendants of both freedmen and *gens de couleur libre* (free persons of color before the Civil War) (7). However, for many years in New Orleans, Creole has meant someone with some degree of African American ancestry (10). This segment of the Creole population is addressed in this chapter.

African Americans living primarily in the Acadiana parishes of Evangeline, St. Martin, and St. Landry (south central Louisiana) also refer to themselves as Creole (11). Living within the Acadiana region and among its ubiquitous Cajun culture, these African American residents have encouraged the use of the term Creole to acknowledge their non-Cajun culture and heritage (11). Many are able to speak or understand Louisiana Creole (French), which differs from the French spoken by their Cajun neighbors.

According to the 2000 US Census, 34,449 Louisiana residents in the Acadiana parishes claimed Acadian/Cajun ancestry. (This does not include individuals who may have selected French or French Canadian ancestry) (12). The 2000 Census did not include a category for Creole in its report of ancestry. Based on the definition for Creole cited previously, the African American or black designation can give some indication of the Creole population. In the 2000 Census, 325,947 residents of Orleans Parish (primarily the city of New Orleans) claimed African American or black ancestry (12).

Diabetes Prevalence

There are no distinct epidemiologic statistics for Cajuns and Creoles within Louisiana's general population. According to analysis of data from the 2000 Louisiana Behavioral Risk Factor Surveillance Survey (BRFSS), diabetes was the fifth leading cause of death in Louisiana (13).

In 2003 the death rate from diabetes ranged from 10.3 to 78.2 (median 36.0) per 100,000 residents in the Acadiana parishes and was 62.4 per 100,000 residents in Orleans Parish; Louisiana's statewide death rate from diabetes per 100,000 people was 38.5 (13,14). The US Department of Health and Human Services initiative *Healthy People 2010* has a goal of no more than 75 deaths per 100,000 people (14).

Risk Factors for Type 2 Diabetes

Obesity

Type 2 diabetes is associated with obesity, family history of diabetes, and race/ethnicity, among other characteristics (15). According to the *2006 Louisiana Health Report Card*, prevalence of adult obesity in Louisiana rose from 16% in 1991 to 27% in 2004 (16). In BRFSS prevalence data (2006) for Louisiana, 35.1% of whites and 36.7% of blacks were overweight (body mass index [BMI] 25–29.9) and 24.3% of whites and 36.1% of blacks were obese (BMI ≥ 30) (17).

Social Factors

Social factors that influence the Cajun and Creole attitudes toward diabetes and the risks associated with it are discussed later in this chapter, in the Traditional Health Beliefs section.

Traditional Foods and Dishes

Roman Catholicism has been the primary religion of southern Louisiana since the earliest days of European settlement, and the religion has shaped the traditional food customs of all residents of the area—including African Americans, whites, Catholics, and non-Catholics. Catholics in this region developed numerous meatless dishes for consumption on Fridays in accordance with strict pre–Vatican II expectations. These dishes featured freshly caught, canned, dried, or salted freshwater or saltwater fish, crustaceans, and mollusks, as well as eggs.

Geographic location dictated the variety of foods available to Cajuns and Creoles. Individuals in close proximity to wetlands included wild fowl and seafood in their diet; whereas those on the prairie or near wooded areas added wild game (18). Indigenous plants—wild plum, muscadine, passion fruit (maypops), black cherry, oyster mushrooms, thistle stalks *(chadron)*, and lotus seeds *(gráin a voler)*—also found their way into the diet of the rural inhabitants (19).

Whether found in rural or urban areas, home gardens provided ingredients for the unique dishes of both cultures in southern Louisiana. Cajuns and Creoles planted *taupinambour* (sunchokes), *mirliton* (chayote), okra, leeks, eggplants, *béné* (sesame) seeds, bay leaves, sassafras (used for *filé* powder, an essential ingredient in certain gumbos), sugarcane, and figs, in addition to more common fruits and vegetables. The practice of breeding livestock yielded pork, beef, poultry, and mutton.

Cajun cuisine is the hearty fare of the southern Louisiana countryside. The foods and food preparation methods reflect French Acadian, French, Native American, German, Spanish, and African influences.

The cuisine found in the homes of the Creole population of New Orleans bears close resemblance to traditional southern or "soul" food. Creoles eat vegetables such as greens, yams, okra, peas and beans; quick breads (cornbread and biscuits); cured and fresh pork; and poultry. Cooking methods are also similar to those used in soul food—one-pot meals, fried foods, and vegetables seasoned with animal fat.

In the New Orleans Creole community, there is a tradition of preparing specific meals on specific days of the week. Some menus are ubiquitous, whereas others are unique to a family or neighborhood. Perhaps the best example of a specific meal for a specific day is Monday's red beans and rice served with a pork chop, fried chicken, or smoked pork sausage. This is included on the menu of virtually every restaurant in the city as well as in hospital cafeterias and most homes. Other examples include serving greens one day of the week, having a spaghetti-and-meatball day, and serving seafood on Friday regardless of religious or cultural background.

Creole cuisine has been distinctively affected by encounters between the Creole population and other immigrant groups that entered the United States through the port of New Orleans. Through these exchanges, New Orleans cuisine has achieved a cosmopolitan quality. For instance, red beans and rice served with a fried pork chop or fried chicken represents both Caribbean and African American or soul influences. Gumbo can be made of many ingredients—chicken *filé;* hen and sausage; shrimp and crab; or squirrel. See Tables 13.1 and 13.2 for more information on traditional foods and dishes. Refer to Appendix A for nutrient analyses.

Table 13.1 · Foods Used in Traditional Cajun and Creole Cuisines

Food Group	Cajun	Creole
Meats and meat substitutes	• Beef—including organ meats, tongue, tripe; sausage; *tasso* (dried, seasoned lean beef strips) • Chicken • Eggs • Guinea fowl • Mutton • Peanut butter Wild fowl (ducks, doves, geese) • Pork—including boudin, *fromage de tete de cochon, gratons, debris, chaudin;* smoked and fresh sausage; ham, bacon, salt pork; *tasso* (dried, seasoned lean pork strips) • Turkey • Wild game (deer, rabbit, squirrel)	• Beef • Canned meats (potted meat, vienna sausage) • Chicken (including liver and gizzards) • Eggs • Peanut butter • Pork—fresh as well as cured products (eg, ham, pickled pork, pickled pigs' feet, bacon); organ meats (eg, chitterlings) • Turkey
Seafood	• Alligator • *Biganeau* (sea snails) • Canned tuna, salmon, sardines • Catfish • Crawfish • Dried or canned codfish • Frog legs • Garfish • Oysters • Pan fish • Shrimp • Turtle	• Canned tuna and sardines • Catfish • Crabs • Oysters • Pan fish • Shrimp • Turtle

(continued)

Table 13.1   (continued)

Food Group	Cajun	Creole
Milk	• "Sour" milk (buttermilk) • *Caillé gouté* (fresh cream cheese); also known commercially as "Creole-style" cream cheese) • Cream • Sharp cheddar cheese • Whole milk	• "Sour" milk (buttermilk) • Cream • Whole milk ("sweet" milk)
Fruits	• Bananas • Blackberries • Canteloupe • Coconut • Figs • Japanese plum (loquat) • Muscadine grapes • Oranges • Peaches • Pears • Persimmons • Raisins • Scuppernong grapes • Watermelon • Wild plums	• Apples • Bananas • Canteloupe • Coconut • Figs • Oranges • Peaches • Pears • Raisins • Watermelon
Starchy vegetables	• Beans (lima, butter, navy) • Corn • Peas (crowder, cream, purple hull, black-eyed) • Potatoes (Irish and red) • Pumpkin • Sweet potatoes • *Taupinambour* (sunchoke)	• Beans (red kidney, lima, butter) • Corn • Peas (black-eyed) • Potatoes (Irish and red) • Sweet potatoes
Nonstarchy vegetables	• Beets • Bell pepper • Cabbage • Carrots • Cauliflower • Cucumbers • Eggplant • Green beans • Greens (mustard, turnip) • Leeks • Lettuce • *Mirliton* (chayote) • Okra • Onions • Tomatoes • Turnips	• Beets • Bell peppers • Cabbage • Carrots • Cucumbers • Eggplant • Green beans • Greens (turnip, mustard, collard) • Lettuce • Okra • Onions • Tomatoes • Turnips

(continued)

Table 13.1 *(continued)*

Food Group	Cajun	Creole
Bread and grains	• Biscuits	• Biscuits
	• Cornbread	• Cornbread
	• Cornmeal	• Cornmeal
	• *Couche-couche* (hot cornmeal cereal)	• French bread
	• Grits	• Grits
	• *Pain ordinaire* (homemade yeast bread)	• Macaroni
	• Rice	• Rice
	• Vermicelli	• White bread
Spices and seasonings	• Bay leaf	• Bay leaf
	• Cayenne pepper	• Cayenne pepper
	• *Filé* (powdered, dried sassafras leaves)	• Garlic
	• Garlic	• Green onions
	• Green onions	• Parsley, flat-leaf
	• Parsley, flat-leaf	• Salt
	• Salt	
Miscellaneous	• Roux (a mixture of fat and flour cooked to varying shades of brown)	• Roux
	• Dry roux (a mixture of half all-purpose white flour and half oil or butter slowly cooked over low heat that changes in both flavor and color from white to blond to brown depending on the cooking time)	• Dry roux
		• Peanuts
	• Cane syrup	
	• Fruit preserves	
	• Hickory nuts	
	• Peanuts	
	• Pecans	

Table 13.2 • Traditional Cajun and Creole Dishes, Beverages, and Desserts

	Cajun	Creole
Dishes	• Chicken fricassee	• Baked macaroni (macaroni and cheese)
	• Court bouillon (fish broth used to poach fish or seafood)	• Crab cakes
	• *Filé* gumbo	• Dirty rice
	• Fried seafood	• Fried chicken
	• Jambalaya	• Fried seafood
	• Okra gumbo	• Oyster dressing
	• Potato salad	• Oyster patties
	• Rice and gravy	• Red beans and rice
	• Rice dressing	• Seafood gumbo (okra-based)
	• Sauce *piquante*	
	• Seafood gumbo (roux-based)	
	• Stuffed *mirliton* (chayote)	

(continued)

Table 13.2   (continued)

	Cajun	Creole
Beverages	• Beer	• Beer
	• Café au lait (half milk/half coffee)	• Coffee
	• Coffee (dark roast)	• Coffee with chicory
	• Sweetened cold beverages including iced tea, soft drinks, powdered drink mixes	• Sweetened cold beverages including iced tea, soft drinks, powdered drink mixes
Desserts	• *'Tites gateaux secs* (tea cakes)	• Beignets
	• Bread with preserves or cane syrup	• Bread pudding with bourbon sauce
	• Cakes with icing	• Cakes with icing
	• Homemade ice cream	• Cobblers
	• *Massepain* (gingerbread)	• Homemade ice cream
	• Old-fashioned banana pudding	• Pecan pie
	• Snowcones or snowballs	• Pound cake
	• *Tarte douce* (sweet dough pies filled with custard or preserves)	• Snowcones or snowballs
		• Sweet potato pie

Traditional Meal Patterns and Holiday Foods

The typical meal pattern in southern Louisiana consists of three meals a day. Residents of the Acadiana region and the Creole population of New Orleans refer to the morning meal as "breakfast." They call the midday meal "dinner" in the Cajun region and "lunch" or "dinner" in the Creole region. "Supper" is the evening meal among Cajuns, but Creoles frequently call this meal "dinner."

Breakfast follows the standard American or southern pattern. Common breakfast foods include biscuits or toast, grits, eggs, bacon or sausage, cold cereal, and milk. Older residents of the Cajun region may eat cornbread or biscuits crumbled into milk or "coffee milk" (similar to *café au lait* but with a higher proportion of milk to coffee) for breakfast. In New Orleans, a light breakfast of french bread, *beignets,* or a biscuit accompanied by coffee is traditional. Fruit or fruit juice is not common at breakfast in either region. Drive-through fast-food restaurants provide breakfast for many working people in both regions.

Although the evening meal is usually the heaviest of the day in both regions, work schedules and the age of the household members may influence this practice. In rural areas and small towns, farmers, the self-employed, and those working close to home still return home for their midday meal. They may consume most of their calories at this time. In the Cajun region, many older people eat the heaviest meal at noon. They eat foods such as *couche-couche* (a hot, dry cornmeal cereal) and milk, cornbread and milk, a peanut butter or cheese sandwich, soup or gumbo, or leftovers from the evening meal. Regardless of when the heaviest meal is consumed, a "complete meal" for Cajuns includes, or consists solely of, rice and gravy or a sauce-based meat or seafood dish. Long-grain and medium-grain rice are both readily available in the region, and most families have a decided preference for one type or the other.

The greater New Orleans area is more culturally diverse (with African American, Italian, German, Jewish, Irish, and Asian residents), and rice and gravy are not the focus of a meal to the same extent seen in the Cajun region. Dishes traditionally and culturally associated with one population are now enjoyed by members of other cultural groups, resulting in a wide variety of foods eaten during meals.

Foods eaten between meals include typical American snack foods (eg, chips, cookies, candy, ice cream, and soft drinks). The most popular brands among the Cajun and Creole are produced by regional companies (eg, Elmer's candies and Cheeweez, Hubig's pies, Zapp's potato chips, Barq's root beer and red pop). In the Cajun region, *boudin* (different types of sausage used in Creole and Cajun cuisine) and *gratons* (crispy cooked pieces of fatty meat, such as salt pork) are popular snack foods that are readily available at neighborhood convenience stores and supermarkets.

Coffee drinks can be a source of significant calories in the Cajun or Creole diet. People in both regions tend to drink coffee throughout the day. Cajuns often serve dark-roast coffee in demitasse cups with sugar and cream, half-and-half, whole milk, or powdered nondairy creamer. Some people use artificial sweeteners. Those in the Creole region enjoy coffee with chicory or dark-roast coffee with the same added ingredients. Sweets are not customarily served with coffee in either region (20).

Just as in other parts of the United States, in Creole and Cajun communities, extended families gather for holiday celebrations. In southern Louisiana, these gatherings are noted for the variety and quantity of regional foods prepared and served with or without traditional "American" fare such as roast turkey and cranberry sauce.

Gumbo (a soup thickened with roux, *filé,* or okra) is served for every holiday in New Orleans. It is sometimes the main course for Christmas dinner in Cajun families. More than one meat-based dish is typically served at every holiday meal in both areas. Pork roast may be the most popular meat eaten during holidays in both cultures. In the Cajun region, pot-roasted wild duck, wild goose, or ham may be served alongside the pork. In recent years, deep-fried turkey injected with Cajun spices has also become popular at holiday meals.

Meat-based accompaniments include rice dressing in the Cajun region and "dirty rice," which has a higher proportion of rice to meat, in the Creole. Smothered eggplant is sometimes added to Cajun rice dressing to make "eggplant dressing." Oyster dressing and oyster patties are also traditional in some families.

Stuffed vegetables—such as *mirliton* (chayote), eggplant, bell peppers, globe artichokes, and cabbage—are very popular in the Creole culture. The vegetables are stuffed with a mixture of well-seasoned rice or bread crumbs and shrimp, crabmeat, ground beef, or pork.

Many Cajun and Creole homes still follow the New Year's Day tradition of serving greens and black-eyed peas to ensure good luck and wealth in the coming year. Soon after the New Year comes the Carnival season (Mardi Gras). It begins on January 6 and runs until the day before Ash Wednesday. The New Orleans tradition of serving king cake is well established throughout southern Louisiana. King cake is a sweet yeast dough ring topped by a powdered sugar glaze and colored sugar crystals. "Filled" cakes with cream cheese, pecan praline, and fruit fillings are arguably more popular than the traditional cinnamon-sugar version, which is similar to a cinnamon roll. Louisiana residents who live in other parts of the United States are no longer deprived of this regional specialty because most bakeries ship king cakes nationwide.

Both cultures continue to follow Lenten traditions regarding food, such as abstaining from meat on Fridays during Lent or on Ash Wednesday and Holy Thursday. On some days during Lent, especially devout individuals may also fast (ie, they consume only one full meal on these days). The influence of pre–Vatican II traditions remains strong in southern Louisiana, and many residents continue to serve seafood in their homes on every Friday throughout the year and not only during Lent. Despite the Catholic Church's relaxation of the rule of abstaining from meat on Fridays, the expectation is that seafood will be included on Friday menus in hospitals, extended care facilities, schools, and restaurants. Refer to Table 13.3 for more information on traditional holiday foods.

Traditional Health Beliefs

In the Cajun and Creole cultures, illness, aging, and death are accepted as inevitable and natural life events. Many believe that whatever happens to one's health is "one's lot in life." When illness or misfortune occurs, Cajuns and Creoles often say "God never sends you more than you can bear," a statement that reflects the strong faith in God and sense of fatalism that residents of south Louisiana possess (8).

People in both cultures often hold beliefs associated with weight that may present a challenge to health care providers. For example, some individuals believe a "thin" person is in poor health or unattractive, when in fact the person is at or near a healthy BMI (21–23).

Table 13.3 · Traditional Foods Consumed During Holidays

Holiday	Cajun	Creole
Christmas	• Candied sweet potatoes • Gumbo • *Macque choux* (smothered corn) • Pork roast • Rice, eggplant, or cornbread dressing • Roast turkey • Roast wild duck	• Baked macaroni and cheese) • Candied sweet potatoes • Dirty rice • Gumbo • Stuffed globe artichokes, bell peppers, eggplant, or *mirliton* (chayote)
New Year's Day	• Black-eyed peas • Greens (smothered cabbage or cole slaw; mustard or turnip greens)	• Black-eyed peas • Greens (cabbage, mustard or turnip greens)
Carnival season (January 6 through Mardi Gras)	• King cake	• King cake
Lent	• Meatless Fridays, Ash Wednesday, sometimes Holy Thursday • Crawfish dishes	• Meatless Fridays, Ash Wednesday, sometimes Holy Thursday • Seafood
Easter	• Baked ham • Candied yams • Gumbo • Rice or cornbread dressing • Roast turkey	• Turtle
Other (Memorial Day, July 4, Labor Day)	• Barbeque (pork and chicken)	• Barbeque (pork and chicken)
Church fairs, festivals, and bazaars	• Barbeque dinners (chicken, white bread, rice dressing, baked beans, slaw) • Gumbo (chicken *filé*) • Jambalaya	

Adults in the Cajun and Creole cultures do not typically participate in regular exercise or lead active lifestyles. Often, adults in these cultures equate a "busy" day with physical activity. However, elementary and secondary school students participate regularly in sports and other physical activities. Anecdotal evidence suggests that parents help students (their children) ensure they have ample opportunities to engage in athletic pursuits. This reflects the seriousness with which adulthood and its family responsibilities are viewed in south Louisiana.

Within the Cajun and Creole regions in Louisiana, diabetes is often called "sugar diabetes," "a touch of sugar," or simply "sugar." These names reflect the belief that diabetes is caused by eating too much sugar and excess starchy foods. In keeping with this assumption, some Creole people believe that diabetes could be avoided by rinsing cooked rice to remove the starch. On the other hand, others associate heredity and obesity with diabetes. However, these individuals may also believe that they have limited, or no, personal control over their health (7,24).

Current Food Practices

When examining current food practices in southern Louisiana, regional variations must be considered. First, the variations remind us that the Cajun and Creole cuisines are different despite common culinary, religious, and geographical influences. Second, regional variation is apparent in the food distribution system, which allows specific foodways to continue in both cultures. Finally, meal composition varies by region.

Cajun and Creole food habits exhibit *inter-* and *intra*regional variations. Gumbo illustrates interregional variation between Cajun and Creole cultures. It is a popular dish in both Cajun and Creole cultures—however, chicken *filé* gumbo is typical of the Cajun region, whereas seafood gumbo is a favorite in New Orleans.

Some foods traditionally associated with one region have gained recognition in the other and are no longer distinctive to just the Cajun or Creole culture. For example, king cake was not known outside New Orleans 30 years ago, but it is now readily available across southern Louisiana. Also, red beans and rice were uncommon outside New Orleans until the Popeye's restaurant chain marketed the dish across the United States.

*Intra*regional variation is more subtle. Using gumbo again as an example, consider the Cajun chicken *filé* gumbo. Known in French as *gombo filé,* it is generally based on a roux. Cajuns who live further north in Acadiana prefer a darker, thicker *filé* gumbo based on a dark roux. However, in some communities near the Gulf, *filé* gumbo is made without any roux (25,26).

An informal food distribution system among families and friends in southern Louisiana has contributed to the retention of Cajun and Creole foodways. This system continues to provide individuals the opportunity to access traditional ingredients. The foods typically provided through the distribution system include wild game and wild fowl, which cannot be purchased commercially in most grocery stores, as well as seafood, crawfish, and freshwater fish. Crawfish, now popular across Louisiana, was previously available in limited supply in rural areas. In New Orleans' Creole neighborhoods, residents use turtle meat provided by family or friends from rural and wetland areas for a traditional Easter dish of turtle cooked in an au jus or tomato gravy. In the Cajun region, wild ducks or geese may be given to a family member or friend who then completes the preparation. The provider of the raw foodstuff then receives a portion of the finished dish or receives an invitation to share the meal featuring their contribution (20,27). Cajuns and Creoles also share the products of animal husbandry and gardening with family and friends.

The women in Cajun families are responsible for transmitting cultural characteristics from one generation to another (20), including the knowledge and skills related to food preparation. While men in southern Louisiana are frequently accomplished cooks, their skills tend to relate to hunting, fishing, and animal husbandry and the preparation of the foods obtained via these means. Men are also involved with cooking at special events such as church bazaars, fundraisers, hunting camp suppers, and local festivals (20).

Sharing meals with family and friends is an integral part of Cajun and Creole cultures. Several generations often share Sunday's noon meal, gathering at the home of one set of grandparents one week and at the other set's home on the following Sunday. Holiday celebrations are also intergenerational events.

In the late spring and early summer, many family gatherings on Friday and Saturday evenings focus on a crawfish boil. Crawfish, corn on the cob, garlic, potatoes, mushrooms, and smoked sausage are typically boiled in water seasoned with spice blends and salt. When cooked, the foods are drained and spilled out onto newspaper-covered tables for guests to enjoy. The children drink soft drinks or powdered drink mixes; the adults often have beer.

Although certainly not consumed by everyone, beer may be the most popular alcoholic beverage in southern Louisiana. It is served at crawfish and crab boils, barbeques, and other cookouts; it often accompanies fried seafood in restaurants and at home; and it is a common beverage to drink with a link of *boudin* or a handful of *gratons.*

Rum and whiskey are consumed perhaps most frequently in mixed drinks. Wine is featured at meals in some homes and chosen to accompany restaurant meals. However, it has never achieved the stature in Louisiana that it has in France, despite the French influence on Louisiana's cuisine and culture.

Cajuns and Creoles are not averse to convenience foods and technological advances in the kitchen, as long as the dishes that reach the table still meet their standards for quality (20). One successful convenience item is the frozen vegetable mix of diced green pepper, onion and celery, which is used in dishes like gumbo and jambalaya. Premade roux and roux flour (browned flour) are available and can save time, but their use is limited if the color of the product does not match the cooks' homemade version. *Filé* powder is another essential ingredient that is commercially processed and sold regionally. Some individuals still produce *filé* powder on a small scale and offer it for sale from their homes.

In the Cajun region the products of *boucherie* (slaughtering of a pig), including *boudin, gratons,* and hogshead cheese, are widely available in convenience and grocery stores and meat markets. Smoked and fresh beef or pork sausages are regularly made on the premises and sold in local meat markets. In addition to fresh fish and raw shellfish, seafood markets sell boiled shrimp, crabs, and crawfish ready for carryout.

All of these foods are considered "convenience" items because they reduce the time required to put a traditional dish on the table. This is important because women, who traditionally prepare meals in the home, are working outside the home more frequently. In an effort to attract these consumers as well as market Cajun and Creole foods outside Louisiana, regional food processors have developed packaged mixes for jambalaya and gumbo that only require the addition of chicken, sausage, or seafood. One major regional brand has developed reduced-sodium versions of several boxed mixes that contain 25% less sodium than original versions (27). Other convenience foods that the Cajuns and Creoles eat include frozen entrées, canned red beans and rice, and canned gumbo. According to managers of grocery stores in both the rural and urban Baton Rouge area, these products are typically used during the work week; however, the dishes are prepared "from scratch" on weekends (28).

Many families continue to use cast-iron and cast-aluminum cookware for certain dishes. Rice cookers are also commonplace. Microwave ovens are found in most homes but are not used to a great extent. Many people claim they can detect the difference between traditional recipes prepared in a microwave as opposed to on the stove (29).

Despite their high standards for well-prepared foods and appreciation for regional specialties, southern Louisiana residents frequently turn to fast foods for their meals. Local and regional fast-food chains and take-out restaurants often put a Cajun or Creole twist on their menu, such as topping a baked potato with crawfish *étouffée*. Popeye's Famous Fried Chicken is one of the best-known examples of a New Orleans restaurant that took their traditional menu and parlayed it into a successful nationwide chain by including special regional Cajun spices.

Counseling Considerations

Adopting a nonjudgmental attitude in nutrition counseling is recommended. To maintain credibility, the RD should demonstrate knowledge of Cajun and Creole food habits and health beliefs. This knowledge should be combined with respect for and acceptance of the validity of these habits and beliefs. The RD should never assume that he or she knows the definitive recipe for a traditional dish because versions vary by region and by family preference. Because many clients are skillful and talented cooks, the RD should recognize that he or she has opportunity to learn about variations within the unique cuisines of southern Louisiana.

Demonstrating Courtesy and Respect

It is considered disrespectful in Cajun and Creole cultures to address adult clients by their first name alone. This is especially true when working with older adults. The RD should initially address the client formally—eg, Mrs. (surname) or Mr. (surname). It may also be acceptable to use "Miss" (given name)—regardless of marital status—or "Mr." (given name), because this is usually the form of address that develops over time.

In counseling sessions, clients may address the RD as *Cher* (French for "darling" or "dear" and pronounced "sha") or *Bay* (a contraction of *bébé*, the French for "baby"), especially if they are from rural areas. "Dah-lin," "honey," or "sweetie," may be forms of address used, particularly by women clients from the New Orleans area. The use of these terms does not mean any disrespect toward the RD; it is merely a custom in most conversations in the area. Women in particular use these terms in a maternal way, especially if the RD is young.

The RD should acknowledge the relatives or companions who accompany the client. This is considered good manners as well as a sign of respect for others. It is appropriate to answer an older adult's questions with "Yes, ma'am" or "Yes, sir."

Interpreting Clients' Nonverbal Communication

Clients may not admit that they do not understand the topics covered in counseling sessions. They may automatically respond "Yes" when asked whether they understand, or "No" when asked whether they have questions. Such responses may reflect a client's embarrassment, feelings of intimidation, low literacy level, anxiety regarding anticipated changes in diet and lifestyle, or inability to read the materials used in session due to vision problems. By asking open-ended questions, you will be more likely elicit a more detailed response and can then tailor the session to the needs of the client.

Inquiring About Clients' Understanding of Diabetes

Given the close family ties that are typical in southern Louisiana, a client may share news of a recent diagnosis of diabetes with others before he or she consults with an RD. As a result, the client may receive inaccurate, incomplete, and/or outdated information regarding diabetes and its treatment from friends or family members (see previous Traditional Health Beliefs section of this chapter). In such circumstances, it is reasonable to expect clients to be overwhelmed by what they perceive as unreasonable expectations.

Therefore, before initiating the diet instruction, try to identify and correct misconceptions by asking the client open-ended questions. These questions can cover topics such as their knowledge of the cause(s) of diabetes, their previous experiences with diabetes in the family or among friends, how they have coped with their own diabetes in the past (if applicable), and what food(s) they have missed since being diagnosed with diabetes.

Discussing Clients' Use of Complementary and Alternative Medicine

Some individuals in Cajun and Creole cultures may assume only limited personal responsibility for their health, believing that control over one's life and health rests ultimately with God. Many people combine orthodox medical care with alternative practices, such as praying novenas or the rosary, attending Mass, having religio-magic treatments, or involving a faith healer or *traiteur*.

The *traiteur* believes he or she possesses a divine gift for healing. *Traiteurs* usually specialize in the treatment of ailments such as sunstroke, bleeding, shingles, headache, worms, warts, and insect and animal bites. *Traiteurs* do not generally treat serious internal ailments, but there are exceptions, and some *traiteurs* may treat disease symptoms. Regardless of the ailment, the treatment always includes prayers and often requires touching the patient. Because both *traiteur* and patient alike believe God to be responsible for healing, failure of the *traiteur* to cure an ailment is seen as a lack of faith on the part of the patient, or as the will of God (30,31).

Although the tradition of the *traiteur* is still alive in many communities, we do not know how widely it is followed. Individuals who consult a *traiteur* do not ordinarily discuss the subject with traditional health care providers. Older adults, less-educated individuals, those with limited access to conventional medicine due to financial limitations or geographical isolation, and those who have not been cured by conventional care may be more likely to seek the assistance of a *traiteur*.

Another type of Cajun folk medicine is religio-magic treatment. This uses objects such as holy water, a scapular medal, or a cloth scapular that has been blessed by a priest (31).

Just as in other cultures, home remedies were traditionally used when professional medical care was not nearby or the cost was prohibitive. Herbal remedies for diabetes centered on decoctions or teas. For example, beech tree bark was used in one decoction. Huckleberry leaf tea was also used (32). See Table 13.4 for more information on alternative treatments. Refer to Appendix C for questions to assess dietary supplement use.

Table 13.4 · Remedies Used by Cajuns and Creoles for Self-Treatment

Name	Description	Used to Treat
Beech bark	Decoction	Diabetes
Honey	Combine with whiskey for cough syrup	Colds (sore throat)
Huckleberry leaves	Tea	Diabetes
Lemon	Hot, sweetened lemon tea	Colds
Whiskey, bourbon	Combine with honey for cough syrup	Colds

Considering Family Demands and Dynamics

Within Cajun and Creole cultures, there are individual family subcultures. Food is, of course, necessary to sustain each family member nutritionally. Beyond this reality lies another—as Nichols State University associate professor of family studies LL Brigham notes, "Each family culture has wrapped in its food, things [events, experiences, concepts] that contribute to their sense of identity and continuity" (unpublished interview; August 29, 2007).

The specific family culture influences what the individuals in a family identify as acceptable or desirable. For example, Brigham indicates that some families will only eat home-raised beef and pork or fruits and vegetables (unpublished interview; August 29, 2007). Some families believe that recipes must be prepared from scratch to show love and concern for one's family members. "Regular" foods may be preferable to "diet" foods.

When one member of the family needs to make dietary modifications, the entire family is affected. The success of the modified diet may depend on which family member is involved. In southern Louisiana, women traditionally take primary responsibility for their family's food preparation and they tend to think of the family first and fulfill its dietary preferences before they address their own dietary needs. A woman with diabetes often puts the health needs of her family ahead of her own. For example, a woman with diabetes may hesitate to modify her family's ways of eating to accommodate her health needs; however, if either her husband or child were affected by diabetes, then she would be more receptive to dietary changes.

Engaging Others in Counseling Sessions

When planning nutrition counseling sessions, ask clients to invite family members (including spouses, in-laws, and older children) who have any or all responsibility for meal planning, food purchasing, and preparation. Women ordinarily prepare daily meals. Men have traditionally planned and prepared meals at special family or community events, and some also prepare family meals as well. Sometimes they are responsible for preparing the protein (meat, fish, or poultry) in a family meal, while the women and/or children prepare the rest of the meal. For example, men may be in charge of frying a turkey for a holiday meal while the rest of the "fixings" are prepared by the family.

Anecdotal evidence suggests that individuals from urban settings may approach counseling situations differently than clients in rural settings. While working for 3 months as a counselor in a Baton Rouge weight-loss clinic, A. Logan observed that her women clients in this urban setting were usually employed outside the home, arrived for appointments alone, and tended to have a professional or business-like demeanor during the session. Logan's previous clients were quite different. She had worked at a weight-loss clinic owned by the same corporation that was located in a smaller urban area bordered by rural countryside known for its Cajun culture. At this clinic, her women clients worked primarily as home-makers. They typically arrived for counseling with family members and expected a personal approach in the sessions (unpublished interview; March 10, 2008).

Lipstate found family support to be very common among her patients with diabetes in south-central Acadiana. Married couples, parents and children, and grandparents with grandchildren often came together to the clinic for counseling. She believes this is a positive feature of the culture (33).

Nutrition Counseling

The National Standards on Culturally and Linguistically Appropriate Services (CLAS) in Health Care state that clients should be provided with health care that is respectful of their culture; understandable, and effective resulting in the client's improved health (34). To provide culturally competent care, RDs should learn as much as they can about Cajun and Creole cultures. Hensley and colleagues found that the more frequently Louisiana clients were seen in a clinic, the more positive the outcome in their overall health (35). Obviously, all health care providers seek this outcome for their clients.

Refer to Appendix B for medical nutrition therapy (MNT) recommendations for diabetes as well as general counseling strategies. In addition, the following culturally specific strategies may be helpful for nutrition counseling of Cajun and Creole clients:

- Encourage clients to share their recipes and methods of food preparation, so you can test them and suggest healthful modifications.
- If you are unfamiliar with Lenten traditions regarding fasting and abstinence, seek explanations from Catholic pastoral counselors, nuns, chaplains, or priests. These individuals may also be able to provide insight if a client expresses fatalism when chronic disease and its treatment are discussed. Catholic and Protestant clergy can also provide information about the role of faith and prayer in healing as experienced by Cajun and Creole clients (36,37).
- Emphasize the importance of portion control for traditional carbohydrate foods such as rice, red beans and rice, french bread, and cornbread.
- Counsel clients about popular sweets, such as king cake, cane syrup, preserves, bread pudding, *tarte á la bouillie,* and tea cakes.
- Demonstrate low-fat methods of food preparation, including the preparation of nonfat roux (such as oven roux, dry roux, or roux flour) and its use in traditional recipes.
- Recommend that clients substitute olive oil or polyunsaturated oils for bacon fat and lard.
- Encourage clients to prepare seafood in *sauce piquante* or bake or broil it, instead of frying. Suggest serving cocktail sauce instead of tartar sauce with seafood or using fat-free tartar sauce.
- Advise clients to limit consumption of *debrís, boudin,* tongue, sausage, chitterlings, and other high-fat meats, as well as fried seafood and poboys with mayonnaise, gravy and or butter.
- Recognize that "average" consumption of alcohol in Cajun and Creole cultures may be more than the moderate amount recommended in most guidelines.

Challenges and Barriers to Nutrition Counseling

In a study of a small sample (n = 10) of self-identified Cajun residents of one southwest Louisiana parish, Waldmeier noted behavior that RDs should consider. Four of the 10 survey participants stated that they obtained health information from television and newspapers. The same number obtained health information from family and friends of Cajun background and indicated that advice from a member of their own community was valued more than advice from a health professional (38).

Many clients, especially older adults, may distrust printed recipes provided at a nutrition counseling session. They may say something to the effect of "My mother/grandmother/ aunt was the best cook I have ever known, and she never measured anything or used a recipe." Be aware that written cooking instructions are not traditional in Cajun and Creole cultures. Instead food preparation techniques and recipes have traditionally been learned by observing and working alongside one's elders.

When working with Cajun or Creole clients, consider the availability of food. Access to food may be restricted by a client's economic status, location, or both.

Finally, the sense of fatalism discussed in other sections of this chapter can be an ongoing challenge to the success of nutrition counseling.

Counseling Tips

When working with Cajun or Creole clients, remember the following essential points:

- Emphasize the importance of portion control.
- Encourage clients to make dietary changes gradually whenever possible. A gradual approach will increase compliance.
- Food preparation demonstrations and "taste parties" may be effective methods of teaching recipe modification because these approaches are in keeping with the hands-on method used by generations in south Louisiana to teach cooking skills.
- Seek information from clergy in the area regarding the role that religion, faith, and prayer play in maintaining health.
- Encourage clients to share their experiences with Cajun and Creole convenience food products. Ask them to bring food labels or packaging to determine if and when these items can fit into modified diets.
- Gardening can contribute to a more active lifestyle and provide fresh fruits and vegetables that can reduce the amount of money spent on groceries.

Resources

Angers WT. *Cajun Cuisine: Authentic Cajun Recipes from Louisiana's Bayou Country.* Lafayette, LA: Beau Bayou Publishing; 1985. (Introductory remarks by Marie Louise Comeaux , home economist and respected authority on Cajun cuisine and culture provide information on traditional cooking methods and ingredients. Recipes are typical of dishes prepared in south Louisiana homes.)

Brasseaux CA. *French, Cajun, Creole, Houma: A Primer on Francophone Louisiana.* Baton Rouge, LA: Louisiana State University Press; 2005. (A scholarly, yet accessible, explanation of the varied cultures in Louisiana).

Chase L, Rivers J. *Down Home Healthy: Family Recipes of Black American Chefs.* Bethesda, MD: National Cancer Institute; 1993. (Difficult to find, but worth the effort for tips on reducing fat and calories in traditional southern recipes that are served particularly in New Orleans.)

Louisiana Department of Health and Hospitals. Office of Public Health. http://www.dhh.louisiana.gov/offices/?ID=79. Accessed March 6, 2009. (Access to Louisiana's parish health profiles.)

Prudhomme E. *Enola Prudhomme's Low-Calorie Cajun Cooking.* New York, NY: William Morrow Cookbooks; 1991. (May be difficult to find, but useful for examples of recipes used in the home.)

Prudhomme P. *Chef Paul Prudhomme's Louisiana Kitchen.* New York, NY: William Morrow; 1984. (While not a cookbook for the calorie-conscious, this volume provides insight into ingredients found in traditional south Louisiana cooking. Includes photos of varied colors of roux.)

Prudhomme P. *Chef Paul Prudhomme's Fork in the Road: A Different Direction in Cooking.* New York, NY: Morrow Cookbooks; 1993. (Suggestions to assist in reducing the fat and calories in traditional south Louisiana cooking.)

University of Michigan Health System Program for Multicultural Health. Cultural Competency Reading List. http://www.med.umich.edu/multicultural/ccp/Reading.htm. Accessed March 6, 2009. (General information on providing health care for diverse populations.)

References

1. Hanna B. UTA to gauge evacuees' willingness to return. *Fort Worth Star-Telegram.* July 18, 2007.
2. Synder M. Katrina: two years later. *Houston Chronicle.* July 1, 2007.
3. Means SP. Katrina documentary praises Utahns for helping hand, harshly criticizes officials. *Salt Lake Tribune.* May 24, 2007.
4. Wind A. Graduating Katrina evacuees have thrived since arriving in Waterloo. *Waterloo Courier.* May 25, 2007.
5. Fortune M. Katrina evacuees still struggling to rebuild. *Chattanooga Times Free Press.* April 26, 2007.
6. Greenlee M. Katrina evacuees: Farewell to Saginaw. *Saginaw News.* February 24, 2007.
7. Brasseaux CA, *French, Cajun, Creole, Houma: A Primer on Francophone Louisiana.* Baton Rouge, LA: Louisiana State University Press; 2005.
8. Brasseaux CA. *Acadian to Cajun: Transformation of a People, 1803–1877.* Jackson, MS: University Press of Mississippi; 1992.
9. Gibson JL, DelSesto S. The culture of Acadiana: an anthropological perspective. In: Gibson JL, DelSesto S, eds. *The Culture of Acadiana: Tradition and Change in South Louisiana.* Lafayette, LA: University of Southwestern Louisiana; 1975:1–14.

10. Powell P. Eccentric, authentic New Orleans. *New York Times Magazine*. October 18, 1992:71–74.

11. Landry R, Allard R, Henry J. French in south Louisiana: towards language loss. *J Multilingual Multicult Develop*. 1996;17:442–468.

12. US Census Bureau. 2005-2007 American Community Survey. Population Finder. http://factfinder .census.gov/servlet/SAFFPopulation?geo_id=05000US22071&_state=04000US22&pctxt=cr. Accessed May 9, 2009.

13. *BRFSS Data and Diabetes in Louisiana, 2006*. Baton Rouge, LA: Louisiana Department of Health and Hospitals; 2006.

14. US Department of Health and Human Services. *Tracking Healthy People 2010*. Washington, DC: US Government Printing Office, November 2000. http://www.healthypeople.gov/Document/ tableofcontents.htm#tracking. Accessed March 9, 2009.

15. National Diabetes Fact Sheet: General Information and National Estimates on Diabetes in the United States, 2005. Atlanta, GA: Centers for Disease Control and Prevention; 2005. http://www.cdc.gov/diabetes/pubs/pdf/ndfs_2005.pdf. Accessed March 9, 2009.

16. 2006 Louisiana Health Report Card. 2007. Baton Rouge, LA: Louisiana Department of Health and Hospitals, Office of Public Health; 2006. http://www.dhh.louisiana.gov/offices/publications/pubs- 275/2006%20LA%20Health%20Report.pdf. Accessed March 9, 2009.

17. *Behavioral Risk Factor Surveillance System Survey Data*. Atlanta, GA: Centers for Disease Control and Prevention; 2006.

18. Leistner CG. *French and Acadian Influences Upon the Cajun Cuisine of Southwest Louisiana* (master's thesis). Lafayette, LA: University of Southwestern Louisiana; 1986.

19. Leistner C, Camel S, Scott B. Health and Cultural Implications of Indigenous Food in South Louisiana. General session presentation at Louisiana Dietetic Association Food & Nutrition Conference, Lafayette LA; April 1, 2007.

20. Gutierrez CP. *Foodways and Cajun Identity* (dissertation). Chapel Hill, NC: University of North Carolina; 1983.

21. Hawkins DB. Cultural attitudes and body dissatisfaction: Morgan State researchers find that perceptions of body image among young African Americans may be life threatening. *Black Issues in Higher Education*. January 27, 2005.

22. Akan G, Greilo C. Sociocultural influences on eating attitudes and behaviors, body image, and psychological functioning: a comparison of African-American, Asian-American, and Caucasian college women. *Int J Eating Disord*. 1995;18:181–187.

23. Molloy BL, Herzberger SD. Body image and self-esteem: a comparison of African-American and Caucasian women. *Sex Roles*. 1998;38:631–643.

24. Leistner CG. *Development of Culturally Appropriate Nutrition Education Materials for Dietetic Practitioners Working in the Cajun and Creole Populations of Southern Louisiana* (dissertation). Tallahassee, FL: Florida State University; 2003.

25. Guidry RJ. *La Cuisine Franco-Louisinaise: Glossaire*. Lafayette, LA: RJ Guidry; 1990.

26. *Recipes of the Gueydan Area*. Gueydan, LA: Gueydan Garden Club; 1979.

27. Zatarin's Web site. http://www.zatarains.com. Accessed August 31, 2008.

28. Ten Eyck TA. Managing food: Cajun cuisine in economic and cultural terms. *Rural Sociol*. 2001;66:227–243.

29. Leistner CG. *Cajun and Creole Food Practices, Customs, and Holidays*. Chicago IL: American Dietetic Association; 1996.

30. Pitre G. Good for What Ails You. Oriol, MD: Cote Blanche Productions; 1998.

31. Ancelet BJ, Edwards JD, Pitre G. *Cajun Country*. Jackson, MS: University Press of Mississippi; 1991.

32. Touchstone SJ. *Herbal and Folk Medicine of Louisiana and Adjacent States*. Princeton, LA: Folk- Life Books; 1983.

33. Lipstate L. Type II diabetes: the Cajun connection. *Diabetes Forecast*. 1996;49:24–26.

34. Department of Health and Human Services, Office of Minority Health. National Standards on Culturally and Linguistically Appropriate Services (CLAS) in Health Care. *Federal Register*. 2000;65(247):80865–80879.

35. Hensley RD, Jones AK, Williams AG, Willsher LB, Cain PP. One-year clinical outcomes for Louisiana residents diagnosed with type 2 diabetes and hypertension. *J Am Acad Nurs Pract*. 2005;17:363–369.

36. Boland CS. Social support and spiritual well-being: empowering older adults to commit to health- promising behaviors. *J Multicult Nurs Health*. 2000;6:12–23.

37. Garg RK, Filozof E, Etheredge GD, Maney E. Health behavior in a Cajun population. *J Cult Divers*. 1998;5:89–93.

38. Waldmeier VP. *Laissez les bon temps rouler* (let the good times roll): can embedded Cajun cultural health beliefs be changed through traditional health education? *J Cult Divers*. 2002;9:113–117.

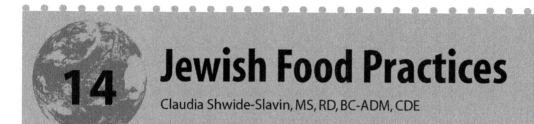

14 Jewish Food Practices

Claudia Shwide-Slavin, MS, RD, BC-ADM, CDE

Introduction

In 2007, there were 6.4 million Jews in the United States (1). In 2001, 85% of the adult Jews in the United States were born in the United States. Among Jews born outside of the United States, the largest group (44%) is from the former Soviet Union, approximately 10% were born in Israel, and another 10% were born in Germany (2,3).

According to the Council of Jewish Federations in North America's 2000 National Jewish Population Survey, 46% of American Jews belong to a synagogue (4). Among those who belong to a synagogue, most belong to one of the three major branches of contemporary Judaism: 38% are part of a Reform congregation, 33% are Conservative, and 22% are Orthodox (4). The following are some distinctions among these groups (5):

- Reform Judaism is the most liberal of the three largest movements. It emphasizes ethics, and its followers may be less likely than Orthodox or Conservative Jews to strictly/ literally adhere to the laws of the Torah.

- Conservative Judaism grew out of tension between the Reform and Orthodox movements. There are many different versions of Conservative Judaism. Conservatives maintain the laws written in the Torah but also believe that Jewish law should change and adapt to modern-day culture.

- Orthodox Judaism describes several different groups with similar beliefs; these include the modern Orthodox, who have largely integrated into modern society while maintaining observance of Jewish law; Hasidic Jews (sometimes called the ultra-Orthodox), who live separately and dress distinctively; and Yeshivish Orthodox. (It can be difficult for anyone who is not Orthodox to understand the differences among the various groups.)

Diabetes Prevalence

The prevalence of diabetes among Jewish Americans is not known. In Israel, the prevalence of type 2 diabetes in the Jewish population is slightly higher than global averages. Between 2003 and 2005, diabetes prevalence in Israeli adults between the ages of 20 and 79 increased from 7.1% to 8.1%, and the prevalence of impaired glucose tolerance increased from 5.4% to 5.9% (6).

Risk Factors for Type 2 Diabetes

US health data rarely include religious affiliation. Therefore, it is difficult to assess diabetes risk factors for Jewish Americans specifically.

In 2006, Benjamins et al conducted a population-based health survey of a representative sample of 201 adults and 58 children selected from 23,000 people in a Chicago Jewish community. The sample population were generally as healthy (or healthier) than average residents of Chicago and the United States. However, many serious health concerns, including obesity, were identified in this community (7).

The Human Genome Project is helping to identify genetic variations that predispose individuals to type 2 diabetes. In 2004, international research teams working on the project identified four genetic variants called single nucleotide polymorphisms (SNPs), which are strongly associated with type 2 diabetes in Ashkenazi Jews (8). This genetic variation alone does not cause diabetes, but, combined with other factors such as obesity or physical inactivity, it increases the risk of diabetes. Generations ago, the Ashkenazi Jewish people living in Poland and Russia endured harsh winters with limited food sources. Survival was probably greater for those with an efficient metabolism and heavier body weight, factors that are known precursors to type 2 diabetes. The gene mutations that were present in the founders of the population remained within the community, increased in frequency, and, over time, increased the risk for type 2 diabetes in the Ashkenazi population (9).

Traditional Foods and Dishes

Historically, Jewish people have lived around the world, and, as a result, traditional dishes reflect the local cooking styles of the regions where they settled, such as eastern and central Europe, Spain, the Mediterranean, the Middle East, Asia, and Africa. Thus, "Jewish food" can refer to many different cooking styles, traditions, and tastes. For example, the Jewish diet may include blintzes and kugels of the Ashkenazi (the Jews who settled in France, Germany, and Eastern Europe), or it may feature falafel and hummus, dishes that originated with the Sephardim (Jews from Spain and Portugal, Northern Africa, and the Middle East). In the United States, dietary practices among Jews are varied: some eat a stereotypically "American" diet and/or explore many ethnic cuisines; others observe kosher dietary laws and/or eat mostly traditional Jewish foods.

Jewish food is often incorrectly equated only with kosher food. "Kosher" *(Kashruth)* means "in keeping with the Jewish dietary laws" written in the Torah, which contains all Jewish teachings. Most modern Jews do not strictly follow the laws of *Kashruth*. Therefore, when discussing modern Jewish cuisine, it is important to distinguish between (*a*) foods and food practices that are directly regulated by religious laws and (*b*) food traditions that have passed down from generation to generation and have become part of daily or special-occasion food habits, regardless of the individual's level of religious observance. (Kosher laws are discussed in greater detail later in this chapter.)

In the United States, Jewish cuisine is often associated with traditional Ashkenazi dishes. A typical Ashkenazi dish is a sweet-and-sour meat and vegetable stew seasoned with sugar, honey, or raisins, as well as vinegar or lemon juice. This flavoring technique is also used for soups and meatless dishes and can introduce hidden carbohydrates in foods usually considered "carbohydrate-free."

Sephardic meals feature a wide variety of salads, cooked vegetables, and *burekas* (small pies filled with feta cheese, spinach, or potato). More aromatic than Ashkenazi dishes, Sephardic cuisine typically includes plant foods that are readily available in the Mediterranean climate, such as lemon, garlic, tomatoes, and olive oil, and spices like cumin and turmeric.

Sephardic dishes vary according to the country of origin. Individuals from the eastern end of the Mediterranean use cinnamon in cooking and as a savory accent in meat dishes, whereas Sephardic Jews from Morocco and other North African countries flavor dishes with cumin, ginger, saffron, and chilies. Dried fruits such as figs, apricots, prunes, and raisins are included in meat dishes and complement the spices. Almonds, walnuts, and olives are also incorporated in many dishes. Turkish Jewish cooking includes meat kebabs, pilafs, and stuffed vegetables (such as grape leaves stuffed with rice, dried fruits, vegetables, spices, and grains). Jews in Morocco eat couscous; in Tunisia, chilies are incorporated into *harissa*, a spicy condiment. Libyan Jewish cooking is influenced by Italian cooking, with its use of tomato paste and sauces, as well as by North African spices, beans, and grains.

Because traditional foods of the Ashkenazi and Sephardic Jews are not identical, RDs should ask each client which traditional foods they eat. Box 14.1 lists foods used in traditional Jewish cuisine, and Table 14.1 identifies traditional Jewish dishes, beverages, and desserts (10–14). See Appendix A for nutrient analyses. Information on kosher dietary laws is provided later in this chapter.

Box 14.1 • Foods Used in Traditional Jewish Cuisine

Starches

Note: In a kosher diet, grains are soaked in water to remove insects.

• Barley	• Noodles
• Buckwheat groats (*kasha or kasha varnishkes*)	• Quinoa
• Bulgur	• Rice
• Couscous	• Wheat
• Millet	

Starchy vegetables

• Peas	• Potatoes
• Corn	• Sweet potatoes
• Legumes (chickpeas/garbanzos, lima beans, lentils)	• Winter squash (acorn, butternut)
	• Yams

Fruit

• Apples	• Honeydew
• Bananas	• Olives
• Carob seed pod (*bokser*; also called St John's bread)	• Oranges
• Dates	• Peaches
• Dried fruit, including apricots, prunes, raisins, fruit compote, fruit soups, and avocado	• Pears
• Figs	• Pineapple
• Grapes	• Pomegranates
	• Watermelon

Nonstarchy vegetables

Note: In a kosher diet, all vegetables are soaked in salted water to remove insects.

• Asparagus	• Mushrooms
• Avocado	• Onions
• Beets	• Radish
• Broccoli	• Salad greens (endive, escarole, iceberg, romaine, arugula, radicchio)
• Cabbage	
• Carrots	• Sorrel
• Cauliflower	• Sour grass (used in *shav* soup)
• Cucumber (pickles)	• Spinach
• Eggplant	• Squash (zucchini, summer squash)
• Kale	• Tomatoes
• Leeks	

(continued)

Box 14.1 *(continued)*

Milk and milk products

Note: In kosher kitchens, separate dairy utensils are required for preparation, cooking, and serving of dairy products.

- Butter
- Cheese (hard and soft types, including cottage cheese and cream cheese)
- Evaporated milk
- Milk and milk derivatives, including sodium caseinate and lactose in candy, cereal, and low calorie sweeteners
- Nondairy products (nondairy substitutes for butter, milk, and cream are allowed in kosher meals with meat)
- Sour cream
- Yogurt

Meats and meat substitutes

Note: Kosher meats include any animal that has cloven hooves and chews its cud, as well as fowl. The animal must be slaughtered in accordance with prescribed Jewish ritual. To remove blood, all meat must be soaked in water for 30 minutes and salted for 1 hour in coarse salt or by sprinkling with salt and broiling. Liver may only be broiled to remove the blood.

- Beef (brisket, pot roast, flanken, sweet and sour meatballs, tongue, corned beef, pastrami, chopped liver)
- Chicken (chopped chicken liver)
- Cornish hens
- Dove, pigeons, squab
- Duck
- Eggs (in kosher kitchens, eggs are opened in a glass bowl to check for blood spots before cooking; if a spot is found the egg is discarded)
- Goose
- Lamb
- Mutton
- Pheasant
- Quail
- Turkey
- Veal
- Venison

Fish

Note: Kosher fish include those with both detachable fins and scales that are removed from the skin before eating. Although fish is *parve* (neutral) and can be consumed with a meat meal, it is an optional course that is served on a separate plate and with separate utensils.

- Bluefish
- Carp
- Cod
- Flounder
- Herring (salted, pickled, smoked, in wine sauce or creamed)
- Pike
- Salmon (lox)
- Scrod
- Sole
- Tuna
- Whitefish

Spices and flavorings

- Chilies (Sephardic)
- Cinnamon (Sephardic)
- Cumin (Sephardic)
- Garlic (Sephardic)
- Ginger (Sephardic)
- Honey (Ashkenazi)
- Lemon (Ashkenazi and Sephardic)
- Olive oil (Sephardic)
- Raisins (Ashkenazi)
- Saffron (Sephardic)
- Sugar (Ashkenazi)
- Tahini/sesame paste (Sephardic)
- Tomato paste (Sephardic)
- Tomato sauce (Sephardic)
- Turmeric (Sephardic)
- Vinegar (Ashkenazi)

All foods listed can be used when creating kosher meal plans.

Table 14.1 · Traditional Jewish Dishes, Beverages, and Desserts

Food	Description
Dishes	
Bagels	Donut-shaped boiled and baked bread with a hole in the middle symbolizing the endless circle of life. Sugar, raisins or honey may be added.
Blintzes	Jewish version of a baked or fried crepe filled with sweetened cheese, potato and onion, apple, cherry and blueberries.
Borscht	Beet soup, often served with sour cream and potatoes.
Brisket	The chest portion of the beef prepared with marinades that can include carbohydrate-containing ingredients, such as cola, wine, honey, ketchup, and onions.
Burekas	Israeli breakfast food made from filo dough triangle filled with cheese or spinach.
Challah	Sweet, golden, eggy bread that is usually braided in a loaf. (Depending on taste, a slice of challah can be as large as 3 ounces, compared with one-ounce packaged bread slices). In addition, sugar content in the recipe may vary as well as the size of the slice with the shape of the loaf.
Chicken soup	Clear broth made with boiled onions, celery, carrots, chicken, noodles, and matzo balls.
Cholent	Stew made from beans, vegetables, beef, barley and sometimes potatoes.
Falafel	Fried chickpea and bulgur patties served in pita bread with lettuce, tomato, pickles.
Gefilte fish	Chopped boiled fish, onions, vegetables, egg, matzo meal and sugar in the shape of a cake or ball. Eaten warm or cold with horseradish.
Hummus	Dip made from chickpeas, tahini (sesame paste), garlic, and lemon.
Israeli salad	Tomatoes, peppers, cucumber, scallion and sometimes kohlrabi diced and mixed together and eaten with hard boiled eggs, cheese and bread for breakfast.
Kasha *varnishka*	Kasha buckwheat groats cooked with onions and chicken stock, mixed with bowtie pasta.
Kishke/stuffed *derma*	Casing made from beef or poultry neck skin stuffed and baked with flour, matzo meal, onions and fat.
Knishes	Baked, crisp dumplings stuffed with mashed potato, onion, chopped liver or cheese.
Kugel	Jewish pudding made from potatoes, eggs, onions, and vegetables.
Lokshen kugel	Jewish pudding made from noodles, fruits and nuts.
Matzo balls	Jewish boiled dumplings in varying sizes made from matzo meal, egg, oil and water.
Matzo *brei*	Pancake made with broken matzo pieces soaked in scrambled egg.
Prakkes	Cabbage leaf filled with meat. Also known as *galuptzi, cholupches, holishkes, holubtsy,* or *galabki.*
Schnitzel	Chicken cutlet breaded with matzo meal.
Strudel	Pastry dough made with high gluten flour, rolled thin and filled with apple, cheese, fruit, poppy seeds, spinach, or savory vegetables.
Tzimmes	Sweet orange colored mix of vegetables and fruit starting with carrots and adding either sweet potatoes, prunes, pineapple, and sugar. Different ingredients are added on different holidays.
Vegetarian chopped "liver"	Salad with mushrooms, string beans, hardboiled egg and onions.
Beverages	
Grape juice	
Sweet wine	
Desserts	
Apple cinnamon kugel	Cake prepared with grated apples, sugar, matzo farfel, egg whites and cinnamon.
Babka	Cake filled with chocolate, cheese or fruit filling of raisins and cinnamon and glazed with a chocolate or fruit-flavored icing.
Candy	Sweets included in dessert selections on Friday night, holidays, and often used as an incentive for children learning.
Halvah	Cooked flour, sugar, spices, oil and nuts, simmered, cooled and cut into squares.

(continued)

Table 14.1   *(continued)*

Food	Description
Fruit compote	Mixed cooked fruit combination of apples, pears, peaches, berries, cherries and added sugar.
Fruit soup	Cold soup made with fruit, sugar and flour that are eaten in summer months.
Hamentaschen	Baked three corner pastry filled with chopped dried fruit, honey, jam, prune concentrate or poppy seeds.
Honey cake	Cake made from eggs, honey, sugar, coffee and flour.
Mandelbrot	Jewish biscotti.
Rugalach	Rolled, baked, crescent shaped filled cookies.

Source: Data are from references 11–14.

Holiday Foods and Meal Patterns

The Jewish calendar is based on the lunar year, which is not the same length as the solar year used by most of the Western world. Although Jewish holidays fall on different dates every year according to our conventional (solar) calendar, the dates do not change from year to year on the Jewish calendar (15).

Holidays are either celebrated both at the synagogue and with home rituals (eg, Rosh Hashanah and Yom Kippur) or take place mainly within the home (Passover, Hanukkah, and the weekly Sabbath). Jewish holidays include those that are described in the Bible (eg, Rosh Hashanah, Yom Kippur, Passover, Shavuos, and Sukkot), as well as rabbinical holidays that were established to remember miracles that occurred during Jewish history (eg, Hanukkah and Purim). In the United States, Jews typically observe Rosh Hashanah and Yom Kippur (the High Holy Days), as well as Passover and Hanukkah. Some Jewish Americans also celebrate other holidays.

Food plays a major part in Jewish holiday meals and landmark events and helps commemorate spiritual history. For example, the holiday meal (Seder) held on the first or first and second nights of Passover celebrates the Festival of Matzos and the liberation of the Jewish people from Egypt's tyranny. The Seder begins after sundown with prayers and a recitation of the holiday's history. Seder rituals include 15 different points throughout the evening when foods are involved, and the main meal may start as late as midnight. Food takes on symbolic meaning during Passover. Yeast breads and other foods made with leaven are prohibited for the length of the holiday. This restriction represents flight from Egypt, when Jews carried the dough on their backs, where it baked into flat, unleavened bread under the hot sun. At the Seder, bitter herbs *(maror)* are eaten to remember the bitterness of slavery, and *haroset* (a mixture of apples, nuts, cinnamon, honey and sweet wine) is served to represent clay and mortar used to make bricks and build the Pharaoh's palaces. A roasted shank bone symbolizes the sacrificial lamb and the rebirth of spring. Parsley *(karpas)* symbolizes the green color of spring and the renewal of faith and hope in the world. A hard-boiled egg is roasted to symbolize life and continued existence.

Sabbath is the most important holiday in the Jewish religion. It is observed every week, starting at sundown on Friday and ending at sundown on Saturday. It includes three main meals: Friday night *(Shabbat)* dinner, Saturday *(Shabbat)* lunch, and a Saturday afternoon meal *(Seudah Shelishit)*. The latter is usually a lighter meal, such as a sandwich, a piece of cake, or fruit. Jewish law prohibits observant Jews from doing any work, including cooking, on the Sabbath. To avoid lighting a flame on the Sabbath, Jews developed stews and dishes that could be started before sunset on Friday and cooked on a low flame or baked slowly. The best-known of these is the Ashkenazi *cholent,* a slow-cooking stew of meat and vegetables. In Sephardic cuisine, slow-baked, single-dish meals called *T'fina* (translated as "buried in the coals") are made from meat, potatoes, chickpeas, and seasonings. The meal is started on Friday night and slowly baked over smoldering coals until it is ready to eat at lunch on Saturday (10). See Box 14.2 for additional description of Sabbath meals and Table 14.2 for information about other holidays (15–23).

Box 14.2 • Traditional Foods Consumed During the Jewish Sabbath

Friday Night *Shabbat*

- Challah
- Fruit (fruit cocktail, grapefruit, melon, fruit soup, applesauce)
- Chicken soup (including any of the following: carrots, celery, potato, noodles, matzo balls)
- Meat course (brisket, boiled beef, chicken, or pot roast, usually prepared with a sweet marinade; chopped liver)
- Fish course (gefilte fish, boiled fish)
- Kugels
- Vegetables (peas and carrots, string beans, broccoli)
- *Tsimmes*
- Salads (lettuce and tomato, tomato and cucumber)
- Dessert (cake, strudel, sponge cake, dates, figs, cookies)

Saturday Lunch (Meat)

- Challah
- Fish (usually gefilte fish; optional separate course)
- *Cholent*
- Cold meats (chicken, beef, chopped liver, cold cuts)
- Salads made from starch (pasta, rice, legumes)
- Salads made from proteins (eggs, tuna fish)
- Salads made from nonstarchy vegetables (greens, cucumber, tomatoes)
- Vegetables
- Dessert (cake, cookies, candy)

Saturday Lunch (Dairy)

- Bagels
- Cheese blintzes with sour cream
- Cooked vegetables (cabbage stuffed with rice, baked potato, sweet and sour cabbage, mushrooms in sour cream)
- Cream cheese
- Eggs (chopped egg and onion, egg salad)
- Fish (lox, baked salmon, whitefish, herring, salads with tuna fish or salmon, fried fish, baked fish)
- Noodle kugel
- Raw vegetables
- Soups (split pea, cold borscht, mushroom barley, cold fruit soup)
- Dessert

Seudah Shelishit"

- Cake
- Challah rolls
- Fruits
- Pizza
- Sandwich
- Tuna salad

Table 14.2 · Traditional Foods Consumed During Jewish Holidays

Holiday/Description	Foods
Biblical holidays	
Rosh Hashanah: Celebrates the Jewish New Year in September or October with a holiday meal before and after the religious services. On the second day, fruits not yet eaten in the new season are served in tandem with a special blessing.	• First meal: round challah; apples dipped in honey; chicken matzo ball soup; gefilte fish with horseradish; *tsimmes;* honey cake; apple cake; strudel; nuts • Second meal: dates, figs, pomegranates, pumpkin, leeks, beets
Yom Kippur: The day to ask forgiveness for one's sins; observed 8 days after Rosh Hashanah. A large, festive, high-carbohydrate, low-sodium meal is recommended before a 25-hour fast. The fast is followed by meat, chicken, or dairy meals (choices vary depending on the family's place of origin). In the United States, the meal is usually similar to a brunch with bagels, lox, cream cheese, herring and other fish, and sweet kugels.	• Meal before the fast: meat (brisket of pot roast stew with potatoes, beans, grains, roast tongue, veal chops, stuffed veal); winter squash (butternut, acorn); soup (lentil, barley); sweet potatoes and other vegetables (fried eggplant, honey carrots, potato stuffing, roast potato) • Breaking the fast: first, a drink (orange juice, sweet yogurt, brandy, coffee, or tea), then a dairy, meat, or chicken meal; typically, a sweet food is followed by a salty food (eg, fruit juice followed by smoked whitefish, smoked salmon, or herring)
Sukkot: The 7-day festival of the Tabernacle is celebrated 5 days after fasting on Yom Kippur. The fall harvest is celebrated by eating fruits, vegetables, and sweets in outdoor booths called *sukkot.*	• Fresh fruits, fall vegetables • Stuffed cabbage (*holishkes, galuptzi, praakes*)—the ingredients and preparation depend on one's grandmother's origins; the Eastern European recipe stuffs cabbage leaves with meatballs in a tomato-based sweet-and-sour sauce • Pomegranates (also called Chinese apples)—eaten at this holiday because of the number of pits in each fruit symbolizes the 613 commandments in the Torah • *Kreplach* (small triangular pieces of dough filled with meat) in soup
Passover: Celebrated in March or April, Passover commemorates the emancipation of Jews from Egypt. It begins with a "spring cleaning" of all products in the house that are made with yeast or any leavening ingredient. All dishes, pots, and other cooking/eating utensils used during the rest of the year are changed. Foods made with leavening (such as bread) are prohibited for the 8 days of Passover. In addition to the ban on leavening agents, wheat (flour), oats, rye, and barley are forbidden. Ashkenazi Jews (but not Sephardic Jews) also prohibit corn, rice, peanuts, and legumes. Some artificial sweeteners (Equal, Splenda, and NutraSweet) are not considered kosher for Passover; others (Sweet 'n Low and Sweetie) are allowed.	• Bitter herbs (*maror*) • Hard-boiled eggs • *Haroset* • Mandelbread (a traditional Jewish cookie combining flavors from sweet cinnamon, orange and chocolate or carob often eaten in the morning with coffee or tea) • Matzo (unleavened bread) • *Matzo brei* (scrambled eggs mixed with broken pieces of matzo and topped with cinnamon sugar or jelly or cooked savory by adding favorite vegetables and fresh herbs, eaten at any meal during the 8-day holiday) • Matzo meal rolls (made by adding beaten eggs to matzo meal and taste similar to popovers especially when eaten fresh out of the oven) • Parsley • Potato starch and flakes in baked goods as a substitute for yeast and as a binder instead of flour • Roasted lamb shank

(continued)

Table 14.2   *(continued)*

Holiday/Description	Foods
Shavuot: Called the Feast of the Weeks and celebrated in May/June when it is harvest season in Israel, Shavuot celebrates when Moses received the Torah on Mount Sinai as well as the first fruit harvest of the new year. Meat is usually avoided and sweet dairy foods like cheesecake and blintzes are eaten to associate sweetness and joy with starting Torah study.	• Sweet dairy foods: blintzes, *lokshen kugel* (dairy noodle pudding with cheese), cheese kreplach, cheese pastries, strudel, cheesecake • Vegetarian foods: beet borscht with sour cream, cucumber soups, *schav* (sorrel soup) • Sephardic dishes include a braided round loaf (*los siete cielos:* the bread of the seven heavens), *kahee* (fried, flat, buttered dough folded into squares and sprinkled with sugar), *atayef* (a filled cheese pancake), *ruz ib asal* (baked rice pudding with honey and rose water), *tortelli dolci* (cheese turnovers filled with ricotta cheese)

Rabbinical holidays

Holiday/Description	Foods
Simchat Torah: Celebrates the finish of one year and the beginning of the next year's reading of the Torah; the celebration includes singing and dancing.	• Sweet foods to celebrate the sweetness of the Torah • Blintzes • Dolmas (stuffed grape leaves) • Orange-colored foods, fruits, candy and sweets • Candy apples
Hanukkah: The 8-day festival of lights in December honors the rededication of the Jewish temple in Jerusalem. Traditional foods are oil-rich to symbolize the miracle that occurred when a lamp filled with only enough oil for one night, burned for 8 days.	• Applesauce • Latkes (potato pancakes) • Sour cream • Doughnuts filled with jelly (Sephardic)
Tu B'Shevat: Celebrates a new year for planting trees. A variety of fruits and nuts are eaten.	• Seven different fruits and grains mentioned in the Bible (wheat, barley, grapes, figs, pomegranate, olives, and dates) are served at a regular meal or a dinner ceremony • Up to 15 fruits may be eaten in one day to celebrate the holiday • Fatty fruits such as avocados, olives, and nuts are eaten first
Purim: A wild holiday celebrated with a feast of foods and wine. The holiday celebrates when the Jewish people in Persia successfully fought and were spared from extermination by the king. Celebrating the holiday involves dressing up in costumes and reenacting history. In addition to a family meal, gifts of food or drink are sent to friends and given to charity.	• Alcohol: drinking to the point of drunkenness is encouraged (pre-holiday counseling on the effect of alcohol on blood glucose is recommended) • *Hamentaschen* (triangular, fruit-filled cookies)

Source: Data are from references 15–23.

Many traditional holiday dishes are high in carbohydrates, and clients may resist suggestions to limit their intake because they feel these foods are essential to their religious observances. Holidays can challenge individuals with diabetes in other ways, too. For example, clients may have difficulty evaluating the carbohydrate content in foods without labels, foods that are infrequently eaten, or atypical portion sizes. In addition, some people may feel uncomfortable about taking diabetes medications in an exposed, social environment. RDs should counsel individuals about healthful ways to participate in holidays, such as limiting the carbohydrates they consume at each meal or adjusting medication doses (if insulin-dependent). See the Nutrition Counseling section later in this chapter for more on this topic.

Fasting is a characteristic of some Jewish holidays. Yom Kippur and Tisha B'Av are major fasts, which begin at sundown and are broken 25 hours later, after a day of prayer and reflection. Even water consumption is not permitted. Minor fasts (from dawn until nightfall) occur five times during the year; each one commemorates a Jewish tragedy. Among Jews, opinions vary about whether individuals with diabetes should participate in fasts. See the Nutrition Counseling section of this chapter for more on the topic of fasting.

Traditional Health Beliefs

Members of the different modern Jewish movements (eg, Orthodox, Conservative, or Reform) vary in their religious beliefs and how closely their behaviors follow the Torah. Differences in religious values affect individual views on health. For example, a person may follow a kosher diet for health reasons or because they believe it is divinely decreed.

Prayers recited on the Sabbath and holidays require a specific amount of food or drink (a *shiur kazayis*). The *shiur* is approximately 4 ounces of liquid or 1 ounce of bread. People with diabetes can choose nontraditional options, such as wine diluted with water or a smaller-than-typical piece of pita bread.

The Kosher Diet

According to the 2001 National Jewish Population Survey, 28% of Jews in the northeastern United States keep kosher at home, compared with 17% in the midwest, and 15% in the west and southwest (24). "Kosher" is defined as follows (25):

- A dietary practice involving the timing of meals, the selection of permitted foods, and the appropriate combination of foods. Kosher laws, for example, mandate that dairy and meat cannot be eaten together.
- A process of food certification that involves an examination of ingredients, the preparation process, and processing facilities.

Kosher Dietary Laws

Kosher foods are either classified as meat, dairy, or *pareve*/neutral foods. Meats must come from animals that were slaughtered according to kosher laws. As noted previously, observant Jews do not combine milk and meat ingredients in the same meal. They also keep separate sets of plates, silverware, cooking utensils, and pots and pans for meat and dairy, and may have a third set for *pareve* foods. *Pareve* foods can be eaten with either meat or milk dishes.

According to kosher laws, the following foods are always forbidden:

- The flesh, organs, and milk of pigs, rabbits, hares, horses, dogs, and cats
- Shellfish (fish with fins and scales *are* permitted)
- Damaged or defective parts of permitted animals
- Meat from animals that died naturally
- Meat from animals whose death was not instant and painless
- Hard cheese made with rennet from nonkosher animals
- Insects (note: fruits and vegetables must be inspected to ensure that insects are not mistakenly eaten)

Kosher Food Certifications

Several kosher symbols may be found on food labels. These symbols are registered trademarks of kosher certification organizations and cannot be placed on a food label without the organization's permission. The symbol is usually near the product name on the label; occasionally it is placed near the list of ingredients. The certifying organization assures consumers that the product is kosher according to the organization's standards. However, standards vary among organizations. If clients observe kosher laws, the RD should ask them which certification system they use. This information can help guide food selection.

The most widely used and recognized kosher symbol is the seal of the Orthodox Union: the letter "U" inside the letter "O." A number of organizations use symbols that incorporate a "K" for *Kashrut*. However, some labels include the letter "K" by itself. A letter of the alphabet cannot be trademarked; therefore, the "K" alone is not a reliable indicator that a product is kosher/rabbinically certified. For example, some foods that contain gelatin (which is not kosher) have labels marked with the letter "K."

In addition to symbols that indicate a food is kosher, labels may also display a "D" for "dairy" or the word *Pareve* or *Parev* (for neutral foods). The letter "P" indicates the food is kosher for Passover.

Counseling Considerations

Demonstrating Courtesy and Respect

According to Smith (26), American Jews rate "thinking for oneself" as the most important value to teach a child. This value can be an asset in counseling situations, where it is important to establish an individualized approach for each client that encourages independent thinking.

When clients follow kosher dietary laws, RDs must understand how to create a kosher meal plan and also respect the time and energy that kosher dietary practices require. By following the kosher laws of the Torah, individuals elevate everyday eating into a religious ritual. They may feel that observing a kosher diet helps strengthen their Jewish identity and community, allowing them to pass on Jewish traditions to the next generation. Also, be aware that many Jewish people do not strictly follow Kosher laws but have "kosher-style" eating practices. Therefore, you should ask respectfully about the specific practices of each individual, instead of simply inquiring whether the client "keeps kosher."

RDs should also respect that religious observances may affect meal planning. Observant Jews stop all normal weekday activities and responsibilities on holidays, including the weekly Friday evening to Saturday evening observance of Sabbath. Businesses and schools close, and all secular activities, such as riding in vehicles, writing, and using electrical devices cease during Sabbath and on holidays. If your clients observe Sabbath or other holidays, ask them about the challenges faced on these days and have them describe practices that can interfere with diabetes management (such as fasting). Also, keep in mind that "sundown" (the beginning of Sabbath) occurs at a different time depending on the season, which can affect the planning and timing of meals.

Interpreting Clients' Nonverbal Communication

If you are a woman, be aware that Orthodox men may avoid direct eye contact or shaking your hand because Jewish law forbids men from touching or being alone with women other than their wives. Respect the client's physical distance, and avoid touching him when talking and working together on diabetes care and education.

Inquiring About Clients' Understanding of Diabetes

It is important to periodically assess each client's knowledge, behaviors, and diabetes self management skills. Ask open-ended questions instead of those that can be answered with a "yes" or "no." Potential questions include the following:

- "How do you define health and wellness?"
- "How do you define diabetes?"
- "How do your religion and beliefs affect your self care and diabetes management?"

Talk with clients about types of diabetes. Some clients may believe that type 2 diabetes is not as serious as type 1 diabetes. Similarly, they may call prediabetes "borderline diabetes" or "a little sugar" and downplay its health risks.

Discussing Clients' Use of Complementary and Alternative Medicine

Like other Americans, Jewish Americans may use complementary and alternative medicine (CAM) to treat diabetes or other conditions. For example, Glucodan Tea is an herbal remedy developed by an Israeli company, Nufar Natural Products (http://www.nufar.co.il), and introduced to the United States in 2006. The company claims that the tea breaks down carbohydrates and fats, thereby reducing and balancing blood glucose levels. RDs should evaluate each client's use of CAM and be prepared to discuss potential risks and benefits. Refer to Appendix C for questions to assess dietary supplement use.

Considering Family Demands and Dynamics

Rates of marriage are comparatively high for Jewish Americans (65% of Jews vs 57% of non-Jews), and divorce rates are relatively low (26). Some Jews believe that a woman's primary obligations and responsibilities are those of wife, mother, and keeper of the household. However, Jewish women determine their own needs and should be asked questions directly even if they are accompanied by their husbands or others.

Orthodox and Hasidic women are regarded as separate from but equal to men. Orthodox men often bring their wives to counseling. However, these men will communicate directly with the RD about their diabetes.

If a client's wife or mother shops and prepare food for the entire family, it important for her to understand the effects of different foods and portions on blood glucose control. Ask the client for permission to include her in counseling sessions.

Among Jews, eating is intimately bound up with family, religion, culture, and ethnic identity. A person with diabetes will often be overwhelmed with information. Use the following tips to help your clients navigate their particular family-related challenges:

- Suggest ways to prepare for the challenges of typical family meals and holiday celebrations. Provide options that recognize the significance of food as a means for introducing children and family to Jewish religion and culture.

- Educate clients about the carbohydrate content of special foods *before* they encounter them at family or holiday celebrations.

- Stress the value of setting a good example for others by caring for one's own diabetes-related needs.

Engaging Others in Counseling Sessions

As noted previously, observance of religious laws, including those related to dietary practices, varies considerably among Jewish Americans. If your client is active in a synagogue or other form of religious community, those institutions may be able to provide insights or resources to inform meal planning and diabetes management. For example, the client's synagogue may be a source of information about fasting practices on holidays or approved kosher certifications.

Nutrition Counseling

Refer to Appendix B for medical nutrition therapy (MNT) recommendations for diabetes as well as general counseling strategies. In addition, the following culturally specific strategies may be helpful for nutrition counseling of Jewish Americans:

- Keep a Jewish calendar on hand and track important dates, such as the High Holy Days. A current calendar is available on the Judaism 101 Web site (http://www.jewfaq.org). Use this calendar when scheduling appointments and to plan for discussions of upcoming holidays.

- In addition to noting the client's usual mealtimes, discuss each holiday individually. Identify which foods are part of their holidays and whether the client intends to fast or restrict foods. Holiday restrictions of food and water are usually observed until after sundown unless there is danger to a human life.

- If the client intends to fast during a holiday, discuss strategies for fasting and breaking fasts safely.
    - Safe use of medication on a fast day depends on the type of oral diabetes agent, its action, and its adverse effects. Some oral agents and fast-acting insulins may be eliminated and dosages of others may be reduced to allow the person to fast. A health care professional should help the client customize the medication regimen before the fast.

- Instruct the client to check blood glucose levels more often when fasting or feasting to maintain blood glucose control.
- To break the fast, advise clients to eat a meal that is light and low in carbohydrates.
- Educate clients that the risk of nocturnal hypoglycemia increases after fasting because the body may be more sensitive to insulin. Advise them to set higher normal blood glucose targets, and encourage them to test blood glucose more frequently to identify problems before they happen.
- Dehydration is a serious and common problem after fasting. Encourage clients to drink plenty of water on the day before, during, and the day after a fast. Clients may believe that they cannot drink during a fast day. However, Jewish laws place health first, so encourage clients to discuss their need for water with their rabbis.
- Be aware that clients may eat melon, grapes, other foods with high water content, and/or hard candy before a fast in an effort to avoid dehydration. However, fruits and candy raise blood glucose levels and cause dehydration. Educate clients about the glycemic index of fruits, grams of carbohydrate in different portions, and how to substitute portions of fruit for the usual carbohydrates eaten. These strategies can help them to control blood glucose levels and avoid dehydration around a fast.

- Prepare clients to navigate stressful pre-holiday periods. For example, advise them to develop an eating plan, adjust recipes, and make shopping lists well before a holiday begins. Also, help them plan ahead so they know how to treat hypoglycemia and/or take medications during holidays.
- Encourage clients to weigh and measure foods in advance of a holiday so they develop experience-based estimates of portion sizes.
- Teach clients to measure the carbohydrate content in recipes—Step 1: Make a list of all ingredients. Step 2: Next to each ingredient; write the amount used in the total recipe. Step 3: Write down the total grams of carbohydrate in each ingredient. Step 4: Add up all grams of carbohydrates in the recipe. Step 5: Divide the total by the number of portions in the recipe to find the total grams of carbohydrate in one portion.
- Ask whether clients have wine or kosher grape juice to make a blessing over food on Sabbaths or holidays. Explain that dry wines are lower in carbohydrate than sweet wines, and find out the carbohydrate content of the wine the client drinks. Discuss diluting wine or juice with water to reduce the carbohydrate and alcohol content. (Acceptable combinations are 60% water to 40% wine or 75% water to 25% wine, depending on the wine's alcohol content.)
- To help clients limit consumption of carbohydrates in holiday foods, stress that sweetness is not just found in food and drink; it can also be found in life, family, friends, and the act of giving.
- If clients need to lose weight, help them find local weight-loss programs that cater to the Jewish community. (Weight Watchers is one possible resource.)
- Teach clients to consider portion sizes and ingredients when eating traditional foods. For example, bagels are made in different sizes, and some are sweetened with sugar while others are not. Similarly, not all types of matzo are the same size or thickness (handmade portions can vary from 30 to 60 g carbohydrate).
- Discuss nonstarchy vegetable substitutions for high-carbohydrate foods. For example, instead of noodles or potatoes, nonstarchy vegetables can be added to soups and kugels or roasted in the oven. Mashed cauliflower is a good substitute for mashed potatoes.
- Advise the client to look for "hidden" carbohydrate-containing ingredients (such as barbeque sauces, sweet marinades, or dried fruits) in traditional fish, meat, and chicken dishes.
- Encourage clients to increase daily activity. Options include taking a walk with the family after the midday meal on Saturday or with a friend while one's children are in school. Orthodox clients may need help to find a gym that is segregated by gender (eg, a women-only facility or a place with times and days reserved for one sex).
- Assess clients' views of blood glucose monitoring on the Sabbath. Some Jews believe blood glucose monitoring to be "an everyday activity," which means it would be prohibited on the Sabbath. In these circumstances, the rabbi may give permission to test blood glucose, or it may be acceptable to write blood glucose records with the opposite hand

(this makes it different from daily activities). Clients may also want to try a blood glucose meter that turns off automatically so testing blood does not violate the law forbidding the operation of any machine.

- Similarly, assess whether clients believe that insulin injections constitute an "everyday activity" prohibited on the Sabbath. Using a separate bottle of insulin on the Sabbath may make taking an injection "different" from the everyday practice. Encourage clients to discuss this option with their rabbi. Also, discuss the use of insulin pens. Because the needle is attached to the pen, the "labor" involved in filling a syringe (forbidden on the Sabbath) is minimized.

- If clients observe the Sabbath, educate them on the risk of hypoglycemia caused by changes in meal timing and amounts of food, increased walking on the Sabbath, and reduced frequency of blood glucose monitoring.

- Note that some Jews will not test for ketones on the Sabbath because the Bible prohibits coloring on the Sabbath, and ketone strips turn colors.

Resources

Bacon JL. *Jewish Cooking from Around the World.* New York, NY: Smithmark Publishers; 1995.
Cohen N. *Enlightened Kosher Cooking.* Nanuet, NY: Feldheim Publishing; 2006.
Cooper J. *Eat and Be Satisfied: A Social History of Jewish Food.* Northvale, NJ: Jason Aronson; 1991.
Friends with Diabetes. http://www.friendswithdiabetes.org. Accessed May 7, 2009.
Jewish Diabetes Association. http://jewishdiabetes.org. Accessed May 7, 2009.
The Jewish Food Mailing List Archive. http://www.jewishfood-list.com. Accessed May 7, 2009.
Leonard LW. *Jewish Cookery.* New York, NY: Crown; 1994.
Marks G. *The World of Jewish Cooking.* New York, NY: Simon & Shuster; 1996.
National Jewish Population Survey (2000-01). http://www.jewishvirtuallibrary.org/jsource/US-Israel/ujcpop.html. Accessed May 7, 2009.
The National Jewish Population Survey 2000-01: Strength, Challenge, and Diversity in the American Jewish Population. http://www.ujc.org/local_includes/downloads/4606.pdf. Accessed May 7, 2009.
Roden C. *The Book of Jewish Food.* New York, NY: Knopf; 1996.
Sternberg R. *Yiddish Cuisine: A Gourmet's Approach to Jewish Cooking.* Northvale, NJ: Jason Aronson; 1993.

References

1. Sheskin IM, Dashefsky A. Jewish population of the United States, 2007. In: Singer D, Grossman L, eds. *American Jewish Year Book 2007.* vol 107. New York, NY: American Jewish Committee; 2007.
2. Jewish Virtual Library Web site. National Jewish Population Survey. http://www.jewishvirtuallibrary.org/jsource/US-Israel/ujcpop.html. Accessed March 18, 2009.
3. United Jewish Communities. Jewish Federations of North America Web site. NJPS: The Jewish Population. http://www.ujc.org/page.aspx?id=46184. Accessed March 18, 2009.
4. United Jewish Communities. Jewish Federations of North America. The National Jewish Population Survey 2000-01: Jewish Connections. http://www.ujc.org/page.html?ArticleID=46194. Accessed May 6, 2009.
5. Rossel S. Judaism today. Basic Judaism Web site. http://www.rossel.net/basic04.htm. Accessed April 28, 2009.
6. International Diabetes Foundation e-Atlas Web site. http://www.eatlas.idf.org. Accessed March 18, 2009.
7. Benjamins MR, Rhodes DM, Carp JM, Whitman S. A local community health survey: findings from a population-based survey of the largest Jewish community in Chicago. *J Community Health.* 2006;31:479–495.
8. Love-Gregory LD, Wasson J, Ma J, Jin CH, Glaser B, Suarez BK, Permutt MA. A common polymorphism in the upstream promoter region of the hepatocyte nuclear factor-4 alpha gene on chromosome 20q is associated with type 2 diabetes and appears to contribute to the evidence for linkage in an Ashkenazi Jewish population. *Diabetes.* 2004;53:1134–1140.
9. Bronstein M, Pisant A, Yakir B, Darvasi A. Type 2 diabetes susceptibility loci in the Ashkenazi Jewish population. *Hum Genet.* 2008;124:101–104. Epub May 31, 2008.
10. Serbe D, Moore E. Jewish Cooking—Foods of the Diaspora. Mama's Kitchen Web site. http://www.inmamaskitchen.com/FOOD_IS_ART_II/food_history_and_facts/Jewish_Cooking.html. Accessed March 20, 2009.

11. Kosher Food.com. http://www.kosherfood.com. Accessed May 7, 2009.
12. Judaism.com. http://www.judaism.com. Accessed May 7, 2009.
13. Kaboose.com Recipes. http://recipes.kaboose.com. Accessed May 21, 2009.
14. Jewish Food Mailing List Archive. Browse the Recipes. http://www.Jewishfood-list.com/recipes/recipe_index.html. Accessed July 22, 2007.
15. Sperber D. *Why Jews Do What They Do: The History of Jewish Customs Throughout the Cycle of the Jewish Year.* Jersey City, NJ: KTAV Publishing House; 1999:43–50.
16. Rich TR. Pesach Seder: How is This Night Different. Judaism 101 Web site. http://www.jewfaq.org/seder.htm. Accessed March 20, 2009.
17. Passover Mandel Bread (recipe). http://emr.cs.iit.edu/~reingold/ruths-kitchen/recipes/passover/passover_mandel_bread.html. Accessed May 5, 2009.
18. Jewish Diabetes Association Web site. http://jewishdiabetes.org. Accessed April 28, 2009.
19. Overview: Shavuot History. My Jewish Learning Web site. http://www.myjewishlearning.com/holidays/Jewish_Holidays/Shavuot/History.shtml. Accessed March 20, 2009.
20. Shavuot on the Net Web site. http://www.holidays.net/shavuot/customs.htm. Accessed April 28, 2009.
21. Kaplan S. Shavuot foods span myriad cultures. Jewish News of Greater Phoenix Online Web site. http://www.jewishaz.com/jewishnews/030530/loopholesside.html. Accessed April 28, 2009.
22. Glazer P. Traditional foods from modern era form Hanukkah menu. LJWorld.com Web site. http://www2.ljworld.com/news/2004/dec/08/traditional_foods_from. Accessed March 20, 2009.
23. Friends with Diabetes. Pesach: Be Prepared! http://www.friendswithdiabetes.org/files/pdf/pesachenglish.pdf. Accessed May 5, 2009.
24. United Jewish Communities. Jewish Federations of North America. Regional Variations in Jewish Connections. http://www.ujc.org/page.aspx?id=46226. Accessed May 5, 2009.
25. Kashrut: Jewish Dietary Laws. Jewish Virtual Library Web site. http://www.Jewishvirtuallibrary.org/jsource/Judaism/kashrut.html. Accessed April 28, 2009.
26. Smith TW. *Jewish Distinctiveness in America: A Statistical Report.* New York, NY: American Jewish Committee; 2005. http://www.jewishdatabank.org/Reports/AJC_JewishDistinctivenessAmerica_TS_April2005.pdf. Accessed May 6, 2009.

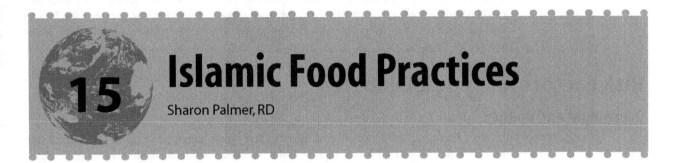

Islamic Food Practices

Sharon Palmer, RD

Introduction

Islam began in Arabia during the 7th century and has grown into a major world religion. At the center of the Islamic faith is Muhammad (c. 570–622), a businessman from Mecca who experienced revelations that Allah was the one god and that Muhammad was his messenger. These revelations were preserved in the Koran. The five pillars of Islam are faith, prayer, fasting, charity, and the Hajj (pilgrimage to Mecca). The term "Islam" means submission to God's will, and "Muslim" refers to a person who submits to his will through a life of faith and dedication to the practices set forth in the Koran. By the beginning of the 16th century, the Islamic community had spread throughout the Middle East; north, Saharan, and sub-Saharan Africa; central Asia, and the Indian Ocean basin. Muslims have subsequently moved throughout Europe, Asia, and North America (1).

There are between 1.1 billion and 1.5 billion Muslims worldwide, comprising 18% to 25% of the world population (2). Some people assume that all Muslims are people of Arab descent and all Arabs are Muslims. In fact, Arabs comprise only 15% of the worldwide Muslim population (3), and some Arabs are Christian or Jewish.

In the United States, 33% of Muslims are South Asian (ie, from Afghanistan, Bangladesh, Bhutan, India, Maldives, Nepal, Pakistan, or Sri Lanka), 30% are African American, 25% are Arab (ie, from one of the 24 Arabic-speaking countries), 3.4% are sub-Saharan African, 2.1% are European, 1.3% are Southeast Asian, 1.2% are Caribbean, 1.1% are Turkish, 0.7% are Iranian, and 0.6% are Hispanic or Latino (3). This chapter primarily explores the health and nutrition-related characteristics of the Arab and South Asian Muslim communities in the United States. Asian Indian and Pakistani cultural food practices are also discussed in Chapter 8. See Chapter 3 for African American food practices.

Diabetes Prevalence

It is difficult to generalize about the prevalence of diabetes in Muslim populations worldwide because they have widely varying ethnic backgrounds, dietary patterns, education levels, socioeconomic factors, and health care. Refer to Salti et al (4) for a population-based study of individuals with type 1 and type 2 diabetes, including data on the frequency of diabetes complications and comorbidities, in 13 countries with Muslim populations (Algeria, Bangladesh, Egypt, India, Indonesia, Jordan, Lebanon, Malaysia, Morocco, Pakistan, Saudi Arabia, Tunisia, and Turkey). Salti and colleagues (4) observe an association between economic development and increasing diabetes prevalence in these countries. Jaber et al (5) report a similar association in Arab communities in the Middle East. See Chapter 8 for a discussion of diabetes prevalence in South Asian populations.

Jaber et al investigated the epidemiology of diabetes in an Arab-American community in Dearborn, Michigan, a Detroit suburb with one of the largest communities of Arab Americans in the United States (5). Compared with white, Hispanic, and African Americans, as well as rural Arab communities, diabetes prevalence among the Arab Americans in Dearborn was high: 41% of the participants age 20 to 75 years had abnormal glucose tolerance (18% had diabetes). The prevalence of abnormal glucose tolerance was greater than 70% in individuals older than 60 years, with diabetes reported in 36% of the men and 54% of the women in this age group.

Risk Factors for Type 2 Diabetes

Overweight and Obesity

In Arab countries, the prevalence of obesity (body mass index [BMI] ≥ 30) is estimated to be between 30% and 40% (6). In Jaber and associates' study of Arab Americans in Dearborn, Michigan (5), 34% of the participants were obese, compared with a rate of 26% for the US population as a whole. Among the Arab Americans in this study, prevalence of obesity increased with age.

For information on obesity and BMI cutoffs for diabetes risk in South Asians, refer to Chapter 8. One study of particular note to this chapter is Griffiths and Bentley's examination of the nutrition transition among women in Andhra Pradesh, India (7). Using data from the second Indian National Family Health Survey (1998–1999), the researchers found that 12% of the women were overweight (BMI > 25) and 2% were obese. Prevalence of overweight and obesity was greater in urban areas compared with rural sites, and in women with higher socioeconomic status. Muslim women were significantly more likely to be overweight or obese than Hindu women. The data did not allow for a definitive explanation of the religious differences, but the authors speculate that diet, activity levels, and socioeconomic status are possible explanatory factors.

Social Factors

Many social factors may increase diabetes risk in the Arab Muslim population. Arabs may regard overweight positively, as an indicator of one's wealth and fertility. Some Arab traditions may specifically affect obesity-related behaviors in women. For example, some traditional women's garments can restrict movement and therefore make it difficult to exercise (6).

In a cross-sectional, population-based study, Jaber et al concluded that a low level of acculturation was a risk factor for diabetes in 520 Middle East–born Arab Americans (206 men, 314 women) living in southeastern Michigan (8). In men, the authors identified significant associations between dysglycemia and (*a*) older age at immigration; (*b*) speaking Arabic with friends; (*c*) being less active in Arabic organizations; and (*d*) more frequent consumption of Arabic food. In women, no significant associations were found between acculturation factors and dysglycemia. However, actual age confounded acculturation effects, and lower acculturation was generally associated with increased prevalence of diabetes.

Traditional Foods and Dishes

Islam promotes abstinence from eating certain foods. The Arabic word *halal* means "lawful" or "permitted." The opposite of halal is *haram,* which means "unlawful" or "prohibited." These terms can apply to all aspects of a Muslim's life, including dietary practices. Certain foods are clearly halal or *haram.* However, the status of some foods can vary depending on their origin, preparation, or ingredients. If a food's status is unclear, it is typically referred to as *mashbooh* (doubtful).

Observant Muslims do not consume *haram* foods, including pork and pork products, animals improperly slaughtered or dead before slaughtering, animals killed in the name of anyone other than Allah, alcohol and intoxicants, carnivorous animals, birds of prey, land animals without external ears, blood and blood by-products, and foods contaminated with any of these products. *Mashbooh* foods include gelatin, enzymes, emulsifiers, and additives that may have an origin from the *haram* list (3,9,10).

The nonprofit Islamic Food and Nutrition Council of America (IFANCA) promotes halal foods and the institution of halal. If IFANCA certifies that a food is halal, the halal certification symbol, the Crescent M, can be printed on the food package (9).

Religious food practices vary among individuals. For example, not all Muslims eat only halal meats, but most do not eat pork. Some Muslims limit fish consumption to fish with scales (10).

Islam is a religion, not an ethnicity. In the United States, specific Muslim communities share food traditions and cuisines that are influenced by their national or regional origins as well as their Muslim dietary practices. See Chapter 8 or reference 16 for more information on South Asian foods and traditions. Refer to Box 15.1 and Table 15.1 for examples of Arab cuisine (3,11–13). See Appendix A for nutrient analyses. It is also important to note that many Muslims living in the United States may be partially or completely acculturated to Western food traditions.

Traditional Meal Patterns and Holiday Foods

Arab Meal Patterns

Arabs typically eat a quick breakfast of bread, dairy products, and tea or coffee. Breakfast pastries and flatbread with olive oil and seasonings are popular. A traditional working-class breakfast is *foul,* a hearty dish of lentils or fava beans. Lunch is usually the main meal of the day and may include a salad and *maza* (appetizers) as a side dish to a portion of meat, poultry, or fish; rice, lentils, bread, or bulgur; and vegetables. The meat and vegetables are typically cooked together. Dinner is usually a lighter meal, which might be as simple as fruit, bread and cheese or dips, pastries, or a kebab (3).

Ramadan

Ramadan is an annual, month-long observance, in which Muslims focus on devotion to God, inner reflection, and self-control. Muslims must fast during Ramadan, because fasting is one of the five pillars of Islam. Exceptions to the fast are made for individuals who are sick or traveling; women who are pregnant, breastfeeding, or menstruating; children younger than the age of puberty; and the elderly, if their physical condition warrants exemption (3,14). Ramadan occurs in the ninth month of the lunar calendar. In the United States, the beginning and end of Ramadan are usually determined by the Islamic Society of North America (3,14).

Fasting during Ramadan begins at the break of dawn and ends as the sun sets. During daylight hours, Muslims abstain from all food, drink, smoking, and sexual relations. Before dawn, they usually have a prefast meal of light, nourishing foods *(suhoor).* After sunset, they traditionally break the day's fast by consuming dates, water, and refreshing juices and soups. Then they have the *iftar,* a festive meal of traditional meat dishes, side dishes, salads, flat breads, and a variety of sweets. The last 10 days of Ramadan are particularly special as a time to come closer to God through good deeds, devotion, reading the Koran, and prayer (3,14,15).

Individuals with diabetes are exempt from the Ramadan fast. Nevertheless, many participate. Salti et al conducted an epidemiologic study of 12,243 individuals with diabetes in 13 Islamic countries and found that approximately 43% of individuals with type 1 diabetes and 79% of those with type 2 diabetes fasted for 15 or more days during Ramadan, with rates varying considerably among countries. Most of those who took diabetes medication or insulin did not adjust their treatment doses (4).

Box 15.1 • Foods Used in Traditional Arab Cuisine

Grains
- Bulgur
- Couscous
- Millet
- Pita bread, made from refined and/or whole-grain flours
- Rice

Starchy vegetables and beans
- Potatoes
- Fava beans
- Garbanzo beans/chickpeas
- Lentils

Nonstarchy vegetables
- Artichokes
- Cabbage
- Cauliflower
- Cucumbers
- Eggplant
- Green beans
- Kousa (type of summer squash; similar to zucchini)
- Okra
- Olives
- Onions
- Spinach
- Zucchini

Milk and milk products
- Butter
- Cream
- Feta cheese
- Goat's milk
- *Jibneh* (cheese)
- *Lebnah* (condensed yogurt)
- Yogurt

Fruits
- Apples
- Apricots
- Bananas
- Cantaloupe
- Dates
- Figs
- Grapes
- Lemons
- Oranges
- Plums
- Pomegranates
- Tangerines
- Watermelon

Meats
- Beef
- Chicken
- Fish
- Lamb

Nuts
- Almonds
- Pine nuts
- Pistachios

Herbs, seasonings, and spices
- Cinnamon
- Cumin
- Garlic
- Mint
- Nutmeg
- Paprika
- Parsley
- Saffron
- Sesame
- Sumac
- Thyme
- Turmeric

Table 15.1 · Traditional Arab Dishes, Beverages, and Desserts

Name	Description
Dishes	
Arayess	Deep-fried lamb sandwich
Baba ghanoush	Char-grilled eggplant, tahini, olive oil, lemon juice, and garlic puree, served as a dip
Bukhari rice	Lamb and rice stir-fried with onion, lemon, carrot, and tomato paste
Falafel	Small, deep-fried patties made of highly spiced ground chickpeas
Fatayer	Pastry pockets filled with spinach, meat, or cheese
Fattoush	Salad of toasted croutons, cucumbers, tomatoes, and mint
Foul	Slow-cooked mash of fava beans and red lentils, dressed with lemon, olive oil, and cumin
Hummus	Puree of chickpeas, tahini, lemon, and garlic, served as a dip with bread
Kabsa	Meat mixed with rice
Kebab	Skewered chunks of meat or fish cooked over charcoal
Kibbeh	Oval-shaped nuggets of ground lamb and bulgur
Koshary	Pasta, rice, and lentils with onions, chilies, and tomato paste
Kouzi	Whole lamb baked over rice so that rice absorbs the juice of the meat
Kufta	Fingers, balls, or flat cakes of minced meat and spices baked or charcoal-grilled on skeweres
Makloubeh	Meat or fish with rice, broad beans, and cauliflower
Mantou	Dumplings stuffed with minced lamb
Markok	Lamb and pumpkin stew
Mouhammara	Ground nuts, olive oil, cumin, and chiles eaten with bread
Moutabel	Eggplant dip made with tahini, olive oil, and lemon juice
Mubassal	Onion pancakes
Musakhan	Chicken casserole with sumac
Mutabak	Sweet or savory pastry turnovers stuffed with cheese, banana, or meat
Shawerma	Cone of pressed lamb, chicken, or beef roasted on a vertical spit where the meat is shaved off and served with bread
Shish taouk	Skewered chicken pieces cooked over charcoal
Tabbouleh	Salad of bulgur, tomato, mint, and parsley
Warak enab (warak dawali)	Stuffed vine leaves
Beverages	
Coffee	
Fruit juices	
Soft drinks	
Tea	
Yogurt drink	
Desserts	
Baklava	Dessert of layered pastry filled with nuts and steeped in honey-lemon syrup
Basboosa	Semolina tart soaked with syrup
Halva	Sesame paste sweet, made in a slab and studded with fruit and nuts
Kunafi	Shoelace pastry dessert stuffed with sweet white cheese, nuts and syrup
Ma'amul	Date cookies
Um ali	Pastry pudding with raisins and coconut steeped in milk

Source: Data are from references 3 and 11–13.

Box 15.2 • Traditional Arab Foods Consumed During Holidays

- Buffalo cream with honey and milk
- *Eid-ul-adha* meat—kebabs, stews, roast, and dishes made of fresh beef, sheep, or goat, including organ meats
- *K'ak al-tamar* (sweet meat)
- Lamb
- Lemon chicken
- Tabbouleh
- Sweets including fruit- and nut-filled pastries, cookies, and crepes

---

Diabetes-related complications of fasting may include hypoglycemia and diabetic ketoacidosis. Other serious complications could include dehydration and thrombosis. Health care providers should evaluate whether clients are at high risk for complications and discuss potential complications with them. If a person with diabetes chooses to fast, management strategies include individualization of the diabetes meal plan, frequent glucose monitoring, appropriate nutrition, and appropriate (but not excessive) exercise. Nutrition considerations include planning for a healthful, balanced diet that meets individual needs and promotes complex carbohydrate intake in the prefast meal and simple carbohydrates in the postfast meal (2). Advise clients to immediately break the fast if hypoglycemia occurs (2).

Other Holidays

Eid-ul-Fitr (the Feast of Fast-Breaking) begins on the first day after Ramadan and lasts for 3 days. Muslims celebrate *Eid-ul-Fitr* by visiting family and friends, dressing in holiday attire, and giving gifts to charity. A midday feast usually features a roasted whole baby lamb, traditional dishes, sweets, and coffee or tea. Depending on the country of origin, other dishes may also be included in the banquet. For example, in South Asia, a dish of fine, toasted vermicelli noodles is served (3,16).

Eid-ul-Adha (the Feast of Sacrifice) is a 3-day celebration of Hajj, the pilgrimage of Muslims to Mecca. Making a pilgrimage to Mecca at least once in one's lifetime is one of the five pillars of Islam. The most important day of the pilgrimage is the ninth day of *Zul-Hijja* (the 12th month of the lunar calendar). The feast starts on the 10th day and commemorates the sacrifice of an animal, whose meat is shared with family, friends, and the poor. In addition, a variety of regional dishes and sweets are eaten (3).

On *Al-Hijra* (New Year's Day), Muslims commemorate Muhammad's migration from Mecca to Medina, which founded the Muslim community. Individuals exchange gifts and share stories of Muhammad's life (17). Considered a day of reflection for most, some Muslims celebrate this day with desserts. Refer to Box 15.2 for additional information on holiday foods (16).

Traditional Health Beliefs

Traditional customs vary among Muslims, and Muslims from different cultural backgrounds may have different views on illness, health, and the role of health care providers. Islam does not recognize a mind-body dualism; preserving spiritual peace is considered an essential part of health. The earthly life is a test to determine one's final destiny, and death returns the soul to the creator. Muslims may consider sickness to be a type of atonement for sin (10). Large body size may be considered a sign of good health.

Preventive health care may not be popular among Muslims with a low educational level. On the other hand, many Muslims respect Western medical practices, and physicians are often held in high regard.

A traditional health system for many Muslims is *Unani* (or *Hikmat*), which is founded on the Hippocratic theory that disease occurs when functions of the vital body forces are imbalanced. The *Unani* practitioner may identify an imbalance and recommend herbal treatments, prayers, and foods to restore equilibrium (18). Foods may be distinguished by their power and digestibility rather than their nutritional merits. For example, "strong" foods include refined sugar, lamb, beef, butter, solid fat, and spices. "Weak" foods, such as boiled rice and cereals, may be reserved for older adults and those who are ill. Raw, baked, and grilled foods may be considered "indigestible" and avoided by the elderly, sick people, and youths (10).

Gender issues and gender roles are often important in Muslim communities and can affect health care. Most Muslims consider modesty in women very important, and women may wear loose garments that cover their head and/or body. Smoking is common among men in Muslim countries, but it is often stigmatized in women. Some Muslims engage in physical activity and go to gyms, but exercise may be taboo in some Muslim families for a variety of religious and social reasons. Because Islam discourages men and women from interacting in public, Muslim women may choose to exercise at women-only gyms or use exercise machines at home. Many Muslim couples have large families, and Islam encourages women to breast-feed babies for 2 years (10).

Current Food Practices

Information about food practices of Muslims in the United States is limited. The annual US market for halal products is approximately $12 billion and has grown more than 70% since 1995 (19). The number of stores and restaurants serving halal food is increasing, and many leading US food companies produce or distribute halal products. Some states have passed laws to regulate halal food labeling (19).

A Web-based study of acculturation patterns in early immigrant and second-generation Arab Americans did not find significant associations between acculturation and sex, age, education, or income. Women and married participants reported stronger Arab ethnic identity and higher levels of religious devotion. Among Muslim participants, integration was not associated with better mental health, whereas religiosity was predictive of better family functioning and less depression (20).

In their population study of Arab American immigrants in southeastern Michigan, Jaber and colleagues used factors that have been shown to influence the adaptation of migrant populations to Western lifestyles, such as socioeconomic status, language use and preference, and ethnicity of friends, to assess the acculturation of participants. Men and women with low acculturation levels ate significantly more Arab food, but adherence to traditional cultural values and attitudes was high for all participants (8).

Counseling Considerations

Muslim clients may not view counseling to be part of medical treatment, and they may not feel comfortable discussing personal issues with people outside of their family and friends. Therefore, counselors may need to investigate additional resources or refer clients to culturally appropriate practitioners (10,21).

Research about effective counseling strategies for Muslim Americans is lacking. Until specific strategies are validated, it is prudent to adapt the following approaches:

- Consider cultural and religious factors.
- Inquire about client's understanding of diabetes.
- Respect Islamic dietary customs and observances.
- Assess the client's use of alternative health care practices.
- Engage others in counseling sessions.

Demonstrating Courtesy and Respect

Before counseling a Muslim client, become aware of your own biases and misperceptions and take time to accurately understand Islamic beliefs, the client's socioeconomic and political background, and culturally appropriate interventions (10,22–24). Individually assess each client's personal, cultural, and religious identity—Muslims' beliefs and practices vary widely.

When greeting clients of the Islamic faith, be courteous and respectful. Note that Muslims may not want to use their left hand to receive food or drink or shake hands.

Keep in mind that Muslim women usually value modesty, and both male and female clients may prefer to work with a health care provider or interpreter who is the same sex they are. Patient confidentiality may also be an important issue to Muslim clients because certain health conditions may be regarded as bring dishonor on the individual or his or her family. Assure clients that you will respect their privacy (22).

Clients may respect physicians more than other health care providers (22). Therefore, it may be helpful to have the physician explain the role of the registered dietitian to the client.

Counseling strategies should consider and respect specific Islamic dietary practices, including halal restrictions and fasting periods such as Ramadan. Additionally, counselors may need to help clients prepare for diabetes management during the pilgrimage to Mecca.

Interpreting Clients' Nonverbal Communication

In client interviews and counseling sessions, observe how clients nonverbally communicate. For example, the client may nonverbally express discomfort when receiving treatment, counseling, or interpretation services from a person of the opposite sex. They may also nonverbally communicate their feelings about (*a*) recommendations from a non-physician health care provider, (*b*) counseling strategies, (*c*) medication regimens, or (*d*) food and nutrition recommendations that do not meet their dietary and religious preferences (22).

Inquiring About Clients' Understanding of Diabetes

Counselors should assess the English-language proficiency of clients and the potential need for a trained interpreter. To determine whether clients comprehend counseling messages, ask open-ended questions instead of questions that can be answered "yes" or "no." Consider that clients may lack understanding of the health care system, or they could privilege medical treatment that includes drugs over counseling and prevention strategies (10). Be prepared to address clients' misperceptions about the etiology and management of diabetes.

Discussing Clients' Use of Complementary and Alternative Medicine

Muslims may use alternative health care practices such as folk medicine, homeopathy, naturopathy, naprapathy, acupuncture, podiatry, and chiropractics (25). (Refer also to the previous section on Traditional Health Beliefs.) Counselors should assess each client's use of complementary and alternative medicine, including whether the client takes herbs or dietary supplements (see Appendix C for assessment questions). Take time to research the potential adverse effects and drug or nutrient interactions, and advise clients about safety and efficacy issues in a culturally sensitive manner.

Considering Family Demands and Dynamics

For many Muslims, the institution of the family is very important. Children are loved and elders are highly respected. The adult male head of the family may be primarily responsible for health care decisions for the entire family (22), whereas women are traditionally in charge of household duties such as cooking (10). However, do not make assumptions about family dynamics. It is important to identify which members of the family are responsible for shopping and cooking.

Engaging Others in Counseling Sessions

With the client's consent, it may be appropriate to engage other family members in counseling sessions. For example, clients may benefit if the male head of the family participates in nutrition education, and it is useful to engage the family members who shop for food and prepare meals.

Nutrition Counseling

Appendix B offers selected medical nutrition therapy (MNT) recommendations for individuals with diabetes and general counseling suggestions that support those recommendations. The following are culturally specific nutrition counseling strategies for Muslim clients:

- Depending on their ethnicity, clients may be accustomed to eating large portions of legumes, breads, rice, and other grains. Suggest that they substitute nonstarchy vegetables, salads, and vegetable soups for some starchy foods and limit portions of high-carbohydrate foods.

- Although Islamic dietary rules include abstinence from alcohol and prohibit the consumption of *haram* foods, dietary practices among Muslims vary. Individually assess each client's diet instead of making assumptions based on their religion.

- Discuss how clients observe Ramadan and other holidays that involve fasts or feasts. If clients choose to fast, provide guidance on glucose monitoring and diabetes management during these periods. (See reference 2 for suggestions.)

Challenges and Barriers to Dietary Adherence

When working with Muslim clients, counselors may find support for nutrition messages in Islamic ideals such as quality, moderation, and fasting. On the other hand, clients may regard plumpness to be a desirable trait and may prefer to be overweight. They may also think it rude to refuse food in social settings, and certain styles of traditional Islamic clothing may interfere with physical activity and exercise (6,21). Other potential barriers include insufficient understanding of nutrition, physical activity, or the etiology and management of diabetes; language barriers; limited literacy skills; and some alternative medicine practices.

Although the Koran exempts sick people from fasting during Ramadan, individuals with diabetes may want to fast, even if the practice poses challenges for glucose control. (Reference 2 provides some suggestions, based on expert opinion, for counseling clients who choose to fast.) The pilgrimage to Mecca also may involve factors that contribute to poor diabetes control, such as traveling to an unfamiliar environment; climate changes; exposure to other illnesses; and limited access to medications, monitoring equipment, and/or medical care (6).

Counseling Tips

In summary, the following tips are essential to counseling Muslim clients:

- Be sensitive to and aware of the client's religious and cultural beliefs and observances. Keep in mind that Muslims come from a variety of regions and bring a diversity of ethnic food practices to the table.

- Identify potential language barriers and use trained interpreters as appropriate.

- With the client's consent, engage family members in counseling sessions.

- Assess clients' alternative health care values and practices.

- Educate clients on the etiology and management of diabetes, and clear up any harmful misperceptions.

- If the client is overweight, emphasize desirable body weight goals.

- Take a detailed diet history, including snacks and portion sizes of typical foods consumed by the client. Then incorporate the client's preferred cultural foods in his or her diabetes meal plan, instead of emphasizing foods that the client is unlikely to consume.

- Instruct clients and their families about appropriate portion control, cooking methods, and meal patterns. Use visual aids such as measuring cups and food samples.
- Teach clients how to read food labels for information on nutrients, ingredients, and serving sizes.
- Recommend healthier substitutions for ingredients in traditional dishes. For example, clients can use nonnutritive sweeteners instead of honey; trade nonfat yogurt and dairy products for full-fat products; use monounsaturated oils instead of butter; or choose leaner cuts of meat.
- Assess the client's cardiovascular disease risk and tailor dietary counseling accordingly.
- Make dietary recommendations as simple and relevant as possible. To improve compliance and comprehension, provide written recommendations at the appropriate reading level.
- Ask clients to keep food diaries. In subsequent counseling sessions, review the diet records and evaluate their progress.
- Refer clients to additional resources if they are needed and available.
- Ask clients to show you examples of food packages and products they regularly consume, as well as recipes and fliers from supermarkets where they shop.
- If possible, encourage patients to take photos of typical meals consumed. Then use these photos to determine portion sizes.

Resources

American Dietetic Association. Nutrition Care Manual. Cultural food practices: Muslim. http://www.nutritioncaremanual.org. Accessed April 9, 2009.

Islamic Food and Nutrition Council of America. http://www.ifanca.org. Accessed April 9, 2009.

Islamic Medical Association of North America. http://www.imana.org. Accessed April 9, 2009.

Southeastern Michigan Dietetic Association. Arabic Food Pyramid. 1998. http://www.semda.org/info/pyramid.asp?ID=1. Accessed April 9, 2009.

Zabihah.com. http://www.zabihah.com. Accessed August 16, 2008. A halal dining guide with more than 19,000 reviews for more than 5,000 restaurants and grocers across the country.

References

1. Islam. In: Wuthnow R, ed. *Encyclopedia of Politics and Religion*. 2 vols. Washington, DC: Congressional Quarterly; 1998:383-393. http://www.cqpress.com/context/articles/epr_islam.html. Accessed June 12, 2008.
2. Al-Arouj M, Bouguerra R, Buse J, Hafez S, Hassanein M, Ibrahim M, Ismail-Beigi F, El-Kebbi I, Khatib O, Kishawi S, Al-Madani A, Mishal A, Al-Maskari M, Nakhi A, Al-Rubean K. Recommendations for management of diabetes during Ramadan. *Diabetes Care*. 2005; 28:2305–2311.
3. American Dietetic Association Nutrition Care Manual. Cultural Food Practices, Muslim. http://www.nutritioncaremanual.org/index.cfm?Page=References&topic=724&s=o. Accessed June 12, 2008.
4. Salti I, B'Enard E, Detournay B, Bianchi-Biscay M, Le Brigand C, Voinet C, Jabbar A. A population-based study of diabetes and its characteristics during the fasting month of Ramadan in 13 countries. *Diabetes Care*. 2004;27:2306–2311.
5. Jaber L, Brown M, Hammad A, Nowak SN, Zhu Q, Ghafoor A, Herman WH. Epidemiology of diabetes among Arab Americans. *Diabetes Care*. 2003;26:308–313.
6. Goenka N, Thomas S, Shaikh S, Morrisey J, Patel V. Providing diabetes care to Arab migrants in the UK: cultural and clinical aspects. *Br J Diab Vasc Dis*. 2007;7:283.
7. Griffiths PL, Bentley ME. The nutrition transition is underway in India. *J Nutr*. 2001;131: 2692–2700.
8. Jaber L, Brown M, Hammad A, Nowak SN, Zhu Q, Herman WH. Lack of acculturation is a risk factor for diabetes in Arab immigrants in the US. *Diabetes Care*. 2003;26:2010–2014.
9. Islamic Food and Nutrition Council of America. What Is Halal? http://www.ifanca.org/halal. Accessed July 21, 2008.
10. English DC. Curbside consultation. Addressing a patient's refusal of care based on religious beliefs. *Am Fam Physician*. 2007;76:1393-1394. http://www.aafp.org/afp/20071101/curbside.html. Accessed May 9, 2009.

11. Southeastern Michigan Dietetic Association. Arabic Food Pyramid. http://www.semda.org/info/pyramid.asp?ID=1. Accessed August 5, 2008.

12. Nolan J. Cultural Diversity: Eating in America. Middle Eastern. Ohio State University Extension Fact Sheet. http://ohioline.osu.edu/hyg-Fact/5000/5256.html. Accessed August 5, 2008.

13. Pellet PL, Shadarevian S. *Food Composition Tables for Use in the Middle East.* 2nd ed. Beirut, Lebanon: American University of Beirut; 1970.

14. Islamic Holidays and Observances. http://www.colostate.edu/Orgs/MSA/events/holidays.html. Accessed August 20, 2008.

15. Kagan S. Ramadan: a holiday of fasting and feasting. Epicurious.com. Aug 22, 2008. http://shine.yahoo.com/channel/food/ramadan-a-holiday-of-fasting-and-feasting-242797/. Accessed August 25, 2008.

16. Food Events. Eid Celebrations. BBC Food Online. http://www.bbc.co.uk/food/news_and_events/events_eid.shtml. Accessed August 20, 2008.

17. Nusseibeh S, Isseroff A. Religious Holidays of the Middle East. Mideast Web. http://www.mideastweb.org/holidays.htm#Muslim%20Festivals. Accessed August 25, 2008.

18. Periyakoil VS, Mendez JC, Buttar AB. Health and Health Care for Pakistani American Elders. http://www.stanford.edu/group/ethnoger/pakistani.html. Accessed August 8, 2008.

19. Agriculture and Agri-food Canada. Agri-food Trade Service. Global Halal Food Market. July 2007. http://www.ats.agr.gc.ca/africa/4352_e.htm. Accessed August 16, 2008.

20. Amer MM, Hovey JD. Socio-demographic differences in acculturation and mental health for a sample of 2nd generation/early immigrant Arab Americans. *J Immigr Minor Health.* 2007; 4:335–347.

21. Yosef AR. Health beliefs, practice, and priorities for health care of Arab Muslims in the United States. *J Transcult Nurs.* 2008;19:284–291.

22. Ahmad N. Arab-American Culture and Health Care. April 15, 2004. http://www.cwru.edu/med/epidbio/mphp439/Arab-Americans.htm. Accessed August 15, 2008.

23. Athar S. Information for Health Care Providers When Dealing with a Muslim Patient. Islamic Medical Association of North America. http://www.islam-usa.com/e40.html. Accessed August 8, 2008.

24. Kobeisy A. *Counseling American Muslims: Understanding the Faith and Helping the People.* Santa Barbara, CA: Praeger Publishers; 2004.

25. Ali ZA, Hussain SH, Sakr AH. Natural Therapeutics of Medicine in Islam. http://www.islam-usa.com/im11.html. Accessed August 15, 2008.

Appendix A

Nutrient Analyses for Selected Ethnic Foods

Navajo Foods

Food	Serving Size	Grams per Serving	Energy (kcal)	Fat (g)	SFA (g)	PUFA (g)	MUFA (g)	Chol (mg)	Sod (mg)	Carb (g)	Fiber (g)	Sugar (g)	Pro (g)	Pot (mg)	Exchanges	Source
Starches																
Blue corn mush with ash (Taa'niil, Gad bil)	0.5 cup	120	65	0.6	0.1	0.2	0.1	0	10	14.1	1.3	0.2	0.8	70	1 Starch	USDA 35130
Blue dumplings (K'ineeshbizhii, naadaa'ak'aan)	0.25 cup	67	73	0.7	0.1	0.3	0.1	0	30	14.6	1.1	0.3	2.1	75	1 Starch	Navajo food composition article
Corn, roasted, dried (Naadaa ditlee sit'e)	2 Tbsp	25	96	1.3	0.2	0.5	0.4	0	26	18.7	2	1.3	2.5	128	1 Starch	USDA 35134
Desert yucca, fresh cooked (Hashk'aan sit'eego)	1.5 cups, mashed	150	75	1.9	0.5	0.6	0.6	0	16	13.3	3.3	4.9	1.2	154	1 Starch	Navajo food composition article
Fry bread (American Indian)	0.5 piece (5" dia)	36	119	4.4	1.7	0.4	1.6	3	118	17.4	0.6	0.7	2.4	28	1 Starch + 1 Fat	USDA 35142
Kneel-down bread, fresh (Nitsidigo'i)	0.33 bread in husk (3"x5½")	35	68	0.8	0.1	0.3	0.2	0	44	13.7	1	1.3	1.5	111	1 Starch	USDA 35140
Tortilla, (flour and baking powder type) (Naneeskaadi)	0.33 piece (6" dia)	25	63	0.1	0	0.1	0	0	153	14	0	0.7	1.8	21	1 Starch	Navajo food composition article
Fruits																
Cantaloupe, dried (Ta'neesk'ani nahineest'aaz)	0.5 strip (10" x 1" x ¼")	15	53	0.1	0	0	0	0	25	12	0.5	10.8	0.9	443	1 Fruit	Navajo food composition article
Navajo banana (mountain yucca), dried (Neesdoig)	0.25 roll (2"dia x 4"long)	20	70	1.8	0	0.1	0.4	0	16	12.3	3	6	1.1	142	1 Fruit	Navajo food composition article
Rhubarb, wild, cooked, unsweetened	1.25 cups	300	63	0.6	0.2	0.3	0.1	0	12	13.6	5.4	3.3	2.7	777	1 Fruit	FNDDS 63147120
Sweets, Desserts, and Other Carbohydrates																
Corn, steamed, dried (coffee creamer) (Lee'shibeezh ts'aalbai)	2 Tbsp	20	71	0.6	0.1	0.2	0.2	0	36	13.7	1.8	1.1	2.7	183	1 Starch	Navajo food composition article
Navajo cake, fresh (Yilkaad, alkaad)	0.5 piece (3" x 3" x 1½")	55	83	1	0.2	0.2	0.5	0	24	15.9	4.2	2.8	2.6	76	1 Carb	Navajo food composition article
Sumac (sour) berry pudding (Tsiitchin toshchiin)	0.25 cup	62	68	0.3	0.1	0.1	0.1	0	21	15.3	0.3	7.5	1	27	1 Carb	Navajo food composition article

(continued)

Navajo Foods *(continued)*

Food	Serving Size	Grams per Serving	Energy (kcal)	Fat (g)	SFA (g)	PUFA (g)	MUFA (g)	Chol (mg)	Sod (mg)	Carb (g)	Fiber (g)	Sugar (g)	Pro (g)	Pot (mg)	Exchanges	Source
Nonstarchy Vegetables																
Squash, yellow, dried (Naayizi nahineest'aaz)	0.33 cup, dry	7	21	0.1	0	0	0	0	9	4.9	0.9	2.5	0.2	188	1 Vegetable	Navajo food composition article
Zucchini squash, dried (Naayizi yazhf nahineest'aaz)	0.33 cup, dry	7	19	0	0	0	0	0	14	4.2	1.1	1.8	0.5	152	1 Vegetable	Navajo food composition article
Fats																
Pinon nuts, roasted, shelled (Neeshch'ff')	2 Tbsp	10	54	3.4	0.3	1.4	1.6	0	31	5.1	4.3	0.3	0.7	46	1 Fat	USDA 35207
Free Foods																
Ash, tumbleweed (Ch'ildeenini bileeshch'ih)	1 Tbsp	8	0	0	0	0	0	0	31	0	0	0	0	51	Free Food	Navajo food composition article
Navajo tea, brewed (ch'il ahwehe nineezigii)	1 cup (8 fl oz)	237	2	0	0	0	0	0	2	0.5	0	0	0	31	Free Food	USDA 14381
Combination Foods																
Blue mush tamale (Be'estl oni)	0.5 tamale in husk (5" x 1" x 1½")	35	73	0.5	0.2	0	0.2	0	18	15.7	0.8	0.3	1.5	15	1 Starch	Navajo food composition article
Mutton stew (Dibe bitsi, shibeezh)	1 cup	252	154	3	1.3	0.3	1.3	58	121	10.6	2.3	1.3	23.7	192	½ Carb + 3 Meat, lean	Navajo food composition article

Northern Plains Indian Foods

Food	Serving Size	Grams per Serving	Energy (kcal)	Fat (g)	SFA (g)	PUFA (g)	MUFA (g)	Chol (mg)	Sod (mg)	Carb (g)	Fiber (g)	Sugar (g)	Pro (g)	Pot (mg)	Exchanges	Source
Starches																
Corn, canned, drained	0.5 cup	82	66	0.8	0.1	0.4	0.2	0	244	15.4	1.6	2.5	2.2	111	1 Starch	USDA 11172
Fry bread (American Indian)	0.5 piece (5" dia)	36	119	4.4	1.7	0.4	1.6	3	118	17.4	0.6	0.7	2.4	28	1 Starch + 1 Fat	USDA 35142
Pancake plain, frozen, reheated	1 pancake (4" dia)	36	81	1.9	0.3	0.4	0.7	6	182	14.1	0.9	3.5	1.9	45	1 Starch	USDA 18288
Pinto beans and salt pork	0.33 cup	59	147	7.8	2.8	1	3.6	8	134	14.1	2.2	5.7	5.1	224	1 Starch + 1 Meat, lean + 1 Fat	FNDDS 41208100
Potato, fresh, mashed, made with milk and fat	0.5 cup	105	106	3	1.4	0.6	0.8	5	266	18.3	1.6	1.4	1.9	310	1 Starch + 1 Fat	FNDDS 71501020
Rice, wild, cooked	0.5 cup	82	83	0.3	0	0.2	0	0	2	17.5	1.5	0.6	3.3	83	1 Starch	USDA 20089
Fruits																
Fresh fruit mixture	0.75 cup, quartered or chopped	120	59	0.2	0	0.1	0.1	0	4	15	2	10	1	128	1 Fruit	Average
Sweets, Desserts, and Other Carbohydrates																
Sport drink (Gatorade)	1 cup	237	62	0	0	0	0	0	92	15.2	0	12.4	0	36	1 Carb	FNDDS 92560100
Wojapi (berry drink)	0.33 cup	79	48	0.1	0	0.1	0	0	2	11.9	1.3	9.1	0.2	31	1 Carb	Recipe
Nonstarchy Vegetables																
Beans, canned, drained (green, wax)	0.5 cup	78	18	0.1	0	0	0	0	204	3.4	1.8	0.6	0.9	87	1 Vegetable	USDA 11056
Tomato, raw (American Indian)	1 medium	123	22	0.2	0	0.1	0	0	6	4.8	1.5	3.2	1.1	292	1 Vegetable	USDA 11529
Zucchini, fresh, cooked	0.5 cup, sliced	90	14	0	0	0	0	0	3	3.5	1.3	1.5	0.6	228	1 Vegetable	USDA 11478

(continued)

Northern Plains Indian Foods *(continued)*

Food	Serving Size	Grams per Serving	Energy (kcal)	Fat (g)	SFA (g)	PUFA (g)	MUFA (g)	Chol (mg)	Sod (mg)	Carb (g)	Fiber (g)	Sugar (g)	Pro (g)	Pot (mg)	Exchanges	Source
Meats and Meat Substitutes																
Bison (buffalo), ground, pan-broiled	1 oz	28	68	4.3	1.8	0.2	1.7	24	21	0	0	0	6.8	97	1 Meat, med fat	USDA 17331
Cheese, American	1 oz	28	106	8.9	5.6	0.3	2.5	27	184	0.5	0	0.1	6.3	46	1 Meat, high fat	USDA 01147
Chicken breast, meat only, cooked	1 oz	28	47	1	0.3	0.2	0.4	24	21	0	0	0	8.8	72	1 Meat, lean	USDA 05064
Luncheon meat	1 oz	28	100	9.1	3.3	1.1	4.3	16	367	0.7	0	0	3.6	57	1 Meat, high fat	FNDDS 25230110
Pork steak (cutlet), cooked, lean and fat eaten	1 oz, boneless, cooked	28	67	3.8	1.4	0.4	1.7	26	111	0	0	0	7.7	100	1 Meat, med fat	FNDDS 22201010
Tripe (callos), honeycomb, cooked	1 oz, cooked	28	26	1.1	0.4	0.1	0.4	44	19	0.6	0	0	3.3	12	1 Meat, lean	USDA 23640
Venison (deer), roasted	1 oz	28	45	0.9	0.4	0.2	0.2	32	15	0	0	0	8.5	95	1 Meat, lean	USDA 17165
Combination Foods																
Beef stew with potato, vegetables	1 cup	238	160	5.2	2.2	0.2	2.3	30	990	17	1.5	3	12.5	414	1 Carb + 2 Meat, lean	Labels + USDA 22905
Macaroni and cheese, made from dry mix (Kraft original)	1 cup	191	410	19	5	5.3	8.4	15	710	49	1	7	9	166	3 Carb + 1 Meat, high fat + 2 Fat	Label + FNDDS 58145114

201

Alaska Native Foods

Food	Serving Size	Grams per Serving	Energy (kcal)	Fat (g)	SFA (g)	PUFA (g)	MUFA (g)	Chol (mg)	Sod (mg)	Carb (g)	Fiber (g)	Sugar (g)	Pro (g)	Pot (mg)	Exchanges	Source
Starches																
Corn, canned, solids and liquid	0.5 cup	128	82	0.6	0.1	0.3	0.2	0	273	19.7	2.2	3.6	2.5	210	1 Starch	USDA 11170
Potato, white, peeled, cooked	3 oz	85	73	0.1	0	0	0	0	4	17	1.5	0.7	1.5	279	1 Starch	USDA 11367
Fruit																
Cranberries, high bush	1.25 cups	119	65	0.2	0	0	0	0	31	14.6	8	4.8	1.3	166	1 Fruit	USDA 35029
Huckleberries	1 cup	150	56	0.2	0	0	0	0	15	13	2.1	9	0.6	116	1 Fruit	USDA 35043
Salmonberries	1 cup	145	68	0.5	0	0.3	0.1	0	20	14.6	2.8	5.3	1.2	160	1 Fruit	USDA 35154
Sweets, Desserts, and Other Carbs																
Agutuk (Eskimo ice cream), with berries, no meat or fish	0.5 cup	88	150	12.9	3.2	4.3	5.3	0	10	7.3	1.9	3.1	0.5	68	½ Fruit + 2½ Fat	Recipe
Nonstarchy Vegetables																
Beach asparagus	1 cup	55	15	0.2	0	0.1	0.1	0	23	2.4	1.3	1.1	1	150	1 Vegetable	Alaska native nutrient value table
Cabbage, fresh cooked	0.5 cup	75	17	0	0	0	0	0	6	4.1	1.4	2.1	1	147	1 Vegetable	USDA 11110
Dandelion greens (tundra greens), cooked	0.5 cup, chopped	52	17	0.3	0.1	0.1	0	0	23	3.4	1.5	0.3	1.1	122	1 Vegetable	USDA 11208
Fiddlehead ferns (tundra greens), raw	0.5 cup	90	31	0.4	0	0.1	0.1	0	1	5	3	1	4.1	333	1 Vegetable	USDA 11995
Seaweed, black, dried	1 cup	13	40	0.3	0.1	0.1	0	0	150	5.5	5.2	0.2	3.8	419	1 Vegetable	Alaska native food values table
Meat and Meat Substitutes																
Caribou, roasted	1 oz	28	47	1.3	0.5	0.2	0.4	31	17	0	0	0	8.4	88	1 Meat, lean	USDA 17163
Moose, roasted	1 oz	28	38	0.3	0.1	0.1	0.1	22	20	0	0	0	8.3	95	1 Meat, lean	USDA 17173
Salmon, coho, wild, cooked by dry heat	1 oz	28	39	1.2	0.3	0.4	0.4	16	16	0	0	0	6.7	123	1 Meat, lean	USDA 15247
Salmon, sockeye (red), cooked, dry heat	1 oz	28	61	3.1	0.5	0.7	1.5	25	19	0	0	0	7.7	106	1 Meat, lean	USDA 15086
Seal, ringed, meat only (no blubber), cooked	1 oz	28	51	1.1	0.3	0	0.6	26	40	0	0	0	8.1	60	1 Meat, lean	Baffin Inuit food comp + USDA 35071
Venison (deer), roasted	1 oz	28	45	0.9	0.4	0.2	0.2	32	15	0	0	0	8.5	95	1 Meat, lean	USDA 17165

(continued)

Alaska Native Foods *(continued)*

Food	Serving Size	Grams per Serving	Energy (kcal)	Fat (g)	SFA (g)	PUFA (g)	MUFA (g)	Chol (mg)	Sod (mg)	Carb (g)	Fiber (g)	Sugar (g)	Pro (g)	Pot (mg)	Exchanges	Source
Fats																
Hooligan (eulachon) grease	1 tsp	5	45	5	1.4	0.1	3.1	0	8	0	0	0	0	0	1 Fat	Alaska Native food comp table
Oil, bearded seal (oogruk)	1 tsp	5	45	5	0.5	1.7	2.4	3	0	0	0	0	0	0	1 Fat	USDA 35057
Combination Dishes																
Moose soup, Alaska native style	1 cup	345	267	1.1	0.3	0.4	0.2	59	134	37	4.6	5.2	26.5	882	2 Starch + 1 Vegetable + 2 Meat, lean	Recipe
Perok (fish pie), Alaska native style	1 slice (⅛th pie)	141	347	16	2.3	8	4.5	64	184	36.2	1.2	1.1	13.5	243	2 ½ Starch + 1 Meat, lean + 2 ½ Fat	Recipe
Wild duck soup (Alaska Native)	1 cup	296	100	0.7	0.2	0.2	0.1	5	63	20.6	3.5	5.6	4.2	367	½ Starch + 2 Vegetable	Recipe

African American Foods

Food	Serving Size	Grams per Serving	Energy (kcal)	Fat (g)	SFA (g)	PUFA (g)	MUFA (g)	Chol (mg)	Sod (mg)	Carb (g)	Fiber (g)	Sugar (g)	Pro (g)	Pot (mg)	Exchanges	Source
Starches																
Baked beans, pork and tomato sauce, canned	0.33 cup	81	76	0.8	0.3	0.2	0.4	6	355	15.2	3.2	4.6	4.2	239	1 Starch	USDA 16011
Corn bread, baked	1 cube (1-3/4")	43	114	3.1	0.7	1.4	0.8	17	283	18.7	1.1	2	2.9	63	1 Starch + 1 Fat	USDA 18024
Corn on cob, fresh, cooked	0.5 ear, large (7-3/4" to 9" long) yiel	59	64	0.8	0.1	0.4	0.2	0	0	14.8	1.7	1.9	2	125	1 Starch	USDA 11168
Grits, cooked	0.5 cup	121	71	0.2	0	0.1	0.1	0	2	15.6	0.4	0.1	1.7	25	1 Starch	USDA 08091
Peas, black-eyed (crowder), cooked	0.5 cup	86	100	0.5	0.1	0.2	0	0	3	17.9	5.6	2.8	6.6	239	1 Starch + 1 Meat, lean	USDA 16063
Rice, white, long grain, cooked	0.33 cup	52	68	0.1	0	0	0	0	1	14.7	0.2	0	1.4	18	1 Starch	USDA 18085
Stuffing (dressing), cornbread, prepared	0.33 cup	66	118	5.8	1.2	1.8	2.5	0	300	14.5	1.9	2.6	1.9	41	1 Starch + 1 Fat	USDA 20045
Fruits																
Watermelon, fresh	1.25 cups	190	57	0.3	0	0.1	0.1	0	2	14.3	0.8	11.8	1.2	213	1 Fruit	USDA 09326
Sweets, Desserts, and Other Carbs																
Sweet potato pie, southern type	1 piece (1/8 of 9" dia)	154	276	13.9	4	3.5	5.4	57	205	32.1	2	13.1	6	253	2 Carb + 3 Fat	FNDDS 53360000
Tea, sweetened iced	1 cup (8 fl oz)	259	52	0	0	0	0	0	8	13.7	0	13	0	91	1 Carb	FNDDS 92302200
Nonstarchy Vegetables																
Beans, canned, drained (green, wax)	0.5 cup	78	18	0.1	0	0	0	0	204	3.4	1.8	0.6	0.9	87	1 Vegetable	USDA 11056
Boiled cabbage and smoked turkey	0.5 cup	88	29	0.5	0.1	0.1	0.3	3	101	5.5	1.8	2.8	2.8	92	1 Vegetable	Recipe

(continued)

African American Foods (continued)

Food	Serving Size	Grams per Serving	Energy (kcal)	Fat (g)	SFA (g)	PUFA (g)	MUFA (g)	Chol (mg)	Sod (mg)	Carb (g)	Fiber (g)	Sugar (g)	Pro (g)	Pot (mg)	Exchanges	Source
Meat and Meat Substitutes																
Beef shortribs, barbecued	1 medium rib (yield after cooking, bo)	66	265	21.2	9	0.8	9.5	48	227	6.5	0.1	4.7	10.9	150	½ Carb + 2 Meat, high fat + 1 Fat	FNDDS 21304210
Chicken, fried (meat and skin), flour coated	1 oz	28	76	4.2	1.1	1	1.7	25	24	0.9	0	0	8.1	66	1 Meat, med fat	USDA 05008
Eggs, scrambled (with added fat)	0.25 cup	55	92	6.7	2	1.2	2.6	194	154	1.2	0	1	6.1	76	1 Meat, high fat	USDA 01132
Fish, fried, cornmeal coating	1 oz	28	65	3.8	0.9	0.9	1.6	23	79	2.3	0.2	0	5.1	96	1 Meat, med fat	USDA 15011
Pork spareribs, barbecued	1 medium rib (yield after cooking, bo)	40	134	8.7	3.2	0.8	3.9	35	174	4.8	0.1	3.4	8.3	119	½ Carb + 1 Meat, high fat	FNDDS 22701040
Fats																
Chitterlings, boiled	2 tbsp	16	37	3.3	1.5	0.2	1.1	44	3	0	0	0	2	2	1 Fat	USDA 10099
Combination Foods																
Chicken and dumplings	1 cup	244	368	19	5.3	4.4	7.5	88	920	21.8	0.7	1.3	26.1	293	1½ Carb + 3 Meat, lean + 2½ Fat	FNDDS 27246100
Coleslaw, deli style	0.5 cup	100	130	7	1	4.1	1.5	5	160	16	2	14	1	179	1 Carb + 1½ Fat	Label + USDA 21127
Hamburger, single patty with condiments, vegetables and bun	1 sandwich	110	279	13.5	4.1	2.6	5.3	26	504	27.3	2.2	6.6	12.9	227	2 Carb + 2 Meat, med fat	USDA 21109
Macaroni with cheese, creamed, homemade type	1 cup	200	416	17.3	7.4	2.7	6	32	356	48.1	2.8	1	16.3	120	3 Carb + 2 Meat, high fat	FNDDS 58147330
Potato salad, with egg	0.5 cup	125	179	10.2	1.8	4.7	3.1	85	661	14	1.6	2.8	3.4	318	1 Carb + 2 Fat	USDA 11414
Spaghetti with meat sauce	1 cup	248	389	13.5	4.3	2.7	4.9	60	908	48.2	4.7	10	17.8	546	3 Carb + 2 Meat, med fat	FNDDS 58132310
Sweet potatoes, candied	0.5 cup	98	141	3.2	1.3	0.1	0.6	8	69	27.3	2.4	21.7	0.9	185	2 Carb	USDA 11659
Turnip and mustard greens with smoked turkey	0.5 cup	96	80	2	1	0.4	0.5	15	109	7	3.1	0.8	9	183	1 Vegetable + 1 Meat, lean	Recipe

Mexican American Foods

Food	Serving Size	Grams per Serving	Energy (kcal)	Fat (g)	SFA (g)	PUFA (g)	MUFA (g)	Chol (mg)	Sod (mg)	Carb (g)	Fiber (g)	Sugar (g)	Pro (g)	Pot (mg)	Exchanges	Source
Starches																
Beans, pinto (frijoles cocidos), cooked	0.5 cup	85	122	0.6	0.1	0.2	0.1	0	1	22.3	7.7	0.3	7.7	371	1 Starch + 1 Meat, lean	USDA 16043
Plantain, ripe, cooked	0.33 cup, slices	51	59	0.1	0	0	0	0	3	15.8	1.2	7.1	0.4	236	1 Starch	USDA 09278
Tamale, Mexican style, meatless, no sauce	1 tamale	72	148	7.8	2.8	1.2	3.3	6	457	17.2	2.2	0.2	2.8	97	1 Starch + 1½ Fat	FNDDS 58103250
Tortilla, corn, ready to bake or fry	1 medium (6" across)	24	52	0.7	0.1	0.3	0.2	0	11	10.7	1.5	0.2	1.4	45	1 Starch	USDA 18363
Tortilla, flour, ready-to-bake or -fry, 7–8 inch diameter	1 tortilla (approx 7"–8" dia)	46	144	3.6	0.9	0.7	1.8	0	293	23.6	1.4	0.9	3.8	71	1½ Starch + ½ Fat	USDA 18364
Fruits																
Mango, fresh	0.5 mango, small (11 oz) yields	104	68	0.3	0.1	0.1	0.1	0	2	17.7	1.9	15.4	0.5	162	1 Fruit	USDA 09176
Papaya, fresh	1 cup, cubes	140	55	0.2	0.1	0	0.1	0	4	13.7	2.5	8.3	0.9	360	1 Fruit	USDA 09226
Milks																
Milk, whole	1 cup	244	146	7.9	4.6	0.5	2	24	98	11	0	11	7.9	349	1 Milk, whole	USDA 01077
Sweets, Desserts, and Other Carbohydrates																
Atole (corn meal-type beverage)	1 cup	249	209	3.8	2	0.4	1	10	47	40.5	0.7	35	4.2	179	3 Carb	FNDDS 92613010
Flan (caramel custard), made with whole milk	0.5 cup	153	223	6.2	2.8	0.6	1.9	138	81	34.7	0	35.4	6.9	181	½ Milk, whole + 2 Carb	USDA 19094
Horchata beverage, almond or chufa "nut" type	1 cup (8 fl oz)	240	245	12.4	1.3	3.9	6.7	0	12	31.8	2.6	27.3	5	149	2 Carb + 2½ Fat	FNDDS 92610010
Milk, sweetened, condensed	1.5 Tbsp	28	91	2.5	1.6	0.1	0.7	10	36	15.5	0	15.5	2.3	106	1 Carb	USDA 01095
Mole poblano sauce	0.25 cup	66	78	5.7	1.4	1.5	2.5	1	152	5.6	1.3	2.5	2.6	140	½ Carb + 1 Fat	FNDDS 28522000
Pan dulce (sweet roll), sugar topping	1 small (2½ oz)	70	237	7	1.6	2	3	30	132	39.5	0.9	15.7	4.3	60	2½ Carb + 1½ Fat	FNDDS 51161270
Pan dulce, crumb topping	1 piece	68	249	7.6	1.5	2.2	3.4	22	109	41.6	1	10	3.9	48	3 Carb + 1 Fat	Nutritionist Pro software

(continued)

Mexican American Foods *(continued)*

Food	Serving Size	Grams per Serving	Energy (kcal)	Fat (g)	SFA (g)	PUFA (g)	MUFA (g)	Chol (mg)	Sod (mg)	Carb (g)	Fiber (g)	Sugar (g)	Pro (g)	Pot (mg)	Exchanges	Source
Nonstarchy Vegetables																
Jicama (yambean, singkamas), cooked	0.5 cup, cubes	78	30	0.1	0	0	0	0	3	6.9	3.1	1.4	0.6	105	1 Vegetable	USDA 11604
Jicama (yambean, singkamas), raw	1 cup, slices	120	46	0.1	0	0.1	0	0	5	10.6	5.9	2.2	0.9	180	2 Vegetable	USDA 11603
Nopales (nopal cactus), cooked	0.5 cup	74	11	0	0	0	0	0	15	2.4	1.5	0.8	1	145	1 Vegetable	USDA 11964
Nopales, fresh	1 cup, sliced	86	14	0.1	0	0	0	0	18	2.9	1.9	1	1.1	221	1 Vegetable	USDA 11963
Tomatillo, fresh	1 cup, chopped or diced	132	42	1.3	0.2	0.6	0.2	0	1	7.7	2.5	5.2	1.3	354	1 Vegetable	USDA 11954
Meats and Meat Substitutes																
Chorizo sausage, Mexican style, cooked	1 oz	28	95	8.5	3	0.5	4.1	20	150	1	0	0	3.5	111	1 Meat, high fat	Label + USDA 07019
Queso anejo (dry or aged Mexican cheese)	1 oz	28	106	8.5	5.4	0.3	2.4	30	320	1.3	0	1.3	6.1	25	1 Meat, high fat	USDA 01165
Queso asadero (Mexican melting cheese)	1 oz	28	101	8	5.1	0.2	2.3	30	186	0.8	0	0.8	6.4	24	1 Meat, high fat	USDA 01166
Queso chihuahua (Mexican or Mennonite cheese)	1 oz	28	106	8.4	5.3	0.3	2.4	30	175	1.6	0	1.6	6.1	15	1 Meat, high fat	USDA 01167
Queso oaxaca (Mexican cheese)	1 oz	28	89	6.2	3.9	0.2	1.8	24	163	0.9	0	0.9	7.3	22	1 Meat, high fat	Latin American food composition table
Fats																
Avocados, raw, all commercial varieties, cubed	0.25 cup, cubes	38	60	5.5	0.8	0.7	3.7	0	3	3.2	2.5	0.2	0.8	182	1 Fat	USDA 09037
Free Foods																
Salsa	0.25 cup	65	17	0.1	0	0.1	0	0	388	4.1	1	2	1	192	Free Food	USDA 06164
Combination Foods																
Enchilada with cheese and beef	1 enchilada	192	323	17.6	9	1.4	6.1	40	1319	30.5	5.2	4	11.9	574	2 Carb + 1 Meat, lean + 3 Fat	USDA 21075
Tamale, meat	1 tamale	70	139	7.9	2.9	0.9	3.5	19	420	11.1	1.5	0.6	6.1	148	1 Carb + 1 Meat, lean + 1 Fat	FNDDS 58103120

Central American Foods

Food	Serving Size	Grams per Serving	Energy (kcal)	Fat (g)	SFA (g)	PUFA (g)	MUFA (g)	Chol (mg)	Sod (mg)	Carb (g)	Fiber (g)	Sugar (g)	Pro (g)	Pot (mg)	Exchanges	Source
Starches																
Arrowroot flour, raw	2 tbsps	16	57	0	0	0	0	0	0	14.1	0.5	0	0	2	1 Starch	USDA 20003
Arrowroot, fresh, cooked	1 cup, sliced	120	78	0.2	0	0.1	0	0	31	16.1	1.6	0.5	5.1	545	1 Starch	USDA 11697
Beans, pink, cooked, no fat or salt added	0.5 cup	84	126	0.4	0.1	0.2	0	0	2	23.6	4.5	0.3	7.7	429	1 Starch + 1 Meat, lean	USDA 1604 1
Beans, red, cooked, no fat or salt added	0.5 cup	88	112	0.4	0.1	0.2	0	0	2	20.2	6.5	0.3	7.7	357	1 Starch + 1 Meat, lean	USDA 16033
Breadfruit, cooked, no fat or salt added	0.25 cup	63	72	0.2	0	0	0	0	1	18.9	3.4	7.7	0.7	307	1 Starch	FNDDS 75208500
Calabaza (winter squash, Spanish pumpkin, auyama), cooked, no salt or fat added	1 cup, small cubes	205	70	0.6	0.3	0	0.1	0	8	16.5	5.9	6.7	2.3	420	1 Starch	FNDDS 73210010
Cassava (yuca, yucca, manioc, mandioca, tapioca), cooked, no fat or salt added	0.33 cup, diced	44	70	0.1	0	0	0	0	6	16.7	0.8	0.7	0.6	107	1 Starch	FNDDS 71930100
Plantain, ripe, cooked	0.33 cup, slices	51	59	0.1	0	0	0	0	3	15.8	1.2	7.1	0.4	236	1 Starch	USDA 09278
Fruits																
Carambola (starfruit), fresh	2 medium (3⅝" long)	182	56	0.6	0	0.3	0.1	0	4	12.2	5.1	7.2	1.9	242	1 Fruit	USDA 09060
Guava (guayabas), common, fresh	2 small (2.5 oz) yields	110	75	1	0.3	0.4	0.1	0	2	15.8	5.9	9.8	2.8	459	1 Fruit	USDA 09139
Mamey (mamey apple, mamey sapote), raw	1 cup, slices	154	79	0.8	0.2	0.1	0.3	0	23	19.3	4.6	14.6	0.8	72	1 Fruit	USDA 9175
Mango, fresh	0.5 mango, small (11 oz) yields	104	68	0.3	0.1	0.1	0.1	0	2	17.7	1.9	15.4	0.5	162	1 Fruit	USDA 09176
Nance	12 cherries	98	65	1.3	0.1	0.6	0.1	0	0	14.2	2.2	12	0.9	218	1 Fruit	Latin American INCAP + USDA 09070

(continued)

Central American Foods *(continued)*

Food	Serving Size	Grams per Serving	Energy (kcal)	Fat (g)	SFA (g)	PUFA (g)	MUFA (g)	Chol (mg)	Sod (mg)	Carb (g)	Fiber (g)	Sugar (g)	Pro (g)	Pot (mg)	Exchanges	Source
Papaya, fresh	1 cup, cubes	140	55	0.2	0.1	0	0.1	0	4	13.7	2.5	8.3	0.9	360	1 Fruit	USDA 09226
Passion fruit (granadilla), fresh, ripe	4 fruits (1¼ oz) yield	72	70	0.5	0	0.3	0.1	0	20	16.8	7.5	8.1	1.6	251	1 Fruit	USDA 09231
Pitaya, sweet, raw pitahaya roja, dragon fruit)	1 small (7 oz) yields	109	59	0.4	0	0.2	0	0	65	14.4	0.7	13.1	1.5	340	1 Fruit	Central American Food comp INCAP
Soursop (guanabana, guyabano), raw	0.33 cup, pulp	74	49	0.2	0	0.1	0.1	0	10	12.5	2.5	10.1	0.7	206	1 Fruit	USDA 09315
Nonstarchy Vegetables																
Chayote squash (mirliton, sayote, christophine), cooked	0.5 cup	80	19	0.4	0.1	0.1	0.1	0	1	4.1	2.2	1	0.5	138	1 Vegetable	USDA 11150
Fats																
Coconut milk, fresh	1.5 Tbsp	22	52	5.4	4.8	0.1	0.2	0	3	1.2	0.5	0.8	0.5	59	1 Fat	USDA 12117
Oil, palm	1 tsp	4	40	4.5	2.2	0.4	1.7	0	0	0	0	0	0	0	1 Fat	USDA 04055
Free Foods																
Tamarind pulp, raw	1 Tbsp	8	18	0	0	0	0	0	2	4.7	0.4	4.3	0.2	47	Free Food	USDA 09322

Caribbean Hispanic Foods

Food	Serving Size	Grams per Serving	Energy (kcal)	Fat (g)	SFA (g)	PUFA (g)	MUFA (g)	Chol (mg)	Sod (mg)	Carb (g)	Fiber (g)	Sugar (g)	Pro (g)	Pot (mg)	Exchanges	Source
Starches																
Boniato (batata, bonita), cooked	0.5 cup, diced	70	80	0.1	0	0	0	0	10	19.1	2.7	0.3	1	466	1 Starch	FNDDS 71941120
Cassava (yuca, yucca, manioc, mandioca, tapioca), cooked, no fat or salt added	0.33 cup, diced	44	70	0.1	0	0	0	0	6	16.7	0.8	0.7	0.6	107	1 Starch	FNDDS 71930100
Name (white yam), cooked, no salt or fat added	0.5 cup	70	80	0.1	0	0	0	0	10	19.1	2.7	0.3	1	466	1 Starch	FNDDS 71945010
Plantain, ripe, cooked	0.33 cup, slices	51	59	0.1	0	0	0	0	3	15.8	1.2	7.1	0.4	236	1 Starch	USDA 09278
Plantains, fried, green (tostones de plantano)	0.5 cup	56	128	6.4	0.9	3	2.1	0	1579	19.3	1.4	9.1	0.8	273	1 Starch + 1 Fat	FNDDS 71901110
Sweets, Desserts and Other Carbohydrates																
Coconut rum eggnog (coquito)	1 small goblet (4 fl oz)	125	299	8.9	6.1	0.4	1.9	68	68	20.4	0.3	20	5	226	1½ Carb + 2 Fat	FNDDS 93301220
Meat and Meat Substitutes																
Pork shoulder roast, Puerto Rican style (pernil)	1 oz, boneless, cooked	28	82	6	2.2	0.6	2.7	25	65	0	0	0	6.5	92	1 Meat, med fat	FNDDS 22411000
Combination Foods																
Beef, ground, seasoned and stewed (picadillo, Puerto Rican style), fat added	0.5 cup	100	302	26.1	7.4	3.5	12.1	52	641	3.9	1	1.9	13.1	331	2 Meat, med fat + 3½ Fat	FNDDS 27118120
Chicken empanada (pastelito, savory pastie), baked, Dominican style	1 empanada	50	117	0.7	0.1	0.3	0.2	6	341	21.6	0.8	0.6	5.2	60	1½ Starch	Recipe
Chicken empanada (pastelito, savory pastie), deep fried, Dominican style	1 empanada	58	166	6.3	0.9	3.3	1.7	7	341	21.6	0.8	0.6	5.2	60	1½ Starch + 1 Fat	Recipe
Chicken fricassee (fricase de pollo), includes sauce and potato	1 cup, boneless	223	428	30.8	6.5	10.2	12.2	80	1354	14.4	2.5	2.6	23.3	624	1 Carb + 3 Meat, med fat + 3 Fat	FNDDS 27348100

(continued)

Caribbean Hispanic Foods (continued)

Food	Serving Size	Grams per Serving	Energy (kcal)	Fat (g)	SFA (g)	PUFA (g)	MUFA (g)	Chol (mg)	Sod (mg)	Carb (g)	Fiber (g)	Sugar (g)	Pro (g)	Pot (mg)	Exchanges	Source
Cod, stewed, Puerto Rican style	1 cup	114	159	4.8	0.7	0.7	2.9	51	2094	5.9	1.7	2.8	22	528	½ Carb + 3 Meat, lean	FNDDS 27151070
Cuban sandwich, with spread	1 sandwich (6" long)	255	696	30.4	10	6.7	12	92	1359	57.8	2.3	7.4	45.1	528	4 Carb + 6 Meat, lean + 3½ Fat	FNDDS 27520410
Green plantains, fried, with cracklings (mofongo)	1 ball (3" dia)	64	223	14.6	3.4	4.4	5.7	19	398	17.5	1.2	8.1	7.1	340	1 Carb + 1 Meat, high fat + 1 Fat	FNDDS 77201210
Oxtail soup or stew	1 cup	244	68	2.5	1.2	0.1	1	0	1159	8.6	0.2	2.4	2.7	32	½ Carb + ½ Fat	FNDDS 28310150
Rice and pigeon pea stew	1 cup	178	242	6.1	1	0.9	3.9	0	911	41.4	2	2.4	5.1	244	3 Carb + 1 Fat	FNDDS 58156610
Soupy rice with chicken (asopao de pollo), Puerto Rican style	1 cup, boneless	263	481	22.1	6	4.4	9.9	92	1612	41	3.2	3.6	28.1	484	3 Carb + 3 Meat, med fat + 1 Fat	FNDDS 58155410
Spaghetti with chicken	1 cup	248	325	5.9	1.5	2.1	1.5	20	461	52.1	5	10.2	14.2	436	3½ Carb + 1 Meat, med fat	FNDDS 58132910
Stew with meat and starchy vegetables (salcocho, sancocho)	1 cup, boneless	245	358	16.2	4.8	3.5	5.9	54	292	35	4.4	7.8	19	1017	2½ Carb + 2 Meat, med fat + 1 Fat	FNDDS 77563010
Tamale, meat	1 tamale	70	139	7.9	2.9	0.9	3.5	19	420	11.1	1.5	0.6	6.1	148	1 Carb + 1 Meat, lean + 1 Fat	FNDDS 58103120

South American Foods

Food	Serving Size	Grams per Serving	Energy (kcal)	Fat (g)	SFA (g)	PUFA (g)	MUFA (g)	Chol (mg)	Sod (mg)	Carb (g)	Fiber (g)	Sugar (g)	Pro (g)	Pot (mg)	Exchanges	Source
Starches																
Arepas (arepa, arepita, cornmeal fritter)	1 fritter (2½" x 2½" x ¼")	40	106	6.9	2.2	2.1	2.2	8	226	8.3	0.4	0.2	2.7	26	½ Starch + 1 Fat	FNDDS 58117110
Mandioca (yuca, yucca, manioc, cassava, tapioca), cooked, no fat or salt added	0.33 cup, diced	44	70	0.1	0	0	0	0	6	16.7	0.8	0.7	0.6	107	1 Starch	FNDDS 71930100
Pao de batata (potato bread)	1 regular slice	34	90	1.1	0.2	0.5	0.2	0	232	17.2	0.8	1.5	2.6	34	1 Starch	FNDDS 51127010
Pao de queijo (cheese bun, bread or roll)	2 buns	50	142	6.7	2.1	2	1.7	40	178	18	0	2.1	2.7	50	1 Starch + 1 Fat	Label + FNDDS 51111010
Quinoa, cooked	0.33 cup	61	73	1.2	0.2	0.7	0.5	0	4	13	1.7	0	2.7	105	1 Starch	USDA 20137
Sweets, Desserts, and Other Carbohydrates																
Arroz doce, arroz dulce (rice pudding, sweet rice)	0.5 cup	112	180	1.9	1.1	0.1	0.5	7	68	37	0.5	25.6	4.1	201	2½ Carb	FNDDS 13210410
Churros, filled with sweetened condensed milk (deep fried dough)	1 churro	26	84	3.7	1.5	0.3	1.9	4	27	11.3	0.1	8.7	1.5	50	1 Carb + ½ Fat	FNDDS 53520200
Panettone (Christmas cake with candied fruit and raisins)	1 piece, large	80	288	9.6	1.1	3.6	4.5	4	216	44	2.7	21	6.4	122	3 Carb + 2 Fat	Label + USDA 18110
Pao de mel (honey cake)	1 square (1½ oz)	45	112	1	0.4	0.1	0.3	21	18	24.1	0.6	5.2	2.2	Miss	1½ Carb	Label
Pudim de leite (milk custard)	0.33 cup	101	162	4.8	2.8	0.6	1.5	91	66	24.7	0	23.4	5.3	211	1½ Carb + 1 Fat	USDA 19094
Meats and Meat Substitutes																
Asado, churrasco, lean beef, grilled or barbecued	1 oz	28	58	2.8	1.1	0.1	1.5	17	22	0	0	0	7.5	83	1 Meat, lean	USDA 13977
Queijo blanco, queso fresco (farmer's fresh cheese)	1 oz	28	57	4.3	2.8	0.2	1.2	17	95	1.9	0	0.2	3.8	37	1 Meat, med fat	FNDDS 14133000

(continued)

South American Foods *(continued)*

Food	Serving Size	Grams per Serving	Energy (kcal)	Fat (g)	SFA (g)	PUFA (g)	MUFA (g)	Chol (mg)	Sod (mg)	Carb (g)	Fiber (g)	Sugar (g)	Pro (g)	Pot (mg)	Exchanges	Source
Fats																
Requeijao, creamy cheese	1 Tbsp	14	41	3.6	2	0.2	1	13	33	0.5	0	0	1.5	17	1 Fat	Label + USDA 01017
Requeijao, creamy cheese, reduced fat (Catupiry brand)	1.5 Tbsp	22	51	4.5	3	0.1	1.3	14	135	0.7	0	0	2.3	38	1 Fat	Label + USDA 43274
Combination Foods																
Coxinha de galinha (deep fried dough filled with chicken)	1 coxinha, appetizer size	40	150	7.4	1.3	3.1	2.7	3	521	16.8	0.8	0.2	3.6	50	1 Carb + 1½ Fat	Label
Empadinha de palmito (mini pie filled with hearts of palm)	1 mini pie	40	94	4.7	2.3	0.8	1.6	0	145	10.4	0.4	0.2	2.4	100	1 Carb + ½ Fat	Label
Empanada (pie type dough filled with meat)	1 turnover, entree size	132	490	36.8	10	7.8	13.8	73	326	27.5	1.5	0.2	14.7	215	2 Carb + 2 Meat, high fat + 3½ Fat	FNDDS 58126110
Esfiha (mini pie filled with meat)	1 mini pie	50	109	3	2	0.3	0.7	6	302	16	1	0.2	5	47	1 Carb + 1 Meat, lean	Label
Feijoada (black beans and pork stew)	0.75 cup	168	289	21.1	8.3	2.2	8.9	56	640	11.2	3.5	Miss	14	303	1 Carb + 2 Meat, med fat + 2 Fat	Brazilian food composition table
Panqueca de carne (savory crepes filled with ground meat)	1 crepe with filling, no sauce	123	200	9.5	3.2	2.1	3.1	73	478	18	1.1	3.2	10.5	257	1 Carb + 1 Meat, med fat + 1 Fat	FNDDS 58120120

213

Asian Indian and Pakistani Foods

Food	Serving Size	Grams per Serving	Energy (kcal)	Fat (g)	SFA (g)	PUFA (g)	MUFA (g)	Chol (mg)	Sod (mg)	Carb (g)	Fiber (g)	Sugar (g)	Pro (g)	Pot (mg)	Exchanges	Source
Starches																
Chappatti (roti, phulka, chapati, chapati, chappathi)	1 small chappatti or roti (6")	27	71	0.4	0.1	0.1	0	0	131	15.1	1.9	0.1	2.6	65	1 starch	FNDDS 52215260
Chickpeas (garbanzo beans), cooked	0.5 cup	82	134	2.1	0.2	0.9	0.5	0	6	22.5	6.2	3.9	7.3	239	1 starch + 1 Meat, lean	USDA 16057
Dhakla, khaman (steamed lentils dish)	1 square (1")	30	104	5	2	1	2	0	539	12	4.8	1	5	111	1 starch + 1 Fat	Recipe
Dhansak (vegetables and lentils)	0.5 cup	120	104	3.5	0.5	1	2	0	137	15	3.3	1.7	4	161	1 starch + 1 Fat	Recipe
Idli (fermented steamed rice and lental breakfast cake)	1 small (1 1/4" dia)	28	77	0.3	0.1	0.1	0.1	0	74	16	1.9	0.6	2.4	79	1 starch	FNDDS 55702000
Matki usal (sprouted moth bean dish)	0.67 cup	114	139	8	5.4	0.7	2	0	257	13.4	2.6	9	4	115	1 starch + 1 Fat	Recipe
Mung dhal (green gram, mung beans), plain, cooked	0.5 cup	101	106	0.4	0.1	0.1	0.1	0	2	19.3	7.7	2	7.1	269	1 starch + 1 Meat, lean	USDA 16081
Naan (flatbread)	0.25 piece (8" x 2")	29	78	2	0.3	0.2	0.8	9	94	12.4	0.5	0.6	2.5	40	1 starch	FNDDS 51108100
Pesrattu, pesrat (lentil pan fried crepe)	1 crepe (9" dia)	75	127	5	1	3	1	0	372	14	4.3	1	5	250	1 starch + 1 Fat	Recipe
Plantain, green, boiled	0.33 cup, slices	51	59	0.1	0	0	0	0	3	15.8	1.2	7.1	0.4	236	1 starch	FNDDS 71901010
Poha (beaten rice dish)	0.5 cup	85	140	6	1	2	3	0	405	18	0.2	0	2	18	1 starch + 1 Fat	Recipe
Puri (poori, puffed bread)	1 puri (approx 4-4/5" dia)	36	107	3.4	0.5	1.3	1.4	0	247	16.8	1.7	0.1	2.7	58	1 starch + 1 Fat	FNDDS 51300180
Rice, white, long grain, cooked	0.33 cup	52	68	0.1	0	0	0	0	1	14.7	0.2	0	1.4	18	1 starch	USDA 20045
Tomato dhal (lentils and tomatoes)	0.5 cup	131	132	3	1.5	1	0.5	0	262	18	7.1	1.3	7	322	1 starch + 1 Meat, lean	Recipe
Toor dhal (pigeon peas, red gram) mature seeds, plain, cooked	0.5 cup	84	102	0.3	0.1	0.2	0	0	4	19.5	5.6	1.7	5.7	323	1 starch + 1 Meat, lean	USDA 16102

(continued)

Asian Indian and Pakistani Foods *(continued)*

Food	Serving Size	Grams per Serving	Energy (kcal)	Fat (g)	SFA (g)	PUFA (g)	MUFA (g)	Chol (mg)	Sod (mg)	Carb (g)	Fiber (g)	Sugar (g)	Pro (g)	Pot (mg)	Exchanges	Source
Sweets, Desserts, and Other Carbohydrates																
Sambar (sambhar) (spicy lentil gravy)	0.5 cup	75	88	1	0	Miss	0.3	0	263	16	5.9	1.3	5	277	1 Carb	Recipe
Nonstarchy Vegetables																
Brinjal (eggplant), plain, cooked	0.5 cup (1" cubes)	50	17	0.1	0	0	0	0	0	4.3	1.2	1.6	0.4	61	1 Vegetable	USDA 11210
Cucumber raita	0.5 cup	90	21	0	0	0	0	0	22	3	0.4	2.6	1	152	1 Vegetable	Recipe
Karela (bitter melon), plain, cooked	0.5 cup (½" pieces)	62	12	0.1	0	0	0	0	4	2.7	1.2	1.2	0.5	198	1 Vegetable	USDA 11025
Mung bean sprouts, seed attached, cooked	0.5 cup	62	13	0.1	0	0	0	0	6	2.6	0.5	1.8	1.3	63	1 Vegetable	USDA 11044
Okra, fresh, cooked	0.5 cup slices	80	18	0.2	0	0	0	0	5	3.6	1.8	1.8	1.5	108	1 Vegetable	USDA 11279
Meats and Meat Substitutes																
Chicken tikka, cooked	3 pieces (1")	31	54	1.6	0.4	0.3	0.6	23	155	0	0	0	8.9	75	1 Meat, lean	Recipe + USDA 05013
Chicken, no skin, roasted	1 oz	28	54	2.1	0.6	0.5	0.8	25	24	0	0	0	8.2	69	1 Meat, lean	USDA 05013
Tandoori chicken, cooked	1 oz	28	75	4	1	1	1.6	25	152	2	0	2	8	69	1 Meat, med fat	Recipe + USDA 05013
Combination Dishes																
Aviyal (vegetables in gravy)	0.5 cup	160	81	2	1	1	0.2	1	412	14	3.2	Miss	2	88	1 Carb	Recipe

Chinese American Foods

Food	Serving Size	Grams per Serving	Energy (kcal)	Fat (g)	SFA (g)	PUFA (g)	MUFA (g)	Chol (mg)	Sod (mg)	Carb (g)	Fiber (g)	Sugar (g)	Pro (g)	Pot (mg)	Exchanges	Source
Starches																
Noodles, egg, cooked	0.33 cup	53	73	1.1	0.2	0.3	0.3	15	3	13.3	0.6	0.2	2.4	20	1 Starch	USDA 20110
Rice vermicelli (noodles), cooked	0.33 cup	53	58	0.1	0	0	0	0	10	13.1	0.5	0.1	0.5	2	1 Starch	USDA 20134
Rice, brown, cooked	0.33 cup	64	71	0.6	0.1	0.2	0.2	0	3	14.8	1.2	0.2	1.7	28	1 Starch	USDA 20037
Sweet potato, baked in skin, skin not eaten	0.5 cup	100	90	0.2	0	0.1	0	0	36	20.7	3.3	6.5	2	475	1 Starch	USDA 11508
Taro root, cooked	0.33 cup, sliced	44	62	0	0	0	0	0	7	15.1	2.2	0.2	0.2	211	1 Starch	USDA 11519
Fruits																
Grapes, fresh, small	17 grapes	85	59	0.1	0	0	0	0	2	15.4	0.8	13.2	0.6	162	1 Fruit	USDA 09132
Mango, fresh	0.5 mango, small (11 oz) yields	104	68	0.3	0.1	0.1	0.1	0	2	17.7	1.9	15.4	0.5	162	1 Fruit	USDA 09176
Persimmon, Japanese, soft, fresh	0.5 fruit (2½" dia)	84	59	0.2	0	0	0	0	1	15.6	3	10.5	0.5	135	1 Fruit	USDA 09263
Pummelo, fresh	0.75 cup, sections	142	54	0.1	0	0	0	0	1	13.7	1.4	9	1.1	308	1 Fruit	USDA 09295
Nonstarchy Vegetables																
Bamboo shoots, cooked	0.5 cup (½" slices)	60	7	0.1	0	0.1	0	0	2	1.2	0.6	0.3	0.9	320	1 Vegetable	USDA 11027
Bitter melon (bitter gourd, balsam-pear, ampalaya, karela), cooked	0.5 cup (½" pieces)	62	12	0.1	0	0	0	0	4	2.7	1.2	1.2	0.5	198	1 Vegetable	USDA 11025
Bok choy (Chinese white cabbage or pak-choi), cooked	0.5 cup	85	10	0.1	0	0.1	0	0	29	1.5	0.8	0.7	1.3	315	1 Vegetable	USDA 11117
Bok choy (Chinese white cabbage or pak-choi), raw	1 cup, shredded	70	9	0.1	0	0.1	0	0	46	1.5	0.7	0.8	1.1	176	1 Vegetable	USDA 11116
Chinese broccoli (gai larn), cooked	0.5 cup	44	10	0.3	0	0.1	0	0	3	1.7	1.1	0.4	0.5	115	1 Vegetable	USDA 11969

(continued)

Chinese American Foods *(continued)*

Food	Serving Size	Grams per Serving	Energy (kcal)	Fat (g)	SFA (g)	PUFA (g)	MUFA (g)	Chol (mg)	Sod (mg)	Carb (g)	Fiber (g)	Sugar (g)	Pro (g)	Pot (mg)	Exchanges	Source
Meat and Meat Substitute																
Chinese-style sausage (pork, soy, spices) fresh, cooked	1 oz	28	101	8.3	2.6	1.1	3.5	24	250	1.9	0	0.9	6	83	1 Meat, high fat	East Asian database + USDA 07064
Preserved egg, thousand-year duck egg, limed	1 egg	63	114	7.3	2.3	0.8	4.1	554	1308	2.6	0	0.6	8.8	323	1 Meat, high fat	East Asian database + FNDDS
Scallops, dried	1 medium	13	44	0.3	0.1	0.1	0	16	56	1.1	0	0	8.6	205	1 Meat, lean	East Asian database + FNDDS
Tofu, soft (nigari)	0.5 cup (½" cubes)	124	76	4.6	0.7	2.6	1	0	10	2.2	0.2	0.9	8.1	149	1 Meat, med fat	USDA 16127
Fats																
Coconut milk, fresh	1.5 Tbsp	22	52	5.4	4.8	0.1	0.2	0	3	1.2	0.5	0.8	0.5	59	1 Fat	USDA 12117
Sesame seeds, dried	1 Tbsp	9	52	4.5	0.6	2	1.7	0	1	2.1	1.1	0	1.6	42	1 Fat	USDA 12023
Tahini (sesame butter or paste)	2 tsp	10	60	5.4	0.8	2.4	2	0	12	2.1	0.9	0	1.7	41	1 Fat	USDA 12166
Combination Foods																
Barbecued pork bun (char siu bao), steamed	1 medium (4 oz)	113	293	8.3	2	1.5	3	20	327	48.4	1.8	16.1	8.3	157	3 Carb + 1 Meat, lean + 1 Fat	Hong Kong food search database
Dumplings filled with meat, poultry, or seafood, steamed	4 dumplings	148	166	3.9	1.1	0.8	1.4	71	644	14.1	0.7	0.8	17.1	278	1 Carb + 2 Meat, lean	FNDDS 58112510
Wontons, meat filled, fried (won ton)	3 wontons	57	161	7.6	2.5	0.8	3.5	59	332	14.2	0.7	0.5	8.6	152	1 Carb + 1 Meat, lean + 1 Fat	FNDDS 58111110

Hmong American Foods

Food	Serving Size	Grams per Serving	Energy (kcal)	Fat (g)	SFA (g)	PUFA (g)	MUFA (g)	Chol (mg)	Sod (mg)	Carb (g)	Fiber (g)	Sugar (g)	Pro (g)	Pot (mg)	Exchanges	Source
Starches																
Cellophane (mung bean) noodles, cooked	0.33 cup, cooked	63	53	0	0	0	0	0	3	13	0.1	0	0	1	1 Starch	FNDDS 56117000
Rice, white, medium-grain, cooked	0.33 cup	61	80	0.1	0	0	0	0	0	17.5	0.2	0.1	1.5	18	1 Starch	USDA 20051
Sticky rice (glutinous), white, cooked	0.33 cup	57	56	0.1	0	0	0	0	3	12.1	0.6	0	1.2	6	1 Starch	USDA 20055
Fruits																
Asian pear, raw	1 fruit (2¼" high x 2½" dia)	122	51	0.3	0	0.1	0.1	0	0	13	4.4	8.6	0.6	148	1 Fruit	USDA 09340
Guava (guayabas), common, fresh	2 small (2.5 oz) yields	110	75	1	0.3	0.4	0.1	0	2	15.8	5.9	9.8	2.8	459	1 Fruit	USDA 09139
Jackfruit, fresh	0.33 cup, sliced	54	51	0.2	0	0	0	0	2	13.1	0.9	10	0.8	165	1 Fruit	USDA 9144
Nonstarchy Vegetables																
Bamboo shoots, cooked	0.5 cup (½" slices)	60	7	0.1	0	0.1	0	0	2	1.2	0.6	0.3	0.9	320	1 Vegetable	USDA 11027
Bitter melon (bitter gourd, balsam-pear, ampalaya, karela), cooked	cup (½" pieces)	62	12	0.1	0	0	0	0	4	2.7	1.2	1.2	0.5	198	1 Vegetable	USDA 11025
Leeks, fresh cooked	0.5 cup	52	16	0.1	0	0.1	0	0	5	4	0.5	0.5	0.4	45	1 Vegetable	USDA 11247
Mung bean sprouts, seed attached, cooked	0.5 cup	62	13	0.1	0	0	0	0	6	2.6	0.5	1.8	1.3	63	1 Vegetable	USDA 11044
Mustard greens, fresh cooked	0.5 cup	70	10	0.2	0	0	0.1	0	11	1.5	1.4	0.1	1.6	141	1 Vegetable	USDA 11271
Meats and Meat Substitutes																
Pheasant (grouse), cooked, meat and skin	1 oz	28	70	3.4	1	0.4	1.6	25	12	0	0	0	9.2	77	1 Meat, med fat	USDA 43283
Pig (pork) feet, cooked	1 oz	28	67	4.5	1.2	0.4	2.3	30	21	0	0	0	6.2	9	1 Meat, med fat	USDA 10173
Pork, ground, cooked	1 oz	28	84	5.9	2.2	0.5	2.6	27	21	0	0	0	7.3	102	1 Meat, high fat	USDA 10220
Squirrel, roasted	1 oz	28	49	1.3	0.2	0.4	0.4	34	34	0	0	0	8.7	100	1 Meat, lean	USDA 17184
Tofu (soybean curd), firm	4 oz	114	80	4.7	1	2	1.4	0	14	1.9	1	0.7	9.3	168	1 Meat, med fat	USDA 16126

(continued)

Hmong American Foods *(continued)*

Food	Serving Size	Grams per Serving	Energy (kcal)	Fat (g)	SFA (g)	PUFA (g)	MUFA (g)	Chol (mg)	Sod (mg)	Carb (g)	Fiber (g)	Sugar (g)	Pro (g)	Pot (mg)	Exchanges	Source
Fats																
Chitterlings, boiled	2 Tbsp	16	37	3.3	1.5	0.2	1.1	44	3	0	0	0	2	2	1 Fat	USDA 10099
Coconut meat (heart), fresh	3 Tbsp, freshly shredded	15	53	5	4.5	0.1	0.2	0	3	2.3	1.4	0.9	0.5	53	1 Fat	USDA 12104
Coconut milk, fresh	1.5 Tbsp	22	52	5.4	4.8	0.1	0.2	0	3	1.2	0.5	0.8	0.5	59	1 Fat	USDA 12117
Lard, pork	1 tsp	4	39	4.3	1.7	0.5	1.9	4	0	0	0	0	0	0	1 Fat	USDA 04002
Combination Foods																
Boiled pork and mustard greens (zaub ntsaub), Hmong-style	1 cup	149	134	6.2	2.1	0.6	2.9	56	64	1.6	1.5	0.1	17.7	357	3 Meat, lean	Recipe

Filipino American Foods

Food	Serving Size	Grams per Serving	Energy (kcal)	Fat (g)	SFA (g)	PUFA (g)	MUFA (g)	Chol (mg)	Sod (mg)	Carb (g)	Fiber (g)	Sugar (g)	Pro (g)	Pot (mg)	Exchanges	Source
Starches																
Rice, Filipino-style	0.33 cup	55	79	2.8	0.3	1	0.5	11	189	11.3	0.7	0.1	2.3	54	1 Starch + ½ Fat	Recipe
Sweets, Desserts, and Other Carbohydrates																
Boiled glutinous rice cake, wrapped in leaves, Filipino-style	1 cake (2 oz)	61	108	7.2	6.4	0.1	0.3	0	557	10	0.1	Miss	1.5	90	½ Carb + 1½ Fat	Recipe
Boiled sweet rice cake flour patties, Filipino-style	1 oz	29	104	4.6	2.7	0.8	0.8	0	22	14.4	1.1	Miss	1.7	78	1 Carb + 1 Fat	Recipe
Glutinous rice with chocolate, Filipino-style	0.67 cup	235	140	8.5	5	0.3	2.8	12	146	14.3	1.6	Miss	4.5	215	1 Carb + 1½ Fat	Recipe
Rice cake, steamed, Filipino-style	1 cupcake	40	104	2.9	1.3	0.2	1.2	35	200	17.4	0	Miss	2.3	44	1 Carb + ½ Fat	Recipe
Meats and Meat Substitutes																
Beef jerky, Filipino-style	1 oz	28	35	1.1	0.4	0	0.4	13	240	1.6	0	Miss	4.7	92	1 Meat, lean	Recipe
Meat Loaf, Filipino-style	1 oz	28	69	5.2	1.7	0.3	2.2	27	85	1.7	0.4	Miss	3.7	71	1 Meat, med fat	Recipe
Roast pork, Filipino-style	1 oz	28	44	2.1	0.7	0.2	1	17	18	0	0	0	5.9	100	1 Meat, lean	Recipe
Combination Foods																
Baked grouper with sweet-sour sauce, Filipino-style	1 fish (3 oz) and sauce (⅓ cup)	175	158	1.4	0.3	0.4	0.3	43	88	11.9	1	Miss	23.6	556	1 Carb + 3 Meat, lean	Recipe
Beefsteak, Filipino-style	1 serving	182	241	14.6	4.5	3.1	5.3	49	453	10.5	2	Miss	17.1	373	1 Carb + 2 Meat, med fat + ½ Fat	Recipe
Eggroll, fried, Filipino-style	1 egg roll	129	232	11.1	1.6	6	2.8	39	341	23.2	1.2	Miss	10.3	207	1½ Carb + 1 Meat, lean + 2 Fat	Recipe
Fresh shrimp coddled in acid stock, Filipino-style	1 serving	466	111	1.3	0.2	0.5	0.2	86	113	11.9	3.5	Miss	14.5	594	2 Vegetable + 1 Meat, lean	Recipe
Fried rice (meat and egg), Filipino-style	1 cup	193	307	11.8	2.4	4.4	3.7	82	488	25.5	0.6	Miss	22.5	296	2 Starch + 2 Meat, med fat	Recipe

(continued)

Filipino American Foods *(continued)*

Food	Serving Size	Grams per Serving	Energy (kcal)	Fat (g)	SFA (g)	PUFA (g)	MUFA (g)	Chol (mg)	Sod (mg)	Carb (g)	Fiber (g)	Sugar (g)	Pro (g)	Pot (mg)	Exchanges	Source
Marinated Chicken Stew, Filipino-style	1 serving (1⅓ cups)	308	297	15.9	4.9	3.7	7.4	85	2623	13.5	0.5	Miss	24.4	429	1 Carb + 3 Meat, med fat	Recipe + FNDDS 28340610
Meat ball soup with noodles, Filipino-style	1 serving (1⅓ cups)	375	207	8.5	2.9	1.4	3.3	26	78	17.1	1.9	Miss	12.1	1047	1 Starch + 2 Meat, med fat	Recipe
Pork barbecue, Filipino-style	1 serving	226	297	10.8	3.8	1.2	4.9	95	1297	14.1	0.2	Miss	34.4	636	1 Carb + 5 Meat, lean	Recipe
Rice and pasta, Filipino-style (Chicken Arroz Caldo)	1 cup	304	128	7.8	0.9	1.7	1.4	14	1173	7.7	0.6	Miss	8.1	136	½ Starch + 1 Meat, lean + 1 Fat	Recipe
Sauteed beef with chickpeas, Filipino-style	1 serving	354	351	15	5	2.6	5.5	145	636	30.1	6.9	Miss	25.3	825	2 Starch + 3 Meat, lean + 1½ Fat	Recipe
Sauteed vegetables, Filipino-style	1 serving	203	135	4.2	1.1	1.2	1.5	46	48	15.2	1.8	Miss	10.3	498	3 Vegetable + 1 Meat, lean + ½ Fat	Recipe
Stewed chicken with ginger, Filipino-style	1 serving	489	251	15.4	0.3	1.1	0.5	82	69	10.2	2.1	Miss	17.6	432	2 Vegetable + 3 Meat, med fat	Recipe

Korean American Foods

Food	Serving Size	Grams per Serving	Energy (kcal)	Fat (g)	SFA (g)	PUFA (g)	MUFA (g)	Chol (mg)	Sod (mg)	Carb (g)	Fiber (g)	Sugar (g)	Pro (g)	Pot (mg)	Exchanges	Source
Starches																
Acorn starch jelly (acorn mook, dotorimuk)	1 piece (2" x 1¾" x ¾")	38	78	4.7	0.6	0.9	3	0	1	8.5	Miss	Miss	1.2	111	½ Starch + 1 Fat	Recipe
Barley, cooked	0.33 cup, cooked	53	65	0.2	0	0.1	0	0	2	15	2	0.1	1.2	50	1 Starch	FNDDS 56200400
Lotus root, fresh, cooked	1 cup	120	79	0.1	0	0	0	0	54	19.2	3.7	0.6	1.9	436	1 Starch	USDA 11255
Mung beans, mature, cooked	0.5 cup	101	106	0.4	0.1	0.1	0.1	0	2	19.3	7.7	2	7.1	269	1 Starch + 1 Meat, lean	USDA 16081
Rice, brown, cooked	0.33 cup	64	71	0.6	0.1	0.2	0.2	0	3	14.8	1.2	0.2	1.7	28	1 Starch	USDA 20037
Rice, white, long grain, cooked	0.33 cup	52	68	0.1	0	0	0	0	1	14.7	0.2	0	1.4	18	1 Starch	USDA 20045
Fruits																
Asian pear, raw	1 fruit (2-¼" high x 2-½" dia)	122	51	0.3	0	0.1	0.1	0	0	13	4.4	8.6	0.6	148	1 Fruit	USDA 09340
Persimmon, Japanese, soft, fresh	0.5 fruit (2-½" dia)	84	59	0.2	0	0	0	0	1	15.6	3	10.5	0.5	135	1 Fruit	USDA 09263
Tangerine, fresh	2 small (2-¼" dia)	152	81	0.5	0.1	0.1	0.1	0	3	20.3	2.7	16.1	1.2	252	1 Fruit	USDA 09218
Yellow melon, Korean, fresh	1 cup, cubes	160	54	0.3	0.1	0.1	0	0	26	13.1	1.4	12.6	1.3	427	1 Fruit	USDA 09181
Nonstarchy Vegetables																
Bok choy (Chinese white cabbage or pak-choi), cooked	0.5 cup	85	10	0.1	0	0.1	0	0	29	1.5	0.8	0.7	1.3	315	1 Vegetable	USDA 11117
Bok choy (Chinese white cabbage or pak-choi), raw	1 cup, shredded	70	9	0.1	0	0.1	0	0	46	1.5	0.7	0.8	1.1	176	1 Vegetable	USDA 11116
Kelp (seaweed), raw	1 cup	80	34	0.4	0.2	0	0.1	0	186	7.7	1	0.5	1.3	71	1 Vegetable	USDA 11445
Mung bean sprouts, seed attached, cooked	0.5 cup	62	13	0.1	0	0	0	0	6	2.6	0.5	1.8	1.3	63	1 Vegetable	USDA 11044
Sesame leaves, fresh	1 cup	91	40	0.7	0.2	0.4	0	0	27	7.7	6.2	0.9	3	417	1 Vegetable	USDA 02065

(continued)

Korean American Foods *(continued)*

Food	Serving Size	Grams per Serving	Energy (kcal)	Fat (g)	SFA (g)	PUFA (g)	MUFA (g)	Chol (mg)	Sod (mg)	Carb (g)	Fiber (g)	Sugar (g)	Pro (g)	Pot (mg)	Exchanges	Source
Meats and Meat Substitutes																
Abalone, cooked	1 oz, cooked	28	59	0.4	0.1	0.1	0.1	48	202	3.4	0	0	9.6	98	1 Meat, lean	FNDDS 26301160
Beef, shortribs, cooked, lean only	1 oz	28	83	5.1	2.2	0.2	2.3	26	16	0	0	0	8.7	89	1 Meat, med fat	USDA 13150
Oxtail, cooked	1 oz	28	72	3.8	1.5	0.1	1.6	30	66	0	0	0	8.8	74	1 Meat, med fat	FNDDS 21301000
Oysters, Pacific type, raw	1 medium	50	41	1.2	0.3	0.4	0.2	25	53	2.5	0	2.5	4.7	84	1 Meat, lean	USDA 15171
Fats																
Oil, brown rice	1 tsp	4	40	4.5	0.9	1.6	1.8	0	0	0	0	0	0	0	1 Fat	USDA 4037
Oil, sesame seed	1 tsp	4	40	4.5	0.6	1.9	1.8	0	0	0	0	0	0	0	1 Fat	USDA 04058
Combination Foods																
Dried pollack and bean sprout soup (bookO kongnamul guk)	1 cup	228	54	2	0.3	1.1	0.4	9	411	3.4	0.5	0.3	7.4	234	1 Meat, lean	Recipe
Kimchi stew (kimchichigae. kimchi jjigae)	1 cup	203	108	5.3	1.3	1.4	1.9	22	397	4.5	1.4	1.5	11.3	306	1 Vegetable + 1 Meat, med fat	Recipe
Mandoo soup (manduguk, Korean dumpling soup)	1 cup broth + 3 dumplings	399	177	5.9	1.8	0.9	2.3	100	689	12.2	1	1.3	18	348	1 Starch + 2 Meat, lean	Recipe
Porridge, abalone (jeonbokjuk)	1 cup	240	147	2.8	0.4	1.1	1.1	19	301	23.3	0.3	0	6	67	1½ Starch + ½ Fat	Recipe

Cajun and Creole Foods

Food	Serving Size	Grams per Serving	Energy (kcal)	Fat (g)	SFA (g)	PUFA (g)	MUFA (g)	Chol (mg)	Sod (mg)	Carb (g)	Fiber (g)	Sugar (g)	Pro (g)	Pot (mg)	Exchanges	Source
Fruit																
Japanese plum (loquat, mayapple), fresh	0.75 cup, cubed	112	53	0.2	0	0.1	0	0	1	13.6	1.9	10.4	0.5	297	1 Fruit	USDA 09174
Persimmon, Japanese, soft, fresh	0.5 fruit (2½" dia)	84	59	0.2	0	0	0	0	1	15.6	3	10.5	0.5	135	1 Fruit	USDA 09263
Nonstarchy Vegetables																
Mirliton (vegetable pear), cooked	0.5 cup	80	19	0.4	0.1	0.1	0.1	0	1	4.1	2.2	1	0.5	138	1 Vegetable	USDA 11150
Oyster mushroom, raw	0.5 large	74	32	0.3	0	0	0	0	13	4.8	1.7	0.8	2.4	311	1 Vegetable	USDA 11987
Meat and Meat Substitutes																
Alligator, tail, cooked	1 oz	28	42	0.6	0.2	0.1	0.3	19	22	0	0	0	9.3	129	1 Meat, lean	Laboratory
Beef tasso	1 oz	28	43	0.6	0.3	0	0.2	22	792	0.8	0	0.8	8.8	67	1 Meat, lean	USDA 13350
Crawfish (crayfish), cooked	1 oz, without shell, cooked	28	25	0.4	0.1	0.1	0.1	39	27	0	0	0	5	67	1 Meat, lean	USDA 15243
Dove, cooked	1 oz	28	62	3.7	1.1	0.8	1.6	33	16	0	0	0	6.8	73	1 Meat, med fat	USDA 43287
Duck, wild, meat and skin, not cooked	1 oz, no bone	28	60	4.3	1.4	0.6	1.9	23	16	0	0	0	4.9	70	1 Meat, med fat	USDA 5144
Frog legs, cooked	2 legs, cooked (yield after bone remov)	48	50	0.2	0.1	0.1	0	34	28	0	0	0	11.3	176	1 Meat, lean	FNDDS 26203160
Hogshead cheese (headcheese, jellied pork)	1 oz	28	45	3.1	1	0.3	1.6	20	236	0	0	0	3.9	9	1 Meat, lean	USDA 07034
Pig's feet, pickled	0.5 foot (yield after cooking, bone rem)	44	61	4.3	1.3	0.3	2.5	36	242	0	0	0	5	6	1 Meat, med fat	USDA 10132
Sausage, beef, smoked, cooked	1 oz	28	88	7.6	3.2	0.3	3.7	19	320	0.7	0	0.7	4	50	1 Meat, high fat	USDA 13357
Sausage, pork, smoked, cooked	1 oz	28	89	8	2.6	1	3.2	17	235	0.6	0	0.3	3.4	137	1 Meat, high fat	USDA 07074
Squirrel, roasted	1 oz	28	49	1.3	0.2	0.4	0.4	34	34	0	0	0	8.7	100	1 Meat, lean	USDA 17184
Turtle (terrapin), cooked, no fat or salt added	1 oz, boneless, cooked	28	30	0.2	0	0.1	0	16	23	0	0	0	6.6	77	1 Meat, lean	FNDDS 26215120
Venison (deer), roasted	1 oz	28	45	0.9	0.4	0.2	0.2	32	15	0	0	0	8.5	95	1 Meat, lean	USDA 17165

(continued)

Cajun and Creole Foods *(continued)*

Food	Serving Size	Grams per Serving	Energy (kcal)	Fat (g)	SFA (g)	PUFA (g)	MUFA (g)	Chol (mg)	Sod (mg)	Carb (g)	Fiber (g)	Sugar (g)	Pro (g)	Pot (mg)	Exchanges	Source
Fats																
Cracklings, pork (gratons), cooked	1.5 Tbsp	9	46	3.6	1.2	0.4	1.6	9	198	0.1	0	0	3.2	48	1 Fat	FNDDS 22704010
Salt pork, cooked	0.25 oz	7	51	5.4	1.9	0.6	2.6	6	91	0	0	0	0.5	4	1 Fat	FNDDS 22621000
Free Foods																
Lotus seeds (Graine a voler), fresh	0.75 oz	21	19	0.1	0	0.1	0	0	0	3.7	1.8	Miss	0.9	78	Free Food	USDA 12205

Jewish Foods

Food	Serving Size	Grams per Serving	Energy (kcal)	Fat (g)	SFA (g)	PUFA (g)	MUFA (g)	Chol (mg)	Sod (mg)	Carb (g)	Fiber (g)	Sugar (g)	Pro (g)	Pot (mg)	Exchanges	Source
Starches																
Challah (egg bread)	1 slice (1 oz)	28	80	1.7	0.5	0.3	0.7	14	139	13.6	0.7	0.5	2.7	33	1 Starch	USDA 18027
Kasha (buckwheat groats), roasted, cooked	0.5 cup	84	77	0.5	0.1	0.2	0.2	0	3	16.7	2.3	0.8	2.8	74	1 Starch	USDA 20010
Matzo (matzoh) crackers, plain	0.75 oz	21	83	0.3	0	0.1	0	0	0	17.6	0.6	0.1	2.1	24	1 Starch	USDA 18217
Matzo (matzoh) crackers, whole-wheat	0.75 oz	21	75	0.3	0.1	0.1	0	0	0	16.8	2.5	0.1	2.8	67	1 Starch	USDA 18219
Matzo ball (knaidel), cooked	2 matzo balls (1¼ oz each)	70	95	3.4	0.9	0.7	1.3	72	24	12.3	0.4	0.2	3.6	39	1 Starch + ½ Fat	FNDDS 52308020
Matzo meal	2 Tbsp	17	66	0.2	0	0.1	0	0	0	14.1	0.5	0	1.7	19	1 Starch	Label + USDA 18217
Noodles, egg, cooked	0.33 cup	53	73	1.1	0.2	0.3	0.3	15	3	13.3	0.6	0.2	2.4	20	1 Starch	USDA 20110
Pancake, broccoli, pre-made (Dr Praeger's)	2 pancakes	114	160	7	0.4	1.8	3.6	0	340	18	4	2	4	244	1 Starch + 1½ Fat	Label
Pita bread, white	0.5 pita (6½" dia)	30	82	0.4	0	0.2	0	0	161	16.7	0.7	0.4	2.7	36	1 Starch	USDA 18041
Potato starch (flour)	2 Tbsp	20	71	0.1	0	0	0	0	11	16.6	1.2	0.7	1.4	200	1 Starch	USDA 11413
Squash, winter, cooked	1 cup, cubes	205	76	0.7	0.1	0.3	0.1	0	2	18.1	5.7	6.8	1.8	494	1 Starch	USDA 11644
Fruits																
Grape juice, bottled	0.33 cup	83	51	0.1	0	0	0	0	3	12.5	0.1	12.4	0.5	110	1 Fruit	USDA 09135
Sweets, Desserts, and Other Carbohydrates																
Eggplant dip (baba ghanoush, ghanou)	0.25 cup	58	97	7.7	1.1	2.9	3.3	0	128	6.6	2.1	1.4	2.4	110	½ Carb + 1½ Fat	FNDDS 75412030
Wine, sweet dessert	1 wine glass (3.5 fl oz)	103	165	0	0	0	0	0	9	14.1	0	8	0.2	95	1 Carb	USDA 14057
Nonstarchy Vegetables																
Carrots, fresh cooked	0.5 cup	78	27	0.1	0	0.1	0	0	45	6.4	2.3	2.7	0.6	183	1 Vegetable	USDA 11125
Meat and Meat Substitutes																
Gefilte fish, no sugar added, frozen, cooked	2 slices (3/8" thick)	52	70	3.5	0.5	1.1	1.2	15	180	3	0.4	0.8	6	122	1 Meat, med fat	FNDDS 27250060
Hummus	0.33 cup	83	137	7.9	1.2	3	3.3	0	313	11.8	5	4.8	6.5	188	1 Carb + 1 Meat, high fat	USDA 16158
Combination Foods																
Gefilte fish, sweet type	2 pieces	84	71	1.5	0.3	0.2	0.7	25	440	6.2	0	Miss	7.6	76	½ Carb + 1 Meat, lean	USDA 15030
Soup, chicken stock	1 cup	240	86	2.9	0.8	0.5	1.4	7	343	8.5	0	3.8	6	252	½ Carb + 1 Meat, lean	USDA 06172
Tsimmes (sweet potato, and fruit, no meat)	1 cup	260	238	2.4	0.6	0.8	0.8	0	92	53.4	4.8	26.8	3	522	3½ Carb	Recipe

Islamic Foods
See also Asian Indian and Pakistani Foods

Food	Serving Size	Grams per Serving	Energy (kcal)	Fat (g)	SFA (g)	PUFA (g)	MUFA (g)	Chol (mg)	Sod (mg)	Carb (g)	Fiber (g)	Sugar (g)	Pro (g)	Pot (mg)	Exchanges	Source
Starches																
Bulgur wheat, cooked	0.5 cup	91	76	0.2	0	0.1	0	0	5	16.9	4.1	0.1	2.8	62	1 Starch	USDA 20013
Couscous, prepared	0.33 cup	52	58	0.1	0	0	0	0	3	12.1	0.7	0.1	2	30	1 Starch	USDA 20029
Foul (fava beans, lemon juice, olive oil, garlic)	0.33 cup	73	147	9.2	1.3	1	6.6	0	197	12.4	3.2	1.1	4.6	179	1 Starch + 1½ Fat	Recipe
Naan masala tandori (tandoori)	1 piece (3 oz)	84	240	3	0.4	1.6	0.6	0	280	44	2	2	8	100	3 Starch	Label
Pita bread, white	0.5 pita (6½" dia)	30	82	0.4	0	0.2	0	0	161	16.7	0.7	0.4	2.7	36	1 Starch	USDA 18041
Taboule (tabouli), prepared	0.5 cup	81	97	2.1	0.4	0.1	1.4	0	193	16.4	3.6	1.5	2.8	55	1 Starch	Label + USDA 20013
Sweets, Desserts, and Other Carbohydrates																
Baklava pastry	1 piece (2" x 2" x 1½")	78	334	22.6	9.5	4.1	7.6	35	253	29.4	2	9.9	5.2	134	2 Carb + 4½ Fat	FNDDS 53441110
Basboosa (seminola tart with syrup)	1 square (3.4 oz)	95	281	9.7	1.5	5.1	2.6	1	28	45.9	1.2	25.7	3.6	67	3 Carb + 1½ Fat	Recipe
Baba ghanoush (eggplant dip, ghanou)	0.25 cup	58	97	7.7	1.1	2.9	3.3	0	128	6.6	2.1	1.4	2.4	110	½ Carb + 1½ Fat	FNDDS 75412030
Mango lassi, low-fat	1 cup	270	148	2.1	1.2	0.1	0.6	7	83	28	2.1	25.4	6.6	449	1½ Fruit + ½ Milk, fat-free	Recipe
Um ali (pastry pudding, raisins, coconut, milk)	1 rectangle (2" x 1")	53	127	7.8	2.5	0.7	2.4	5	121	11.4	0.5	4.2	2.7	76	1 Carb + 1½ Fat	Recipe
Meats and Meat Substitutes																
Cheese, feta, regular	1 oz	28	75	6	4.2	0.2	1.3	25	317	1.2	0	1.2	4	18	1 Meat, med fat	USDA 01019
Falafel (spiced chickpea and wheat patties)	3 patties (approx 2¼" dia)	51	170	9.1	1.2	2.1	5.2	0	150	16.2	2	3	6.8	298	1 Carb + 1 Meat, high fat	USDA 16138
Hummus	0.33 cup	83	137	7.9	1.2	3	3.3	0	313	11.8	5	4.8	6.5	188	1 Carb + 1 Meat, high fat	USDA 16158
Shawarma (pressed meat)	1 oz	29	65	4.9	2.1	0.4	2.2	15	59	1.2	0.2	0.5	3.8	66	1 Meat, med fat	Recipe

(continued)

Islamic Foods *(continued)*

Combination Foods

Food	Serving Size	Grams per Serving	Energy (kcal)	Fat (g)	SFA (g)	PUFA (g)	MUFA (g)	Chol (mg)	Sod (mg)	Carb (g)	Fiber (g)	Sugar (g)	Pro (g)	Pot (mg)	Exchanges	Source
Alu chole (curried garbanzos and potatoes)	1 container (9.2 oz)	262	350	6	0.5	Miss	Miss	0	620	65	9	3	12	Miss	4 Starch + ½ Fat	Label
Chicken biryani (chicken, vegetables, brown rice)	1 container (10 oz)	283	390	12	1.5	Miss	Miss	20	1080	54	4	7	16	Miss	3 Starch + 2 Vegetable + 1 Meat, lean + 1½ Fat	Label
Coconut curry samosa	1 serving	82	170	3	1	Miss	Miss	15	520	26	1	Miss	8	Miss	2 Carb + 1 Meat, lean	
Dal bahaar (lentils, vegetables, tofu, brown rice)	1 container (11 oz)	312	360	8	1	Miss	Miss	0	500	61	8	5	13	Miss	3½ Starch + 2 Vegetable + 1 Fat	Label
Fatayer (spinach pastry-type appetizer)	1 pastry	68	157	9.3	0.9	2.2	5.8	0	211	16	1.2	1	2.7	151	1 Starch + 2 Fat	Recipe
Fattoush salad (pita, romaine, tomato, feta)	1 serving	161	214	14.5	4	1.4	8.5	15	359	16.9	2.3	3	5.4	264	½ Starch + 2 Vegetable + 3 Fat	Recipe
Kabsa (Arabian rice and chicken)	1 serving (⅛ recipe)	347	365	12.4	5	1.8	4.4	64	511	42.8	3.3	7.9	20.9	542	2 Starch + 2 Vegetable + 2 Meat, med fat	Recipe
Koshary (grains, lentils, tomato chili sauce, onions)	1 cup	260	296	7.8	1.6	1.3	3.6	0	249	46.3	8.1	5.3	11.1	528	2½ Starch + 2 Vegetable + 1 Fat	Recipe
Palak paneer (spinach and cheese)	1 container (9.2 oz)	262	380	15	6	Miss	Miss	35	640	46	6	6	14	Miss	3 Carb + 2 Meat, med fat + ½ Fat	Label
Warak enab (warak dawali, stuffed vine leaves)	4 stuffed leaves	96	118	5.2	0.7	0.8	3.4	0	180	16.4	2.9	2	2.5	164	1 Starch + 1 Fat	Recipe

Sources

General

US Department of Agriculture, Agricultural Research Service. 2007. USDA National Nutrient Database for Standard Reference, Release 20. Nutrient Data Laboratory Home Page. http://www.ars.usda.gov/ba/bhnrc/ndl. Accessed August 29, 2008.

USDA Food and Nutrient Database for Dietary Studies, 3.0. 2008. Beltsville, MD: US Department of Agriculture, Agricultural Research Service, Food Surveys Research Group. http://www/ars/usda.gov/Services/docs.htm?docid=12089. Accessed November 11, 2008.

Navajo Foods

Wolfe WS, Weber CW, Arviso KD. Use and nutrient composition of traditional Navajo foods. *Ecol Food Nutr*. 1985;17:323-344 (blue dumplings; dessert yucca; tortilla, flour and baking powder type; cantaloupe, dried; Navajo banana; corn, steamed, dried; Navajo cake; sumac berry pudding; squash, yellow, dried; zucchini, dried; ash, tumbleweed; blue mush tamale; mutton stew).

Northern Plains Indian Foods

American Dietetic Association and American Diabetes Association. *Northern Plains Indian Food Practices, Customs, and Holidays*. Ethnic and Regional Food Practices series. Chicago, IL: American Dietetic Association; 1999 (wojapi recipe).

Alaska Native

Nobmann E. *Nutrient Value of Alaska Native Foods*. Anchorage, AK: US Department of Health and Human Services, Indian Health Services; 1993 (beach asparagus; seaweed, black, dried; hooligan (eulachon) grease).

Kuhnlein HV, Soueida R. Use and nutrient composition of traditional Baffin Inuit foods. *J Food Comp Anal*. 1992;5:112–126 (seal, ringed, meat only, cooked).

Hunt D, ed. *Native Indian Wild Game, Fish and Wild Foods Cookbook*. Edison NJ: Castle Books; nd (wild duck soup recipe).

American Dietetic Association and American Diabetes Association. *Alaska Native Food Practices, Customs, and Holidays*. Ethnic and Regional Food Practices series. Chicago, IL: American Dietetic Association; 1998 (perok [fish pie] recipe; moose soup recipe; agutuk with berries, no meat or fish [Eskimo ice cream] recipe).

African American Foods

Tibbs KE. *Healthy Food, Healthy Soul, African American Cooking*. 2nd ed. Lansing, MI: Michigan Public Health Institute and the Michigan Department of Community Health; 1998 (boiled cabbage and turkey recipe; turnip and mustard greens recipe).

Mexican American Foods

Oficina Regional de la FAO para America Latina y el Caribe. Tabla de composición de alimentos de America latina. http://www.fao.org/REGIONAL/LAmerica/bases/alimento. Accessed April 21, 2009 (queso Oaxaca).

Central American Foods

Leung WTW, Flores M. *INCAP-ICNND Food Composition Table for Use in Latin America*. Guatemala: Institute of Nutrition of Central America and Panama (INCAP), Interdepartmental Committee on Nutrition for National Defense (ICNN); and Bethesda, MD: National Institutes for Health; 1961 (nance [#320]).

Institute of Nutrition of Central America and Panama Americas (INCAP). Table of Food Composition of Central America (after 2000). http://www.tabladealimentos.net/tca/TablaAlimentos/antecedentes.html. Accessed August 18, 2008 (pitaya).

Caribbean Hispanic Foods

Aunt Clara's Kitchen: Dominican Cooking. http://www.dominicancooking.com/Forums/starters-buffet-food/1298-empanaditas-pastelitos-savoury-pasties.html. Accessed November 12, 2008. (empanaditas/pastelitos [savoury pasties], baked, adapted recipe; empanaditas/pastelitos [savoury pasties], deep-fried, adapted recipe).

South American Foods

Núcleo de Estudos e Pesquisas em Alimentação—NEPA. Universidade Estadual de Campinas—UNICAMP. Tabela Brasileira de Composição de Alimentos TACO. 2nd ed. Campinas, SP. 2006. http://www.unicamp.br/nepa/taco/contar/taco_versao2.pdf. Accessed November 10, 2008 (arroz doce/arroz dulce [+ FNDDS 13210410]; churros [+ FNDDS 53520200 and USDA: sweetened condensed milk]; feijoada; panqueca de carne [+ FNDDS 58120120]; pastel de carne).

Philippi ST. Tabela de Composição de Alimentos: Suporte para Decisão Nutricional. ANVISA, FINATEC/NUT-UnB, Brasília, DF; 2001. http://www.ANVISA.gov.br/rotulo/rotulo_categoria_producto_LST.asp. Accessed November 10, 2008 (pudim de leite [+ USDA]).

Asian Indian and Pakistani Foods

American Dietetic Association and American Diabetes Association. *Indian & Pakistani Food Practices, Customs, and Holidays*. Ethnic and Regional Food Practices series. Chicago, IL: American Dietetic Association; 2000 (includes nutrient analyses for 11 recipes: aviyal, sambar, dhansak, dhakla, matki usal, pesrattu, poha, tomato dhal, tandori chicken, chicken tikka, and cucumber raita; however, recipes are *not* available).

Chinese American Foods

US Department of Health, Education, and Welfare, and Food and Agriculture Organization of the United Nations (FAO). Food Composition Table for Use in East Asia. 1972. http://www.fao.org/docrep/003/X6878E/X6878E00.htm. Accessed August 24, 2008 (dried scallop [#1460]; Chinese sausage [#1145]; preserved egg [#1181]).

Centre for Food Safety. The Government of the Hong Kong Special Administrative Region. Nutrient Information Inquiry. http://www.cfs.gov.hk/english/nutrient/presearch3.shtml. Accessed August 25, 2008 (BBQ pork bun [char sin bao], steamed).

Hmong American Foods

American Dietetic Association and American Diabetes Association. *Hmong American Food Practices, Customs, and Holidays*. Ethnic and Regional Food Practices series. Chicago, IL: American Dietetic Association; 1999 (boiled pork and mustard greens [zaub ntsaub] recipe from Sawyer S. *Hmong Recipe Cook Book*. South St. Paul, MN: New Citizens' Hmong Garden Project, First Presbyterian Church; 1986).

Filipino American Foods

Elefano-Quirante R, Serraon-Claudio V, eds. *Filipino American Cookbook for Calorie Controlled Diets*. Port Arthur, TX: Filipino American Dietetic Association; 1993 (recipes for all 21 Filipino foods).

Korean American Foods

Korean National Tourism Organization. Asia Food: The Wonderful World of Korean Food. http://www.asiafood.org/jeonbok.cfm. Accessed November 12, 2008 (abalone porridge recipe).

Korean Foods NYC Recipes. http://207.228.230.125/koreanfood/HTML/recipe_026.htm. Accessed December 3, 2008 (dried pollack and bean sprout soup recipe).

About.com: Korean Food. Spicy Kimchi Soup. http://koreanfood.about.com/od/soupsandstews/r/Kimchichigae.htm. Accessed November 12, 2008 (kimchi stew recipe).

Recipes Wiki. Mandoo Guk. http://74.125.113.132/search?q=cache:caVT4YIXBz0J:recipes.wikia.com/wiki/Mandoo_guk_(Korean_dumpling_soup)+korean+dumpling+soup&hl=en&ct=clnk&cd=4&gl=us. Accessed Dec 3, 2008 (mandoo soup recipe).

Cajun and Creole Foods

Moore's Extended Nutrient (MENu) Database. Baton Rouge, LA: Pennington Biomedical Research Center (alligator tail, cooked).

Jewish Foods

AOH Food: Sweet Potato-Carrot Tsimmes. http://artofhacking.com/aohfood/60000/60048-sweetpotatocarrottsimmes.htm. Accessed November 11, 2008 (tsimmes—sweet potato, carrot, and fruit, no meat—recipe).

Islamic Foods

Newgent J. *The All-Natural Diabetes Cookbook*. Alexandria VA: American Diabetes Association 2007 (mango *lassi*, low-fat, recipe).

Baydoun LC, Halawani NM. *Jordanian Cooking Step by Step*. Beirut, Lebanon: Arab Scientific Publishers; n.d. (adapted *foul* recipe; adapted *shawarma* [pressed meat] recipe).

Cooks.com. http://www.cooks.com/rec/doc/0,1842,150162-236206,00.html. Accessed November 15, 2008 (*koshary* recipe).

Recipe Zaar. http://www.recipezaar.com/Basboosa-74312. Accessed November 15, 2008 (*basboosa* recipe).

Food Geeks.com. http://foodgeeks.com/recipes/recipe/20114,middle_eastern_spinach_pies_fatayer .phtml. Accessed November 17, 2008 (adapted *fatayer* [spinach pastry] recipe).

Insalata's Restaurant. http://www.insalatas.com/html/syrian_fattoush_salad.html. Accessed November 15, 2008 (adapted *fattoush* salad recipe).

Recipes.com. http://ricerecipe.org/al-kabsa-traditional-saudi-rice-chicken-dish. Accessed November 17, 2008 (adapted *kabsa* recipe).

LebGuide: Your Touristic Guide to Lebanon. http://www.lebguide.com/lebanon/lebanese_cuisine/ lebanon_lebanese_cuisine_warak_enab.asp. Accessed November 17, 2008 (*warak enab* recipe).

Group Recipes. http://www.grouprecipes.com/21656/um-ali.html. Accessed Nov 17, 2008 (um ali recipe).

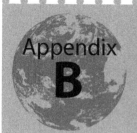

General Counseling Tips for Medical Nutrition Therapy Recommendations

	Recommendations	Counseling Tips
Energy	Prescribed calorie intake should allow client to attain or maintain a reasonable body weight. Weight loss should be recommended to all overweight and obese adults who have or are at risk for diabetes.	• Emphasize portion control and demonstrate appropriate serving sizes using food models and measuring tools. • Suggest reduced-calorie substitutions and cooking methods for traditional dishes. • Promote consumption of water in place of beverages with added sugar. • Encourage physical activity and planned and leisure-time activities.
Optimal macronutrient balance	Encourage consumption of macronutrients based on the DRIs for healthy adults: 45%-65% of total energy from carbohydrates, 20%-35% from fat, and 10%-35% from protein.	• Separate myths from facts regarding popular/fad diets. • Help clients create an individualized meal plan appropriate for managing their diabetes and related conditions.
Carbohydrate	Carbohydrate should provide 45%-65% of total daily energy. Total carbohydrate intake is a strong predictor of glycemic response; use of the glycemic index or glycemic load may provide a modest added benefit over that observed when total carbohydrate is considered alone.	• Emphasize benefits of whole grain foods, such as whole wheat and whole grain breads and cereals. • Encourage consumption of whole fruits and vegetables instead of fruit or vegetable juices. • Help clients plan ahead for social situations and special occasions when foods made with refined sugars (eg, birthday cake) will be served. Teach clients to have these foods as part of a meal, rather than on their own. • Emphasize that the total amount of carbohydrate consumed is more important than types of carbohydrates.
Fat, cholesterol, and cardioprotective nutrition therapy	Total fat intake should be 20%-35% of daily energy intake prescription. Limit saturated fats to < 7% total energy intake and minimize intake of *trans* fats. Cholesterol intake < 200 mg/d. Two or more servings of fish per week (not including commercially fried fish filets) are recommended. Also encourage interventions to improve blood pressure.	• Encourage clients to use heart-healthy fats, such as nuts, avocados, olive oil, and canola oil, while emphasizing portion control to prevent weight gain. • Encourage clients to eat fewer fried foods and reduce the amount of oil or fat added in food preparation. • Promote lower-fat cooking methods, such as boiling, steaming, and baking. • Advise clients to cut off visible fat from meat, remove skin from poultry, and discard fat from commodity meats, if they are part of their diet. • Educate clients about low-fat and nonfat milk and milk products, including substitutions they can make in traditional dishes that use whole milk, cream, or other high-fat dairy.

(continued)

(continued)

	Recommendations	Counseling Tips
		• Identify types of high-fat meats, such as canned meat, bologna, other luncheon meats, hot dogs, sausage, and bacon, and encourage clients to limit consumption of these foods. • Teach clients to select lower-fat foods in regular and fast-food restaurants. • Offer a list of foods high in fat. • Provide tips for reducing sodium intake, such as label reading and ways to add flavor to foods without using salt.
Protein	The RDA for protein in adults is 0.8g/kg-1.0g per kilogram of body weight. Usual protein intake (~ 15%–20% of daily energy intake) does not need to be changed for individuals with diabetes and normal renal function.	• Provide a list of leaner cuts of meats. • Emphasize the appropriate portion size for meats (typically, two 3-oz servings/d). • Explain that dried beans and peas are low-fat sources of protein.
Fiber	Individuals with diabetes should meet the DRI for fiber (14 g/1,000 kcal) by eating a variety of fiber-containing foods. Evidence is lacking to recommend a higher fiber diet for diabetes management.	• Encourage consumption of minimally processed grains, fruits, and vegetables. • Advise clients to choose whole grain foods (eg, brown rice instead of white rice) and increase the amount of dried beans, peas, and lentils in their diet. • Encourage the use of whole fruits instead of fruit juice, fruit nectars, and fruit drinks. • Encourage clients to eat more nonstarchy vegetables.
Nonnutritive sweeteners	Consumption of nonnutritive sweeteners within the levels set by the FDA is safe.	• Teach clients how to read food labels and identify nonnutritive sweeteners on ingredient lists. • Discuss labeling terms and explain that "sugar-free" and "no-added sugar" do not mean a food is calorie-free or carbohydrate-free. • Explain types of nonnutritive sweeteners and their uses. Discuss recipe substitutions for sugar.
Dietary supplements	There is no clear evidence of benefit from vitamin or mineral supplementation in people with diabetes (compared with the general population) who do not have underlying deficiencies. A daily multivitamin supplement may be appropriate for older adults, especially those with reduced energy intake. Routine supplementation with antioxidants, such as vitamins E and C and carotene, is not advised. Chromium supplementation is not recommended.	• Discuss the risks and benefits of using dietary supplements.
Alcohol	If adults choose to consume alcohol, they should limit intake to < 1 drink/d for women and < 2 drinks/d for men. 1 drink (15 g alcohol) = 12 oz beer, 5 oz wine, or 1.5 oz distilled spirits. To reduce the risk of nocturnal hypoglycemia, individuals using insulin or insulin secretagogues should only consume alcohol with food.	• Promote abstinence from alcohol. • Explain the dangers of excessive alcohol consumption (eg, adverse effects on glucose control and diabetes management). • If clients use insulin or diabetes medications, discuss the associated risks of alcohol use (eg, hypoglycemia). • Advise clients to only consume alcohol with food. • On the other hand, remind clients to consider the calorie and carbohydrate content of mixed drinks, beer, and wine and realize that drinking alcohol may increase the likelihood they will overeat.

Abbreviations: DRI, Dietary Reference Intake; RDA, Recommended Dietary Allowance; FDA, Food and Drug Administration.

Source: Data are from (*a*) American Diabetes Association. Nutrition recommendations and interventions for diabetes: a position statement of the American Diabetes Association. *Diabetes Care.* 2008;31(Suppl 1):S61-S78; and (*b*) American Dietetic Association Evidence Analysis Library. Diabetes Type 1 and 2 Evidence-based Nutrition Practice Guideline for Adults. http://www.adaevidencelibrary.com/topic.cfm?cat=3251. Accessed May 28, 2009.

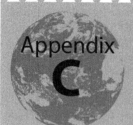

Appendix C

Dietary Supplement Intake Assessment: Questions to Ask Clients[1]

As part of any nutrition assessment, health professionals should ask clients questions about dietary supplement intake. The following questions are designed to gather information that will help clients make informed decisions about supplement use. Ask your clients to bring supplement packages to an appointment to help answer these questions.

Note: For questions marked with an asterisk, ask the question for each supplement taken and check labels.

- What supplements do you use? (Be sure to explain that supplements include vitamins and minerals, herbals, amino acids, protein, fiber, fatty acids, etc.)
- What are your main reasons for taking this supplement?* (Suggest reasons, such as to prevent a disease, to help treat a disease or condition, general health, energy, weight loss, pregnancy, mood, muscle-building, etc.)
- How long have you used this supplement?*
- How long do you plan on using it?*
- How often do you take this supplement?*
- What brand of supplement do you take?
- What form of supplement do you take?*
- How much of the supplement do you take?*
- Do you ever take more than the dose shown on the label?*
- How much money do you spend on supplements? Does this cost make it hard to afford food?
- Have you had any changes in your health or medical condition since you started taking this supplement?*
- Since you started using this supplement, have you had any bad reactions?* (Give examples of adverse effects, such as rash, stomach problems, mood changes, or nervousness.)
- Are you allergic to any foods, insects, plants, or flowers? Are any of your supplements made from things that give you allergies? (To answer the second question, it may be necessary to read supplement labels. For example, if a patient has an allergy to bee stings or honey, he or she may react to bee pollen supplements.)
- What other drugs do you take? (Ask about both prescription and over-the-counter medications.)
- Do you drink alcohol or drinks with caffeine (coffee, tea, cola)? Do you drink these when you take supplements?

---

[1]This appendix is reprinted with permission from Sarubin Fragakis A, Thomson C. *The Health Professional's Guide to Popular Dietary Supplements.* 3rd ed. Chicago, IL: American Dietetic Association; 2007:662–663.

Index

Page number followed by *b* indicates box; *f*, figure; *t*, table.